THE HERMEN
AND THE PHENC

INTERNATIONAL LIBRARY OF ETHICS, LAW, AND THE NEW MEDICINE

Editors

DAVID C. THOMASMA, *Loyola University, Chicago, U.S.A.*
DAVID N. WEISSTUB, *Université de Montréal, Canada*
THOMASINE KIMBROUGH KUSHNER, *University of California, Berkeley, U.S.A.*

Editorial Board

SOLLY BENATAR, *University of Cape Town, South Africa*
JURRIT BERGSMA, *Rijksuniversiteit Utrecht, The Netherlands*
TERRY CARNEY, *University of Sydney, Australia*
UFFE JUUL JENSEN, *Universitet Aarhus, Denmark*
GERRIT K. KIMSMA, *Vrije Universiteit, Amsterdam, The Netherlands*
EVERT VAN LEEUWEN, *Vrije Universiteit, Amsterdam, The Netherlands*
DAVID NOVAK, *University of Toronto, Canada*
EDMUND D. PELLEGRINO, *Georgetown University, Washington D.C., U.S.A.*
DOM RENZO PEGORARO, *Fondazione Lanza and University of Padua, Italy*
ROBYN SHAPIRO, *Medical College of Wisconsin, Milwaukee, U.S.A.*

VOLUME 5

The titles published in this series are listed at the end of this volume.

THE HERMENEUTICS OF MEDICINE AND THE PHENOMENOLOGY OF HEALTH

Steps Towards a Philosophy of Medical Practice

by

Fredrik Svenaeus

*Department of Health and Society,
University of Linköping, Sweden*

KLUWER ACADEMIC PUBLISHERS
DORDRECHT / BOSTON / LONDON

Library of Congress Cataloging-in-Publication Data

Svenaeus, Fredrik.
 The hermeneutics of medicine and the phenomenology of health : steps towards a philosophy of medical practice / by Fredrik Svenaeus.
   p. cm. -- (International library of ethics, law, and the new medicine ; 5)
 Includes index.

 1. Medicine--Philosophy. 2. Medical ethics. 3. Hermeneutics. I. Series.

R723 .S845 2001
610'.1--dc21

00-052051

ISBN 978-90-481-5632-0

Published by Kluwer Academic Publishers,
P.O. Box 17, 3300 AA Dordrecht, The Netherlands.

Sold and distributed in North, Central and South America
by Kluwer Academic Publishers,
101 Philip Drive, Norwell, MA 02061, U.S.A.

In all other countries, sold and distributed
by Kluwer Academic Publishers,
P.O. Box 322, 3300 AH Dordrecht, The Netherlands.

Printed on acid-free paper

All Rights Reserved
© 2001 Kluwer Academic Publishers
Softcover reprint of the hardcover 1st edition 2001
No part of the material protected by this copyright notice may be reproduced or
utilized in any form or by any means, electronic or mechanical,
including photocopying, recording or by any information storage and
retrieval system, without written permission from the copyright owner.

TABLE OF CONTENTS

Preface	vii
Acknowledgements	ix
Introduction	1

PART 1: THE CLINICAL ENCOUNTER — 11

1.1	The Rise of a Western Tradition of Medicine	12
1.2	The Doctor-Patient Relationship in Pre-Modern Western Medicine	16
1.3	The Birth of Modern Medicine	22
1.4	Medical Technology	29
1.5	The Modern Medical Meeting – Success and Crisis	33
1.6	Research on the Clinical Encounter in the Twentieth Century	39
1.7	The Social and Cultural Background	44
1.8	Philosophy of Medicine	51

PART 2: THE PHENOMENOLOGY OF HEALTH AND ILLNESS — 59

2.1	The Ancient Tradition	59
2.2	The Biostatistical Theory – Boorse	62
2.3	The Holistic Theory – Nordenfelt	68
2.4	Husserl's Phenomenology	75
2.5	The Phenomena of Health and Illness	78
2.6	Heidegger's Phenomenology	83
2.7	Health as Homelike Being-in-the-World	90
2.8	Homelikeness as the Rhythm of Life	94
2.9	Ability to Act and Attuned Understanding	100
2.10	The Lived Body and the Broken Tool	106
2.11	Health and Phenomenology – Medicine and Hermeneutics	114

PART 3: THE HERMENEUTICS OF MEDICINE

3.1	Explanation and Understanding	121
3.2	Hermeneutics – The Choice of Gadamer	130
3.3	Medicine and Hermeneutics	134
3.4	Ricoeur – Textuality and Narrativity in Medicine	140
3.5	The Medical Meeting – Interpretation Through Dialogue	146
3.6	Lifeworlds and Horizons in the Medical Meeting	153
3.7	The Goal of the Medical Meeting(s)	158
3.8	The Hermeneutics of Medicine – A Recapitulation and Discussion	163
3.9	Between Facts and Norms – Descriptive and Normative Analysis in the Philosophy of Medicine	166
3.10	Concluding Remarks and Future Projects – To Approach Medical Ethics from Attunement	173

Summary	177
References	183
Index of Names	193
Index of Subjects	197

PREFACE

Fredrik Svenaeus' book is a delight to read. Not only does he exhibit keen understanding of a wide range of topics and figures in both medicine and philosophy, but he manages to bring them together in an innovative manner that convincingly demonstrates how deeply these two significant fields can be and, in the end, must be mutually enlightening. Medicine, Svenaeus suggests, reveals deep but rarely explicit themes whose proper comprehension invites a careful phenomenological and hermeneutical explication. Certain philosophical approaches, on the other hand – specifically, Heidegger's phenomenology and Gadamer's hermeneutics – are shown to have a hitherto unrealized potential for making sense of those themes long buried within Western medicine. What results from his 'reading' of those themes is a bold and important ontology and epistemology of medicine – from central concepts such as 'health' and 'illness', to what is mostly termed the 'physician-patient relationship', to a constructive interpretation of the prominent 'methods' and 'goals' of medicine.

As the author makes quite clear, moreover, it is medicine's own rich historical traditions that itself demonstrates the need for the kind of phenomenological approach he engages. The most prominent characteristics of that history, he rightly appreciates, are, first, that the fundamental point of medicine is the *encounter* or 'meeting' with patients; therefore, second, medicine must be understood as a specific kind of *practice*. While it is true that medicine's centerpiece, so to speak, is the clinical event, Svenaeus argues that very few of those who have written about medicine focus on the encounter, the meeting of doctor and patient, itself. What has instead captured most attention are the results or outcomes of that meeting – health, compliance, satisfaction, autonomy. However interesting such matters are, and Svenaeus does not dispute this, the fact is that medicine has only rarely been apprehended in light of the ontological and most important epistemological themes which, more than anything else, reveal what medicine is.

Svenaeus clearly appreciates as well how deeply contemporary medicine has been influenced by the close relationships it has developed over the past 100 years with the biomedical sciences. As he suggests, however, such sciences are themselves specific types of human activity that impact not only medicine but the everyday world as well. Not only must this influence be critically appreciated, but a fuller phenomenology of medicine, he appreciates, must include critical explications of the central orientations and concepts of the biomedical and natural sciences. Although he does not engage in the latter, beyond a number of intriguing suggestions arising from his central concern with medicine as a clinical practice, it is clear that he understands this wider thematic quite well.

One of his more creative analyses is found in the way Svenaeus utilizes the key notions developed by Heidegger, especially in *Sein und Zeit*, to work his way through the major features of the clinical practice – that is, the medical encounter. It is in his quite fascinating 'reading' of Gadamer, however, that readers will be treated to perhaps the most innovative and intriguing features of this important book. After a careful critique of Ricoeur and other, more recent, discussions of hermeneutics, Svenaeus concludes that none prove entirely adequate or pertinent to the dimensions of clinical practice – whose major characteristic is not 'text', but rather *dialogue.* Suggesting how Gadamer's main notions are commensurate with Heidegger's ontology, Svenaeus then embarks on his own phenomenological explication of the clinical encounter – and here, as I've suggested, is his native air, the place he knows best and where his innovation and insight are clearest.

To help make his case as clear and compelling as possible, it is evident that he understands what is needed: a *'praxical'* discussion of actual clinical encounters. There are a number of clinical examples provided, each chosen because it illustrates some paradigmatic features of the clinical encounter, and in these discussions Svenaeus's wonderfully articulate 'feel' for actual clinical life is the clearest and most interesting.

I first came to know Fredrik Svenaeus during his extended visit at our Center for Clinical and Research Ethics at Vanderbilt University Medical Center. His excitement over what became available to him here was obvious, as was his quick intelligence and, more, his completely natural sense for, and his ease in, clinical encounters. He was, if I may so express it, very much 'at home' – not unlike the way in which he assimilates Heidegger's key notions of the 'homelike' (and 'un-homelike') 'attunement' in order to understand the special aspects of meetings and encounters which present people as ill, injured, or compromised by social or genetic circumstances.

This book is a pleasure to read, for it sheds important light on hitherto only rarely understood features of medicine as a clinical practice. Unusually articulate and well read in the important literatures of both fields, Svenaeus shows a sound knowledge both of medicine and phenomenology. His innovation and insights will doubtless make this book a standard against which future studies in the philosophy of medicine will be judged.

Nashville, Tennessee, August 2000

Richard M. Zaner

ACKNOWLEDGEMENTS

This book is a slightly revised version of my doctoral dissertation which I finished and defended in Linköping in April 1999. At the defence Wim Dekkers from the Catholic University of Nijmegen acted as opponent and I would like to thank him for the interesting and enjoyable dialogue which we enjoyed on this occasion. Wim performed a critical and insightful reading of my work, and his comments were one of the main sources for the amendments which I have made since then, mainly in Part 2 of this book. I hope that this new edition will find its way to more readers than the original dissertation manuscript published by Linköping University Press, and that the changes I have carried out make my theses on medicine and hermeneutics clearer and more plausible.

It seems to me that the course culminating in a doctoral dissertation is, in many ways, the entire, lengthy path wandered during the intellectual journey of one's life. The path is, of course, not meant to end there, but where did it really begin? And who is responsible for the itinerary in question? If this work stems from me, then I am myself certainly made up by others. Thus, I will begin these acknowledgements by going back to my own beginnings.

I would like to thank my mother, my father and my sister. Among many other things, my mother gave birth to me, which, I have heard, was a far from pleasant experience. My father introduced me into the art of philosophical thinking and dialogue, which, I hope, was more enjoyable. My sister, finally, has been there ever since the beginning offering me a kind of reversed mirror image of what is important in life. We are very much alike and yet so different.

It is not easy to find good teachers and supervisors as one makes one's way forward through the philosophical scrub. Good pathfinders are indispensable in this terrain. Alexander Orlowski introduced me to phenomenology and hermeneutics, and during the first half of the 1990s, I had the opportunity to take part in the meetings of the phenomenology seminar at the Department of Philosophy at Stockholm University led by him. Although my visits to the seminar, due to lack of time, have become less frequent during the last years, it has certainly been crucial for my knowledge and image of continental philosophy, and I am indebted to its members for offering me this opportunity, rare in the Swedish philosophical community, otherwise so one-sidedly dominated by analytical philosophy. In this connection I would also like to thank the members of our private, nameless, nomadic philosophical seminar, which convened evenings during many years to read and discuss different masters of suspicion over a cup of tea.

The academic year 1992-93 I was awarded a scholarship by DAAD, which made it possible for me to spend two semesters at the Free University in Berlin. This year was crucial for my orientation in the German philosophical tradition, and I would particularly like to mention the excellent seminars led by Milan Prucha and Michael Theunissen, which opened my eyes to many new perspectives. During that year I also met David Fopp and Ludger Hagedorn with whom I had many stimulating philosophical discussions. These friendships have proved lasting and our discussions, renewed during my visits to Germany and theirs to Sweden, inexhaustible. In the context of this book I would especially like to thank David, who has scrupulously read every part of it and provided very helpful as well as sharp criticism.

In 1994 I was accepted as a graduate student at the Department of Health and Society, University of Linköping. Tema Hälsa och samhälle has ever since then been my second home, and I would like to thank, not only the professors and graduate students, but also the administrative staff, for creating such a relaxed and effective environment for pursuing good research. The librarians at the now sadly closed Tema Library should here also be remembered. They and their colleagues at the Royal Library in Stockholm, of which I have also made extensive use, have offered valuable help in finding books and articles, not obscure perhaps, but still hard to get hold of in this country.

Although I have chosen to organize these acknowledgements chronologically instead of hierarchically I cannot resist to single out one person as the most significant when it comes to the writing of this book. It is of course customary to recognize one's supervisor as the first person to thank, but Lennart Nordenfelt not only had the courage to accept me as his student, although my field of philosophy was not his speciality, but also to let me cultivate phenomenology and hermeneutics within the philosophy of health and medicine in my own way. He has always supported me and believed in the value of what I am doing, and his critique of my manuscript at different stages has been very productive. Lennart has not only been a good pathfinder in the philosophy of medicine and health, but has also taught it to me in the manner of sharpening my own machete, rather than borrowing his. For being given the opportunity, ability and responsibility of pruning the underbrush into my very own garden I am greatly indebted to him.

Another significant intellectual partner in the work on this book has been Nils Uddenberg at the Institute for Futures Studies in Stockholm. We have met at different stages of the development of this work to discuss drafts and ideas, and these conversations have meant a great deal for the present form and contents of this study. Our dialogue has, however, not only been helpful in the process of creating arguments, but also immensely stimulating and encouraging in itself, simply an excellent example of the joy of doing philosophy together.

My Vergil in the world of clinical medicine has been Mikael Thyberg from the University Hospital of Linköping. I would like to thank him for his administrative as well as intellectual labours in initiating me into the basics of modern medicine. I would also like to thank Lars Perers, head of Ekholmen Primary Care Centre, for allowing me to follow and study him and his colleagues in their daily clinical work.

The interdisciplinary world of Tema has offered a number of seminar series which have given me the chance to learn, think about, and discuss different aspects of health and health care. The meetings of the seminar on the philosophy of health care were my major home during the years 1994-97, and the seminar series 'Meetings and Lifeworlds' during 1998-2000. In some of these seminars I have presented drafts of different parts of this manuscript. For offering able and important criticism in these seminars I would especially like to thank Jennifer Bullington, Per-Erik Liss, Sonja Olin Lauritzen, Ingemar Nordin, Jan Perselli, Bengt Richt, Gunilla Tegern, Per-Anders Tengland, Sofia Torstensson and Annika Törnström.

A scholarship from the Swedish Institute made a stay at the University of Vanderbilt in Nashville during the academic year 1997-98 possible. Richard Zaner kindly invited me as a visiting graduate student to his Center for Clinical and Research Ethics, and I would like to thank him for offering me so much of his valuable time in reading and discussing, not only the different parts of this book, but also his own pioneering work in the phenomenology of medicine, as well as that of other significant contributors to this field. I am also greatly indebted to the members of the seminar for clinical philosophy at the Center, where I presented parts of this work, as well as to many others at the Department of Philosophy at Vanderbilt, where I visited seminars on other themes. I would especially like to mention three of them here: Gregg Horowitz, who gave a brilliant seminar series on psychoanalysis and philosophy through which I was able to develop some of the thoughts put forward in this study; and Marian Shug McBay and Jason Winfree, who both offered valuable comments on different parts of the manuscript.

Per Sundström acted as opponent at a final seminar on the entire manuscript in Linköping in September 1998, during which he offered a qualified and interesting critique. I would like to thank him and the following persons for reading and commenting upon the entire manuscript or parts of it: Håkan Forsell, Per-Anders Forstorp, Lars-Erik Hjertström, Roger Qvarsell, Eva Åhrén Snickare, Jan Sundin and Jan Willner. For scrutinizing and improving my English I would like to thank Thomas Masterman.

The most important people behind a dissertation, however, are not one's academic partners in discussions on the manuscript, but one's family. My last thanks thus go to my wife and love, Lina, who has always supported me in my work on this book in every possible way. Our first son, Agaton, is equally old as my first thoughts on medicine and hermeneutics – six years now – and our second son, Osvald, was born only nine months ago. I dedicate this book to them.

This research project on medicine and hermeneutics has received financial support from Vårdalstiftelsen.

Stockholm, August 2000

INTRODUCTION

'Though this be madness, yet there is method in it.'[1]

Misunderstanding is a very real possibility, not only in the conversations of everyday life, but also in the more specific encounters between a text and its readers in academic institutions. Although there is no possibility of a total safeguarding of one's work from this kind of violence, there are some things one *can* do in order to guide the reader and make his journey safer and more comfortable, as well as, to as great extent as is possible, appealing and interesting. The latter goal, no less than the former, certainly seems crucial, since it is clear that the greatest risk you run in presenting a work is not to be misread, but not to be read at all. The purpose of this introduction is therefore to provide the reader with appropriate guidance in the reading of this book and to awake some interest for the matters I am going to pursue there. It will consequently mainly be devoted to methodological issues, but I will, in the process of presenting these issues, make use of some illustrative quotations and metaphors to create a stage setting for the arguments and theories that are going to be performed later on. I therefore beg the reader who finds the representations and metaphors of philosophy and medicine in this introduction too crude and daring to remember that they are only meant as illustrations, as an introduction to the far more sober and specified arguments to come.

The best way to start this guide to *The Hermeneutics of Medicine and the Phenomenology of Health: Steps towards a Philosophy of Medical Practice* might be to state explicitly what it is *not*. It is not, despite its title, a book about clinical method or the art of diagnosis. My aim is not to propose yet another method for the general practitioner or for other health-care personnel to be applied in their clinical work. Others are far better equipped to write such books than I am. This is not to say that what I have to contribute could not be of use in the clinic – I indeed hope it will prove to be of relevance precisely for people who meet the ill in their everyday work – but this use will be of an indirect kind and demand some reflection.

Neither is this an empirical work; that is, it is not a psychological, sociological, or anthropological empirical study of recorded clinical encounters or interviews with health-care personnel and patients. The examples of medical meetings which I make use of in this study are based on participating observation in the clinic and on real-life encounters taken from books, but the cases have often been altered in order to be particularly illustrative and fitting for the arguments and theories that I put forward

---

[1] Shakespeare, *Hamlet, Prince of Denmark* (1985, p. 127).

here. The point of the case studies is not to prove empirically that the theory is right – whatever that would mean – but to make it possible for the reader to better follow my arguments. Nevertheless, the examples are meant to be typical in the sense that they represent common cases in everyday clinical practice, and in that they are chosen in order to cover as much as possible of the very diverse area of clinical medicine. My hope is that persons working in and visiting health-care institutions will recognize themselves in these examples and find them plausible.

Finally, what I present here is not a historical study of medical practice. The first part of this work indeed deals with this history, but the purpose is here again to provide a background to my main thesis and make it emerge with greater sharpness and urgency. Although I partly base my thesis on historical research, it does not therefore itself represent any such research.

So what *is* the main thesis of this work? In acute compression it can be put like this: Clinical medicine is not a theory, not even an applied theory, but a practice. This practice, I will claim, can best be understood as an interpretive meeting between health-care personnel and patient with the aim of healing the ill person seeking help. Hermeneutics will in this work be used to further explicate what is understood by 'an interpretive meeting', and phenomenology will be put to work to better understand the meaning of 'health' and 'illness'.

What kind of thesis is this? It is best understood as a philosophical thesis; more specifically, as a thesis belonging to the sphere of the philosophy of medicine. The question that this thesis provides an answer to is thus a philosophical question; more specifically, the question, 'What is medicine?', and also – as a variation on this first question – the possibly more restricted question, 'What is medical knowledge?'. In what sense then are these questions to be understood as *philosophical* questions? What does it mean that they are philosophical, rather than, let us say, historical, psychological, sociological, or anthropological questions? To start with, it surely means that they belong to a discipline with a long academic history, which could be questioned and quoted for advice and support in this matter. Does it also mean something more than this? Are there one or several specific methodological approaches that characterize philosophy in contrast to other disciplines? Let us, in an attempt to answer this question, go back to what is considered the starting point of Western philosophy – classical Greece – to one of the first great representatives of the activity of philosophizing, Plato, and his dialogue the *Theaetetus*. The question pursued in this dialogue concerns the nature of knowledge:

> Theaetetus: Then I think that the things Theodorus teaches are knowledge – I mean geometry and the subjects you enumerated just now. Then again there are the crafts such as cobbling, whether you take them together or separately. They must be knowledge, surely.
>
> Socrates: That is certainly a frank and indeed a generous answer, my dear boy. I asked you for one thing and you have given me many; I wanted something simple, and I have got a variety.
>
> Theaetetus: And what does that mean, Socrates?

INTRODUCTION

Socrates: Nothing, I dare say. But I will tell you what I think. When you talk about cobbling, you mean just knowledge of the making of shoes?

Theaetetus: Yes, that is all I mean by it.

Socrates: And when you talk about carpentry, you mean simply the knowledge of the making of wooden furniture?

Theaetetus: Yes, that is all I mean, again.

Socrates: And in both cases what you are doing is to define what the knowledge is of?

Theaetetus: Yes.

Socrates: But that is not what you were asked, Theaetetus. You were not asked to say what one may have knowledge of, or how many branches of knowledge there are. It was not with any idea of counting these up that the question was asked; we wanted to know what knowledge itself is. Or am I talking nonsense? (p. 146c-e).

Today, within most disciplines outside of philosophy, the answer to Socrates' last question to poor Theaetetus would indeed be yes: Yes, you are talking nonsense, your approach to the matter is too general, there is not one but a multitude of types of knowledge which may be enumerated but not fitted together under one simple definition or criterion. Therefore, the first, quickly dismissed suggestion of Theaetetus for a definition of knowledge quoted above – pure enumeration – is precisely the one that would lie closest to hand if one were seeking an answer to the question of the nature of knowledge outside the discipline of philosophy. The three ensuing proposals in the *Theaetetus* for a definition of knowledge – sense perception, true judgment, and true judgment accompanied by an account – represent milestones on the way to a theory of knowledge in philosophy, but in most other disciplines they would be regarded as too abstract and general to be of any use.

In a way the reason for this rejection in fields outside philosophy is that the question of the nature of knowledge is not really *their* question. It might make sense within, for example, the field of psychology to ask what the psyche is, or what is meant by psychological knowledge. But why address the question of being and knowledge in general? Such a level of abstraction and generality seems to represent a maddening ambition and a project beyond common sense. But even the more modest abstractions, well within the theoretical grasp of a discipline might, to many participants of this discipline, seem too general to be sensible. Medicine is a good example. Would not most doctors today think that the attempt to provide univocal answers to the questions, 'What is medicine?' and 'What is medical knowledge?', represents an impossible project, given the vast variety of activities in the clinic?

And yet these are the very questions of this work. Indeed I think that the philosophical madness of generality represents a healthy antidote, rather than a maddening impossibility, for the discipline of medicine, which has become increasingly specialized as it has made rapid progress in the understanding of the structure and function of the healthy and the diseased organism. What Pollonius says about Hamlet in my opening quotation can thus be taken as a characterization of the nature of philosophy: it might be madness, but there is surely system – method – to it. Indeed, the very generality of philosophical questions makes it into a largely meta-methodological enterprise. Philosophy is all about the way – *meta hodos* – to truth and not about any truth in particular.[2]

I will soon say a bit more about this methodology, exemplified by the philosophical theories of phenomenology and hermeneutics, but first I would like to extend my medical metaphors by offering another one to characterize the relationship between medicine itself and philosophy. As we will see in the first part of this work, which deals with the history of medical practice, medicine and philosophy enjoyed a rather close partnership until the emergence of modern medicine around 1800. What happens at that point can be envisaged as a radical *philosophectomy* in medicine. Philosophy is cut off as a useless and even dangerous speculative approach to questions of health and illness – questions which can only be answered through sober empirical research.

During the last three decades of this century we have, in contrast to this attitude, witnessed a gradual rebirth of philosophy in medicine. It seems a general consensus is developing that medicine cannot solve all its problems with the help of empirical science, but rather needs a more reflective, theoretical approach, which can be provided by philosophy, as well as other disciplines, in the expanding field of medical humanities. The most obvious example of this is the booming interest in medical ethics, which deals with the question not of what can be done, but rather what *should* be done with the exploding arsenal of new medical knowledge and technologies, today and in the future, particularly in light of the limited resources in the health-care sector.

The questions to be answered in this work are not primarily ethical – rather, they are ontological and epistemological – but still the example of the rebirth of medical ethics is useful for expanding upon the metaphor of philosophectomy employed above. It seems like the operation that modern medicine *believed* it had performed around 1800 was much like an appendectomy – the excision of an ancient, now useless and possibly even infective part of the body of medicine. But what actually proved to have been excised was rather a more vital part of the gastro-intestinal tract: the rebirth of philosophy in medicine today is related exactly to the latter's inability to digest new knowledge and absorb it in an appropriate way. Thus the mission of a contemporary philosophy of medicine can be visualized as a re-establishing of these digestive functions in the organism of medicine. My attempt to carry out this mission in this work represents a methodology aimed at re-discovering and activating this resected part through a close examination and explication of the activities of clinical practice. It is consequently not a question of transplantation – application of ready made philosophical matrices to the body of medicine – but rather an attempt to find and explicate the philosophy of medicine in and through medicine itself. Thus, to conclude my metaphorical illustration of the relationship between philosophy and

---

[2]See Ritter and Gründer (1980, vol. 5, p. 1303).

medicine, with the arrival of modern medicine, the philosophy of medicine was – in the language of intestinal surgery – not so much *resected* as *defunctioned* and *concealed*; that is, medicine was temporarily dispossessed of a vital part and function, which is now to be re- activated.

Consequently my answers to the questions, 'What is medicine?' and 'What is medical knowledge?', in a curious way will *articulate* what every experienced medical practitioner already *knows*. The emphasis on articulation is vital here, because even if the experienced practitioner knows that illness is not only disease, but rather a life-form, and that medicine is not only science, but primarily dialogue and understanding, he presently lacks a language for articulating this knowledge in a systematical way.[3] It is precisely for this purpose I will show phenomenology and hermeneutics to be of great value. Rather than being classified as belonging to the ill-defined realm of the 'art of medicine', the 'unscientific' aspects of medicine can through the concepts of these theories emerge with clarity and reclaim a central role in the medical enterprise.

This sounds very ambitious indeed, and I would like to make the immediate disclaimer that what I have managed to do in this work only represents a few steps on the way to such a hermeneutical and phenomenological theory of medical practice. Yet I think that the general *direction* taken on in this work is absolutely correct and of great importance. As I said above, medicine today needs the antidote of philosophy in order not to wander astray in the maze of details, and in order not to blind itself to the temptations and risks of *hubris*, given the impressive progresses of medical science during the second half of this century. Thus, as the reader might already have noticed, the focus upon medical ontology and epistemology rather than on medical ethics in this work does not exclude a normative standpoint. Description and norm, 'is' and 'ought', are related, since the project of explicating and articulating a hidden structure of clinical practice also operates with the underlying premise that this structure *should* be paid attention to in order to facilitate the goal of this practice – the restitution of the health of the patient.

There remains to be said something more about phenomenology and hermeneutics before we take off on our journey towards a philosophy of medical practice. If philosophy can be characterized as a peculiar madness of thought in its implacable drive towards generality, this madness indeed needs to be controlled in order to, so to say, stay healthy. Plato's world of ideas, abstracted from any particular time or place, is a suitable illustration of the risks that philosophical thinking is faced with. There is indeed no thought without time and place, no sound philosophy performed from the ivory tower, as many philosophers from different schools have pointed out after Plato. Phenomenology and its adherent, phenomenological hermeneutics, are

---

[3]Though I acknowledge that, through the unreflective use of linguistic conventions, one often runs the risk of recapitulating the biases of patriarchal society, in this work, the masculine pronoun will, nevertheless, be used to avoid the cumbersome 'he or she', 'him or her', 'him- or herself', etc., in contexts in which the subjects are not specified by gender. I originally considered using feminine pronouns instead, but given the regrettable paucity of female actors throughout the history of medicine, this would have had an unintended comical effect.

good representatives of a more earth-bound manner of philosophizing, since their starting point is human experience with all its lifeworld characteristics – embodiment, culture, sociality, history etc.[4] This is consequently a type of philosophy that preserves the drive towards generality, concept and abstraction, but nevertheless acknowledges its relation to other disciplines which carry out more specific and empirical research.

It would be hard here to give even a very brief account of phenomenology and hermeneutics and their basic points of departure and terminology. I have chosen to save these introductions for Parts 2 and 3, where I will be able to provide a broader account of the theories and integrate the introductions in examinations of the concepts of health and medicine. Nevertheless, at this early juncture, I would like to stress one basic concept of phenomenology – namely, *explication* of the meaning of experience. As mentioned above, my theory will only be able to explicate, to find and articulate, in medical practice what is already *there* – and thus, in a sort of unreflected way, is already known by the participants of the clinical encounter. In a way similar to the conceptual analysis of everyday language use in analytical philosophy, phenomenology explicates the meaning and structure of the activities carried out in the everyday world.

Thus it is indeed in a way not very informative merely to say that health and medicine are phenomenological and hermeneutical occurrences, since everything related to human experience and activity can be analysed phenomenologically. What is important is that the theories of phenomenology and hermeneutics are particularly *suitable* for this kind of analysis in the case of health and medicine, since they manage to explicate features that would otherwise have remained hidden in an exclusively natural scientific approach to the subjects. The mode of attention of the medical phenomenologist is thus different than that of the medical scientist, and they consequently succeed in uncovering different things in their investigations of the same phenomena – illness and healing – or, as the medical scientist would prefer to designate them – disease and cure.[5] Medicine today, as everybody knows, certainly does

---

[4] The hermeneutical theory that I will make use of in this book is the philosophical, phenomenological hermeneutics developed mainly by Martin Heidegger and Hans-Georg Gadamer. This form of hermeneutics represents a continuation of the phenomenological project initiated by Edmund Husserl. Consequently, in this introduction, I sometimes take the liberty of talking only about 'phenomenology' when referring to this tradition of phenomenology and hermeneutics.

[5] The contrast and relation between the concepts of 'disease' and 'illness' will be laid out in detail in what follows; I will not, however, in this work make use of any sharp distinction between 'curing' and 'healing'. The first term is commonly used in a more biomedical sense than the second, which often indicates a more 'holistic' view upon matters of health. It is certainly true that my own proposals for theories of health, illness and medicine, which I will develop in Parts 2 and 3, emphasize psychological, cultural and social perspectives in addition to the biological perspective, and that they are thus holistic and based on healing rather than cure in this sense. Nevertheless, I think there lies a danger in regarding the concepts of 'curing' and 'healing' as a form of dichotomy, as it is often done in so-called 'alternative medicine'. The general practitioner in most cases does indeed not only cure, but also heals the patient, since his profession is not only to deal with biology, but with the *persons* (often) affected by a deviant biology.

INTRODUCTION 7

not suffer from a general lack of theory, but rather, as I will try to make evident in what follows, from a lack of phenomenological and hermeneutical theory.[6]

Curiously enough, as we will see, not many seem to have realized the appropriate place for phenomenology and hermeneutics in medicine. These theories have mainly lived a life restricted to the humanities. Part of the reason for this will be given by our historical investigation of the path of modern medicine in Part 1 of this work. Negligence of the 'human' side of medicine has been fostered and fed by a focus upon medical scientific research and its biological objects, as existing in a relation of opposition to, instead of connecting with, the encounter between doctor and patient with its specific 'lived' characteristics.

This work adopts the opposite approach and finds its point of departure in the experienced clinical encounter, instead of in medical science. Thus, it is vital to remember that, in what follows, the term 'medicine', if not otherwise specified, always means 'medical practice'. Another terminological issue which I would like to address at this point is that concerning the 'subjects' of medical practice (as opposed to the 'objects' – that is, the patients). I will most often use the terms 'doctor' or 'physician' for the professional party of the clinical encounter. This is not meant to exclude other members of the clinic, such as, for instance, nurses, who also, of course, take part in medical meetings. The relation between different professional groups in clinical practice will indeed, to some extent, be explicitly discussed in the text. My paradigm subject is, however, the general practitioner, in contrast not only to the nurse, but also to the specialized physician. Other medical actors are regarded as embodying or carrying out only parts of the structure which I will explicate as fundamental to clinical practice.

From the beginning, in working on this study, it has been my aim to write a book that can be read not only by philosophers, but also by other people involved in clinical medicine by way of research or profession. As I have gradually come to realize this is truly in many ways a maddening ambition, and reading through my work at this point I fear I have partly failed. The theoretical horizons of the different groups of potential readers identified above have often been too different to allow a solution suitable to everyone. It is hard to provide adequate introductions to every philosophical theme made use of if one's text is going to stay within manageable propor-

---

[6] As I have pointed out above in discussing methodology, philosophy represents a kind of 'meta-meta' perspective on things. This is evident when it comes to the issue of the meaning of 'theory'. The difference between a philosophical theory and a scientific theory is often that the former represents a theory about some other theory, like in the philosophy of science. A scientific theory is a theory about the world, philosophy of science is theory about the scientific theories. But in the case of phenomenology and hermeneutics the 'meta-meta' character carries another meaning. Phenomenology is not a theory about other theories, but rather a theoretical enterprise which tries to take a step *back* from other theories in order to free itself from prejudices and be able to study 'the things themselves' as they become manifest in their 'self-showing', in accordance with Husserl's famous credo, interpreted by Heidegger in *Sein und Zeit* (1986, pp. 27-28). Thus the difference between the theories of medical science and the theories of phenomenology and hermeneutics is not that the latter are about the former, but rather that the latter provide a framework in which science can be seen to attain its *specific* meaning. We will return to this matter – the relation between science and lifeworld – many times in this work.

tions. Thus this book includes introductions to the philosophical theories of phenomenology and hermeneutics, as well as a brief one to the philosophy of medicine, but none – except the tentative illustrations in this section – to the subject of philosophy itself. Nor have I found it possible to abstain from some rather theoretical discussions of and with other philosophers in my text.

My main reason for keeping the discussion on a rather theoretical level is that I have found the philosophical apparatus of phenomenology and hermeneutics necessary in order really to say something new and interesting about clinical practice. Thus I do not recapitulate the vocabulary out of a desire to be faithful to preceding philosophers, but rather out of a desire to be faithful to the age old human phenomena of medicine, illness and health themselves. Consequently I am not primarily exploring what previous phenomenologists and hermeneuticists have thought and written about medicine, but rather in what way their work can be used in building a theory about illness and clinical practice. My work is therefore to be understood as thematic and critical, rather than historical, and the extent to which I am employing the vocabulary of the phenomenological movement is indeed directed by that which *I* want to say. Further parts of the philosophical theory and vocabulary might indeed have been removed in favour of a more ordinary idiom, but the price paid would, in many cases, have been a lack of clarity and precision. I have not been willing to make this sacrifice in order to facilitate further accessibility in this work.

Instead of sacrificing the philosophical terminology, I will here suggest a compromise, in the form of a reading strategy based on the three parts of this work. Inevitably, this compromise will not please every reader; but my hope is that it will enable a greater number of readers to accompany me to the end of this work and prevent them from abandoning me halfway. The second part – *The Phenomenology of Health and Illness* – is probably the part most difficult to grasp for the reader untrained in the tradition of philosophy. Martin Heidegger, whose theories play a central role in the framework I there develop in order to understand the goal of medical practice – regained health – is not known to be the most accessible of modern philosophers. Though the rumours of his incomprehensibility, created in the Anglo-American philosophical community, are certainly false, following the line of reasoning I pursue while providing an introduction to his philosophy and then working critically within it in order to understand better the phenomena of health and illness, might, nonetheless, prove to be a formidable task for the philosophical beginner. The reader not primarily interested in health theory and the ways of phenomenological analysis could therefore move on to the last part of my book immediately after finishing the first one. This strategy will probably not enable the reader to follow all the arguments of Part 3 – *The Hermeneutics of Medicine*, since the proponent of the theory I am going to make use of there, in order to understand the structure of the medical meeting – Hans-Georg Gadamer – is a student and follower of Heidegger; but such a jump is nevertheless possible, as well as advisable, for the reader mainly interested in clinical practice. The philosopher merely interested in phenomenology and hermeneutics and in the philosophical analysis of health and clinical practice, on the other hand, might skip the historical background provided in Part 1 – *The Clini-*

cal Encounter – and move on immediately to Part 2 after having finished this introduction. To the readers choosing to adopt either of these leaping strategies, I would certainly recommend a reading of the concluding sections of Parts 2 respectively 1. They will make the omissions possible.

By way of ending this introduction, let me return to my opening lines concerning the risks of misunderstanding. I hope these introductory pages will help somewhat in providing a way for understanding the arguments and theories I want to communicate in the following pages. However, let me also say that I would indeed be greatly indebted to the reader who succeeds in finding more in my text than I thought I had put into it. Only through dialogue – so runs one of the main theses of this work – are truth and health to be attained.

PART 1

THE CLINICAL ENCOUNTER

'In pathology the first word historically speaking and the last word logically speaking comes back to clinical practice.'[7]

As mentioned in the introduction, we will begin this work by providing a historical sketch of medicine in the Western world. For obvious reasons, it will not be possible, in the context of this book, to present a comprehensive survey of the development of the theory and practice of medicine in the West. Nor is this my aim. I will not even mention most of the physicians and scientists whose great discoveries resulted in the examination and treatment methods which characterize modern medicine today. I will instead focus upon medical *practice*: the way physicians and patients get and got together in what is usually referred to as the 'clinical encounter' or 'consultation' – what I will often call the 'medical meeting'. The theories and techniques of medical science, however, as we will see, certainly have had an impact upon that meeting, and from that point of view they will also be dealt with here.

What I will be doing in this first part of my work must not be confused with an empirical, historical study of the clinical encounter. I will rather rely on standard works on the history of medicine and already existing empirical research on clinical practice from which I will try to extract a sketch of the development of Western medicine. My aim is to provide a historical framework which will make the topic of this book understandable and urgent. My focus upon medical practice instead of upon medical science and technology is motivated by the ontological claim introduced above, which I will try to defend and make lucid in this work: medicine is an interpretive meeting, which takes place between two persons (the doctor or some other clinical professional and the patient) with the aim of understanding and healing the one who is ill and seeks help. Clinical medicine – and this is the sense in which the term 'medicine' will be used in this book unless otherwise specified – is thus first and foremost a practice and not a science. Medical science must be viewed as an integrated part within the clinical interpretive meeting and not as its true substance; that is, not as the core mode of clinical practice, which is here merely 'applied' in contrast to the pure science of the laboratory.

---

[7]Canguilhem, *The Normal and the Pathological* (1991, p. 226).

1. THE RISE OF A WESTERN TRADITION OF MEDICINE

Having provided this historical sketch I will then in this first part of my work take a brief look at existing theories dealing with the medical meeting from different points of view (mainly psychological, sociological and anthropological theories), and begin developing a philosophical theory about the meeting as an interpretive activity with a specific goal. The following two parts of this study will be dedicated to developing this phenomenological and hermeneutical theory of medicine.

1. THE RISE OF A WESTERN TRADITION OF MEDICINE

There is good reason to believe that people have cared for their ill fellow beings ever since prehistoric time. Illness has always belonged to the human condition and the attempt to heal people is probably very old. Caring for the ill and seeking cures for diseases and other maladies could be as old as man himself. Although historical evidence from the times that precede the ancient civilizations and the invention of writing is extremely meagre, some additional support for this view can be gathered from the few remaining groups of human beings who still live in societies which remain on a Stone Age level.[8] The members of these societies have developed knowledge about herbs and plants that cure or bring relief in different types of illness, and they also master some basic surgical techniques (Ackerknecht 1982, p. 10 ff.). This 'primitive' medical knowledge is integrated into a supernatural cosmology which explains disease as being caused by spirits, ghosts or sorcerers. The healer in primitive medicine is accordingly not only a doctor but, first and foremost, a kind of spiritual healer who possesses supernatural knowledge and powers. The 'medicine man' or 'shaman' heals his patients not only with drugs but also with amulets and by expelling evil spirits from their bodies. Treatment of illness is designed according to a cosmology which provides it with meaning and prescribes different magical 'cures' in different cases.

Despite the religious, magical character of this activity, there exists in these primitive societies a distinct form of relationship that we could call medical – the relationship between the medicine man and his client. The trust, care and making sense of the illness that this relationship provides have, incontestably, in many cases, a curative effect; although, from a modern biological point of view, most of the treatment methods would be considered ineffective mumbo-jumbo and their benefit would be attributed to the placebo effect. One should not, however, underestimate the success of the different therapies. The medicine man is mainly faced with chronic diseases, such as rheumatic diseases, digestive disturbances and skin diseases, and to deal with these he is rather well equipped. The relative absence of epidemic diseases and the low life expectancy of his clients add to his reputation (Ackerknecht 1982, p. 16). The members of these tribes do not expect to live a long life free from pain and

---

[8]See Ackerknecht (1982) for an introduction to paleopathology and paleomedicine; that is, the study of teeth and bones (often fossilized), and mummies, which contain traces of disease. Another possible source for the medical prehistorian is prehistoric works of art.

other medical nuisances, and consequently, the demands and standards of medical success do not resemble those of modern Western society.

The founder of Western medicine is said to have been Hippocrates who lived in ancient Greece about 400 B.C. Large parts of the Hippocratic oath are still meant to capture the duties of a physician today.[9] Although most of what belongs to the Hippocratic Corpus was not written by a man called Hippocrates, and although the very disparate collection can, in all probability, be traced to several authors with very different medical ideas, there is certainly some truth to the claim that people in ancient Greece around 400 B.C. witnessed the birth of what we today in the Western world call medicine.[10] The theories of health and illness that we find in the Hippocratic Corpus and in other philosophical texts from this time are probably not entirely 'new' – that is, independent from the theories of healing in, for example, ancient Egypt. And they are not entirely rational in the sense of being free from all religious conceptions and practices. Nevertheless, the followers of Hippocrates, the 'Asclepiads' of Cos, Cnidos and Rhodos, were much more similar to the physician of today than the Egyptian magician in their rejection of supernatural explanatory models for most diseases, in their willingness to engage in rational arguments in matters of health and disease, and in their systematic gathering of empirical evidence, which aimed at giving a prognosis and finding a cure for different illnesses (Amundsen and Ferngren 1983, pp. 11-13).

The Hippocratic physician considered his patient as placed in a world order – a *kosmos* – which was essentially mirrored in the makeup of the individual. Illness was due to imbalance between the elements that compose the body. Once one knew wherein this imbalance consisted – for instance, in the excess or lack of a certain fluid in the body, such as blood, bile or phlegm – one could prescribe a diet which aimed at re-establishing balance.[11] This knowledge of cosmological balance gathered through experience and argument was the speciality of the Hippocratic physician. He was neither a magician nor a scientist, but rather a craftsman who offered his services in return for payment.[12] The German historian Ludwig Edelstein gives a rather down-to-earth picture of the celebrated Hippocratic physician, the first representative of Western medicine:

> The medical craft is not under any restrictions. Anyone can practice it without having to pass an examination and without being accredited by any authority. As a craftsman, the physician of antiquity is classified socially as a businessman. While the modern doctor, in spite of the payment he receives, is not on the same social level as the other craftsmen who, like him, are paid for their services, the ancient physician is the equal of the other craftsmen and thereby occupies a low position in society. These circumstances determine the attitude of the patient to the physician and, consequently, the at-

---

[9] For a historical and philological interpretation of the different parts of the oath, see 'The Hippocratic Oath: Text, Translation and Interpretation', in Edelstein (1967).

[10] See 'The Genuine Works of Hippocrates', in Edelstein (1967).

[11] See Nutton (1995a).

[12] But a craftsman who often possessed considerable theoretical knowledge. For a discussion of the relation between theory and practice, *theoria* and *techne*, as well as *phronesis* in Greek medicine, see 'Greek Medicine as Science and Craft', in Temkin (1977).

titude of the physician to the patient. For the patient, the physician is not the doctor, the educated man to whose knowledge he defers and whom he recognises as an authority in his field; on the contrary, the physician is a craftsman who must prove that he knows his business and that he is just as eager to do his work well as to earn money.[13]

The meeting between doctor and patient in Hippocratic medicine, according to Edelstein, is more reminiscent in a contemporary scenario of the dealings of a deceptive automobile mechanic with his customers, than of the modern doctor's relation to his patients. However, other historians, on the basis of essentially the same material – the Hippocratic Corpus and other contemporary texts – give a totally different picture of the Hippocratic physician.

Pedro Lain Entralgo, a Spanish medical historian, has a more sympathetic (or one might say idealized) view on the subject. He sees the relationship between doctor and patient in ancient Greece as characterized by a special form of friendship – 'medical philia' – which he regards as having been essential to Western medicine up until the present day:

> Let us imagine a typical medical event. Apart from his economic and professional interests, the doctor is moved by desire to give technical help to the invalid. The invalid, on his part, has consulted the doctor chiefly because he wants to be cured. Yet in spite of the obvious difference between the two motives, the Greeks had the perspicacity to give them the same name: both were generally described as *philia*, or 'friendship'. 'The sick man loves the physician because he is sick,' says Plato in the *Lysis* (217a). 'Where there is *philanthropia* (love of man), there is also *philotechnia* (love of the art [of healing])', declares a famous Hellenistic passage in the Hippocratic *Praecepta* (L.IX,258) (Lain Entralgo 1969, p. 17).

The two different views on the doctor-patient relationship, as either a business transaction or as an encounter based on an urge to understand and help, seem to have been with us, both in practice and in theory, ever since Hippocrates, up until today. But in the case of Edelstein and Lain Entralgo, the two positions might, at first sight, appear to be more in conflict with each other than they actually are. Lain Entralgo does not deny that there existed an economic aspect to the consultation in ancient Greece; he only deems it secondary to the ambition to help and to cure. On the other hand there is nothing, in principle, that prevents the honest and loving physician from practising in the workshops of Edelstein's market place in competition with the hawkers. He could certainly be successful in the competition for clients precisely through his excellent techniques and friendly attitude.

Hippocratic medicine is, according to both historians, a handicraft – an art and a practice – which aims at curing the patient through the doctor's skills. These skills are developed by experience and rational argument and are based on certain theories of health and illness as balance and imbalance in the constitution of human beings. According to both Edelstein and Lain Entralgo, medical practice takes place in a meeting between doctor and patient – a medical meeting – in which the doctor must study and interpret the situation of the patient – his state of ill health – in order to find a cure. The doctor basically has two sources for this interpretation: the story told

---

[13]'The Hippocratic Physician', in Edelstein (1967, p. 87).

by the patient and his physical appearance. The patient on the other hand must attempt to place trust in the physician in order to be able to tell him his story, show him his body and follow his prescriptions. Friendship or egoistic striving for survival might or might not be the ultimate source of the strategies of the two parties of the consultation; in either case there must arise a basic trust between the two individuals present in the medical meeting if the practice is to be successful.

As I mentioned in the introduction to this work, medicine and philosophy were more closely united in the ancient world than they are in the contemporary clinic. There exists a general analogy between medicine and philosophy in ancient philosophy: the former aims at curing the body and the latter strives to provide arguments to heal the soul from its suffering. Martha Nussbaum has examined this analogy at length in her book *The Therapy of Desire: Theory and Practice in Hellenistic Ethics* (1994). According to Nussbaum, it was Democritus who first developed the analogy between medicine and *philosophy*, although there exists an even older tradition in Greek thinking in which an analogy is drawn between medical treatment of the body and *logoi* (speech and argument) as a *pharmakon* for the soul (1994, p. 51). Lain Entralgo, in *The Therapy of the Word in Classical Antiquity* (1970), has also studied the connection between verbal therapy and medicine in Greek philosophy. He traces the development from Homeric charms (*epodai*) to the power of philosophical argument in Plato and Aristotle and claims that philosophical discourse was thought to have a healing effect on the psyche: it was thought to produce temperance (*sophrosyne*).[14] The close relationship between medicine and philosophy in the ancient world thus bears a twofold significance. Not only did the theories employed in medical practice have a philosophical origin;[15] but also, philosophy in the ancient world, just like medicine, was a practice rather than a theory, and it had a therapeutic, educating mission.

If we agree to view the meeting of Hippocratic medicine as the origin of the modern doctor-patient relationship, it is important to point out at the same time the many differences between the two historical positions. The theories of modern medicine do not have very much in common with the ancient ones, and this of course means that physical examination and therapies are very different if one compares Hippocratic to modern medicine. The Hippocratic physician did perform bonesetting and some surgery, but the basic form of therapy was pharmaceutical, or rather, it was related to diet and life style (Nutton 1995a, p. 26; Temkin 1977, p. 147). It is also important to call attention to the fact that slaves and free men were regarded very differently in ancient Greece: the medical treatment of slaves was not the activity of the real physician, but rather 'a sort of veterinary service for men' (Lain Entralgo 1969, p. 31). A third important difference between the Hippocratic

---

[14] Lain Entralgo's book (1970) pursues a slightly different course than Nussbaum's (1994) – it omits the Epicureans and Stoics for example – and tends to stress the medical rather than the ethical effect of the word. It is nevertheless strange that Nussbaum does not mention this important book. Particularly interesting is Lain Entralgo's discussion of *katharsis* in Aristotle's poetics and its similarity to medical purging.

[15] We will come back to this issue in Section 8 of this part and in Section 1 of Part 2.

and the modern medical meeting is the lack of privacy inherent in the former (Edelstein 1967, p. 88). The Hippocratic meeting between doctor and patient took place in front of an audience consisting of the pupils of the physician, the friends and family of the patient, and other curious bystanders. The idea of privacy in the meeting – the medical meeting of two individuals protected from the gazes and opinions of others – is something that did not come into being until the birth of modern medicine around 1800 – that is, more than two millennia later.[16] Despite these major differences between the Hippocratic medical meeting and the modern clinical encounter, they share a focus upon the health of the individual and upon the duties of the physician towards his patient, which has made it customary to talk about a coherent tradition of Western medicine – a tendency reflected in the persistent reference to the Hippocratic oath as the source of medical ethics.

2. The Doctor-Patient Relationship in Pre-Modern Western Medicine

The general picture of the development of medicine after Hippocrates and Galen in the Western world is one of decay. No essential progress seems to be made until about A.D. 1600, when a scientific revolution is initiated that will result in the birth of modern medicine around 1800.[17] The ancient theories of humours, elements and qualities continued to exert their influence until the birth of the modern clinic and pathological anatomy paved the way for a different understanding of the body and its diseases. In the following I would like to qualify this general statement and bring to light certain aspects of ancient medical practice which withstood the benightedness of 'the Dark Ages'.

We have taken a brief look at the activities of the Hippocratic physician in his workshop. Did he have other competitors than his colleagues in the healing profession? Certainly. From the beginning physicians have had to contend with the hard competition of magicians and other lay healers. Self-devised cures and healing within the family have, in addition to this, probably always been the most common forms of treatment for diseases, especially for minor ailments.

It is important to realize that little distinction was made between the physician – *iatroi, medici* – and other healers in the ancient world, since there were no official schools of medicine or special certificates issued for physicians (Edelstein 1967, p. 87). Not until the thirteenth century and the rise of the universities in Europe was a medical doctorate established which licensed the physician and placed him in starker contrast to other healing professions, such as, for example, surgeons (Nutton 1995c, p. 153 ff.). Medicine in the Hellenistic world was not uniform, but was rather divided into different schools or 'sects' which advocated different healing strategies and had different theoretical outlooks. These sects were later, by medical historians, assembled into two main groups, the dogmatics and the empirics. The former stressed *a*

---

[16] I will return to the question of the privacy of the meeting and to the issue of the patient as subject (person) and object in and of the clinical encounter in the two following sections.

[17] See for instance the famous work by Shryock (1948) for such a view.

priori etiological theories of illness, the latter the clinical experience of the individual patient (Nutton 1995a, p. 36). After Greek medicine had conquered Rome, the dogmatics and the empirics were joined by new sects like the 'pneumatists' and the 'methodists' in the first century A.D. (Nutton 1995a, pp. 41-44).[18]

The unification of medicine was to a great extent the work of one man and the effect of the tremendous influence he came to enjoy: Galen of Pergamum (129-c. 216). Galen, through his work and books, was successful not only in diminishing the influence of competing schools such as the methodists, but also in reviving Hippocrates and establishing him as the father of medicine, the only medical theorist worth studying except Galen himself (Nutton 1995a, p. 58 ff.). The corpus of medical literature which was studied in medieval Europe consisted almost solely of Galen and the works of Hippocrates which he had commented upon. The works of Galen, which treated such topics as the qualities of pulses and inspection of urine and which included a human anatomy based on dissections of apes and pigs, were to exert their influence for a very long time.

With the rise of Christianity and the fall of the Roman Empire, the development and tradition of ancient medicine not only came to a stand-still, but was also, to a great extent, actually forgotten. The Christian religion provided illness and suffering with a new meaning: they were punishments from God for the sinfulness of human life and should accordingly be endured in thankful silence and penitent prayer. Those who sought cure in medical therapy and not in prayer risked being looked upon with suspicion and contempt (Lain Entralgo 1969, pp. 78-79). Even the Greeks had viewed the attempt to cure the *incurable* illnesses as *hubris*: medicine should work with, not against, nature. But the Christian interpretation of illnesses as punishment sent from God meant that *all* illness could be considered the result of a sinful life. Thus the attempt to cure illness by physical means could be looked upon not only as useless, but also as potentially sinful – a rebellion against the will of God.

Even though illness was often interpreted as carrying a religious meaning, most people surely went on seeking relief and cure for it. Not everybody is a saint, and accordingly he has neither the strength to endure illness without lamenting or seeking relief for it, nor the faith in or prospect for a miracle. Doctors still carried out their profession and made a living during the Middle Ages, even if they were not held in high esteem.

---

[18]Richard Zaner has, in his book *Ethics and the Clinical Encounter* (1988), analysed the basic differences in medical outlook between the empirics and the dogmatics. Zaner comes to the conclusion that the empirical school should be considered the true origin of clinical medicine today rather than the dogmatical: the former highlights the importance of focusing attention on the individual patient and the context of his illness, whereas the latter proceeds from general theories of disease and then simply applies them to the individual case. This is a quite complex matter, however, since total resistence toward general statements about disease would result in the sceptic position of not being able to learn anything from one case which could be applied to another. The empiric doctor's experience from one patient (and other empiric doctors' experiences which are related to him) must in some sense make him more capable of curing new patients, if there is to be any point in adopting the empiric outlook. Zaner, in his book, tries to show how this indeed was the case among some of the empirics.

The advent of Christianity also meant a new attitude towards the poor, which had the opposite result of what one would expect from the principle of non-intervention based upon religious faith. To care for the poor, ill and suffering – for one's neighbour – was the duty of a good Christian. This did not mean that medical theory and therapeutics made any progress, but it certainly meant that a loving care that brought relief for the ill and dying was exercised. The first hospitals for this purpose – hostels – were built in the fourth century A.D. (Nutton 1995c, p. 153 ff.).[19] These hostels were run by people from the church and the role of the lay physician was consequently gradually taken over by the 'priest physician' (Lain Entralgo 1969, p. 61 ff.). The rise of the monasteries meant that the monks combined the care of the soul with the care for the illnesses of the body, and it was in these monasteries that various elements of the knowledge of ancient medicine were preserved during the Middle Ages, c. 600-c. 1100, in Europe.

The monks, as well as the few lay physicians who still worked in private practices or in the houses of kings and other rich men, were under the obligation to care first and foremost for the souls of their patients (Lain Entralgo 1969, p. 98 ff.). The worst thing that could happen to a doctor (and to a patient) was that the latter died without confessing his sins to a priest. The eternal life of the soul was far more important than the temporary sufferings of the body. The consoling, spiritual conversation was therefore an important part of the meeting. Besides this conversation between doctor and patient, physical examination and treatment were generally limited to the feeling of the pulse, inspection of urine, dietetic prescriptions and possibly blood-letting, bone-setting, simpler surgery and purging (Lain Entralgo 1969, p. 80 ff.; Nutton 1995b, pp. 83-87). These activities could, however, also be carried out by surgeons, wise women and other healers.

An essential turn in the medical tradition takes place with the revival of ancient medicine, mediated, enriched and returned to Europe by way of the Islamic medical tradition, from c. 1100 and onwards.[20] The famous school of Salerno in southern Italy was founded even earlier, by, according to popular tradition, a Roman, a Jew, an Arab, and a Greek who brought with him the writings of Hippocrates (Nutton 1995c, p. 139). The truth was that most of the lost texts of Galen and Hippocrates were translated from Arabic, rather than re-discovered in the Greek original. The development of the school of Salerno and the rise of the first universities in Europe – in Bologna c. 1180, in Paris c. 1200, in Salamanca c. 1218 and in Padua c. 1222 – gradually improved the position of the lay physician, reintroduced the theories of ancient medicine, and established the practice of human dissection.[21]

---

[19]Historical predecessors to the Christian hospital were the healing shrines of Asclepius where the ill went to live for a time and seek cure in devotion, and the Roman military camps in which the wounded were looked after by doctors in special tents (Nutton 1995a, pp. 49-52). For a history of the hospital, see also Granshaw (1993).

[20]See Conrad (1995a).

[21]See Ottosson (1984), a study of the teaching and theories of medicine in late medieval and early Renaissance Italy. For introductions to the history of anatomical dissection with adequate references, see French (1993) and Johannisson (1997).

The medical doctorate provided the physician with a license which distinguished him from surgeons and other healing professions.[22] The university-trained doctor, however, was a physician for the elite – the rich and educated residents of the big cities; the majority of doctors still carried out their practice without any university studies or licenses. Gradually, societies for physicians were also established. The Royal College of Physicians in London, for example, received its royal charter in 1518. But again, these were societies for the 'elite physicians' with university degrees and not for the country doctors. Unlicensed practitioners looked after the poor, most often in the homes of the latter, but occasionally in hospitals, which become larger and more numerous as we approach the Renaissance and as lay physicians begin to reconquer the domain of medical practice from the healers of the Church (Granshaw, p. 1184 ff.).

The Renaissance in Italy with the return to classical sources meant the rediscovery and re-introduction of ancient medical texts in the original Greek language – mainly Hippocrates and Galen – and also a renewed study of human anatomy through public dissections of executed criminals. Andreas Vesalius (1514-64) and others succeeded in proving false many of the anatomical and functional theories of Galen, who had mainly based his works upon the dissection of animals. Paracelsus's (1482-1546) focus upon chemistry instead of humoral pathology was another source for a growing anti-Galenic wave in medicine. Paracelsus attempt to describe diseases without making appeal to the humoral state paved the way for the voluminous disease catalogues of physicians like Thomas Sydenham (1624-89), based upon empirical studies of patients, rather than ancient texts of medicine. The formulation of a modern mechanistic philosophy in the seventeenth century, inagurated by thinkers such as René Descartes and Francis Bacon, which laid the foundation for the coming scientific revolution, obviously had repercussions for medicine, though they did not become apparent at once.[23]

---

[22] See Gelfand (1993).

[23] In the case of Descartes the influence of his philosophy on medicine has been quite significant not only when it comes to a general modern, scientific, 'anti-metaphysical' way of thinking. A dualistic picture of the human being based upon the influence of Cartesian philosophy seems to be prevalent even today in medicine, making itself apparent in labels like 'psycho-somatic'. The mind might no longer be thought of as a non-extended substance conjoined to the body by the pineal gland, but the prevailing opinion among doctors seem to be that dualism, of some sort, is the only alternative to a reductionistic, materialistic worldview content to jettison the psyche altogether. Hans Jonas's *The Phenomenon of Life: Toward a Philosophical Biology* (1966), a highly significant work in this context, describes the transition from an animated 'pan-vitalistic' world view to a mechanistic one. This transition takes place, he claims, in part on account of the impact of Cartesian dualism, which allows a study of nature in itself freed from any animated teleology. If, according to the pre-Cartesian world view, the dead body was an enigma because everything was essentially 'alive', today the living body has become the real problem since we are 'under the ontological dominance of death'; that is, 'only when a corpse is the body plainly intelligible' (1966, p. 12). As I will try to show in this study phenomenology and hermeneutics provide better tools than dualism for thinking about the ill as something more than molecules, tissues and organs. An important work which discusses Descartes's influence on contemporary medicine and attempts to present an alternative based on the phenomenology of embodiment is Drew Leder's *The Absent Body* (1990a). Leder traces the roots of Descartes's dualism to the lifeworld of his (and our) time, in which the body is seen as an obstacle and source of error for abstract thinking, philosophy and science. That the body as a consequence of

Now, what did Renaissance and later, classical medical discoveries – such as William Harvey's book on the circulation of the blood and the function of the heart in 1628, or Antoni van Leeuwenhoek's (1632-1723) identification in his self-built microscope of what we now know to have been bacteria and red corpuscles – mean for the doctor-patient relationship? What indeed did they mean to medical practice – to the examination and treatment methods which were applied in the meeting? The answer seems to be, not much, if anything. Diagnosis in the seventeenth century was still carried out in an essentially Galenic manner:

> To determine the nature of the illness, he (the seventeenth century physician) relied chiefly on three techniques: the patient's statement in words which described his symptoms; the physician's observation of signs of the illness, his patient's physical appearance and behaviour; and, more rarely, the physician's manual examination of the patient's body.[24]

I will comment upon these three parts of the procedure of diagnosis – taking the patient's statement, the physician's observation, and his examination – in reverse order. Examination of the patient's body was rare in pre-modern medicine. This was the case for several reasons. Religious chasteness played a role, especially when women were involved; but perhaps more importantly, the doctor had to rely on a theoretical approach in order to avoid being confused with other healers like surgeons: 'The physician, by contrast (to the surgeon), was a thinker, not a toucher' (Porter and Porter 1989, p. 75). The theories of pre-modern medicine did not view the body as a functional mass which could be palpated and opened up in search for pathologies. Humoral pathologies were rather detected through the general appearance, behaviour and character of the patient, as well as through the signs that could be discerned by feeling his pulse and temperature and by examining his stools and urine. Sometimes, in addition to this, the physician would also examine the tongue and the eyes of the patient, smell his breath, and in some cases study spots on his skin. The most important aid in making a correct diagnosis was, however, the patient's own history. Only the patient had direct access to his own symptoms and these were crucial to the diagnosis. The patient's own feelings and thoughts upon his illness thus, in an obvious way, occupied the centre of pre-modern medicine. This is probably the main difference between pre-modern and modern medical practice. How are we to understand this focus upon the patient as *person* rather than object of investigation in pre-modern medicine?

The influence of the patient in the medical meeting of pre-modern medicine must first be considered against the background of the low prestige of doctors in these times (Shorter 1985, p. 51). Even the few distinguished university-trained physicians

---

this distrust is freed from spirit means that it is literally surrended to and opened up for modern science; although, as we shall see in the next section, this development was delayed until around 1800. An interesting fact that does not appear to be well known is that Descartes studied medicine himself. He practised dissection of animals, wrote on physiology, treated himself and gave medical advice to ill friends. For details see Lindeboom (1979).

[24]Reiser (1978, p. 1). For a survey of the art of diagnosis in pre-modern medicine see also Bynum and Porter (1993a); Nicolson (1993a); Porter and Porter (1989); and Shorter (1985).

who enjoyed a good reputation had patients who often occupied a higher position in society than themselves, such as aristocrats or the rising wealthy bourgeoisie. Patients could thus often dominate the meeting in a sense that would be impossible today. The establishing of a diagnosis often had the form of a negotiation between doctor and patient, during which the latter would suggest causes and explanations for his illness, which he wanted the doctor to confirm (Porter and Porter 1989, p. 78). If the doctor refused the patient might simply call for another doctor who was easier to convince.

The doctor's chief task, then as now, seems to have been to prescribe a cure. The patients appear to have been more interested in treatment than diagnosis, since they soon found out that there were nearly as many diagnoses as doctors. The general low prestige that the doctor struggled against was, however, certainly also due to the very doubtful effects that the therapy he applied had on illness. Most treatment was oriented toward evacuation – towards making the patient bleed, defecate, sweat or salivate (Porter and Porter 1989, p. 160; Shorter 1985, p. 44). The lancet, used for inducing bleeding, and various strong – sometimes poisonous, but more often simply useless – drugs were accordingly the main therapeutic means of the pre-modern doctor. No wonder he had problems in the competition with surgeons, pharmacists, wise women and other healers. He most often did not possess any better therapies for illness than they did. The difference between doctor, surgeon and pharmacist was consequently far from obvious in the times when doctors' standard therapies were to bleed their patients and mix their own patent drugs (Porter and Porter 1989, p. 27).

As we touched upon in the foregoing section, despite the central place of the patient's account, feelings and opinions in the pre-modern medical diagnosis, the *privacy* of the medical meeting is essentially a modern phenomenon. The encounter before the nineteenth century took place amidst an assembly of family and friends, who listened and commented upon the diagnosis and treatment. Often several doctors and other healers were gathered around the sickbed and quarrelled about the correct diagnosis (Porter and Porter 1989, pp. 79-83; Wear 1995, p 238). It was also quite common at this time to arrive at a diagnosis based simply on a written account of the patient's illness; that is, the doctor prescribed a treatment without actually having met the patient (Nicolson, 1993a, p. 809; Porter and Porter 1989 pp. 76-78). Although the doctor in pre-modern medicine without doubt attached significance to the patient's account of his life and illness to a greater extent than is usually the case in modern medicine, it would thus nevertheless be misleading to draw the quick and easy conclusion that the patient, as the subject of the diagnosis, was, to a greater extent than is the case today, considered an individual *person*. The Enlightenment not only brought about an objectifying positivism, but also, to some extent, as we will see, witnessed the birth of a modern, human, autonomous self that transformed the character of the medical meeting.[25]

---

[25]See Taylor (1989) for a historical-philosophical study of the sources and development of the modern self.

The history of medical practice in the West, the outlines of which I have traced so far, shows that the medical meeting before the dawning of modern science took place between two *equals* in a more pronounced sense than at the present day, when the doctor is generally the party in command of the meeting. As I have tried to show, however, it would be a hasty conclusion to say that this made the meeting more 'humane' than is the case in the contemporary clinic. Apart from the useless and often painful therapies for illness sprung from faulty premises on the design of the human body, pre-modern human beings – patients as well as doctors – had a different sense of private self and human value than we do today. Human life was not accorded any absolute moral respect, neither in theory nor in practice. Human beings were thought to be part of a grand design, but they were not thought to be at the centre of this design – a belief which formed the basis of a system of values very different from our modern world view. This applies for the thinking of antiquity as well as for the Christian cosmology of pre-modern Europe.

However, it is not easy to arrive at any certain or conclusive views upon the differences in the sense of selfhood experienced by the people in the Greek *polis*, in contrast to that experienced by the monks in the monasteries of Middle Age Europe, or by the doctors in the universities of Renaissance Italy, or indeed by the people in the modern clinic of today. What we can learn from a historical study of medicine is, nevertheless, that medicine always was and probably always will be first and foremost a *meeting* and a *practice*. Medicine is not only science and technology, as the state of modern medicine today might mislead us into thinking. Medical science is a rather new invention. The medical meeting, which is the focus of the present study, certainly preceded and has indeed survived the birth of modern medicine and science, although the patient, as the consequence of this development, as we will now see, in a new sense becomes the *object*, and not only the subject, of diagnosis and treatment.

3. THE BIRTH OF MODERN MEDICINE

In spite of the difficulties involved in pinpointing a time and place for the birth of modern medicine, two so entirely different medical historians as Richard Shryock and Michel Foucault seem to agree that it took place in Paris in the turbulent years following the revolution of 1789.[26] They also agree upon the course of events and significant factors involved in this process; what marks the significant difference between their views are the theories with the aid of which they attempt to explain and make sense of this transition in the history of medicine.

Modern medicine essentially arose through the unification of two phenomena: the medical clinic and pathological anatomy. Neither of these were invented in Paris around 1800, but they were systematically brought together there in a way that created a new approach towards the human body and its diseases. The closing down of

---

[26]See Shryock (1948, p. 129) and Foucault (1994a, p. 146). For a study of the dawning of modern medicine in Paris, see also Ackerknecht (1967).

the universities in France after the Revolution and the development of a new medical educational system centred around the hospitals, which to a far greater extent favoured bedside studies of patients, meant a new focus upon systematical empirical studies of diseased bodies. Patients were classified through an investigation based primarily, not on what they told the doctor about their symptoms, but rather on the signs detected through inspection of their bodies – through touching, looking and listening. Systematical records were kept through which the course of illness for different patients with similar signs of disease could be compared. The modern teaching and research clinic of the Paris school admittedly had predecessors, such as the schools in Vienna and Edinburgh in the second half of the eighteenth century; but, in Paris, to this systematic, empirical approach to the diseases of *living* patients in the hospitals was linked a study of their *deceased* bodies by means of dissection. It is at this point that the subjection of medicine to what the philosopher Hans Jonas calls 'the ontological dominance of death' commences (1966, p. 12). The patient's body is viewed as a functional space that can be opened up for inspection:

> To establish these signs (of disease) . . . , is to project upon the living body a whole network of anatomo-pathological mappings: to draw the dotted outline of the future autopsy. The problem, then, is to bring to the surface that which is layered in depth; semiology will no longer be a *reading*, but the set of techniques that make it possible to constitute a *projective pathological anatomy* (Foucault 1994a, p. 162).

Nor pathological anatomy, however, was an invention of the French clinic. It suffices to mention the works of Giovanni Battista Morgagni (1682-1771), who developed a morbid anatomy of organs and emphasized the importance of post-mortem dissections to reveal disease lesions. What was then the essential step, taken by the French physician Xavier Bichat, 'often cited as the founder of modern medicine', which enabled him to surpass Morgagni? (Shryock 1948, p. 130). Shryock gives an answer which is similar to the account given by Foucault:

> Only by correlating bedside observations and subsequent pathological findings could physicians arrive at distinctions between different disorders. Only by improving clinical observations and, at the same time, probing deeper into pathological anatomy, could medical men sketch out the rational nosography so necessary to further progress in the medical sciences. That the young Frenchmen of 1800 went farther in this direction than Morgagni, was due to their consistent pursuit of these two ideals – to Bichat's more searching investigations in gross pathology, and to the improvement made by his colleagues in the technique of clinical observation (Shryock 1948, p. 132).

Bichat, Pinel, Louis, Laënnec – they all shared this conviction of the importance of linking clinical observation to post-mortem dissection. The body of the patient was looked upon as a functional space where the disease resided. Bodily function, localized to systems of organs and tissues (and later to cells and molecules), and the diseases that interfered with these functions (or rather the effects of these diseases in organs and tissues), could be studied through observation, palpation and auscultation of the living body of the patient, and through a dissection of the dead body as soon as the patient had passed away. Diseases were then found in form of morbid changes in the tissues which were thought to have given rise to signs and sounds on the surface of the diseased body when the patient was still alive.

What effect did this new approach to disease have for the patient and to what extent did it change the nature of the doctor-patient relationship? Different historians provide us with different answers here. To start with, it is important to realize that the activities in the modern clinic had a relatively slow impact upon the practice of private physicians, who continued either to receive patients in their offices or call upon them in their homes. The hospital was, until the twentieth century, mainly a place for the very poor patients, who did not possess the means to pay a private physician. Edward Shorter, who has studied the history of the doctor-patient relationship, dates the advent of the modern doctor with his new diagnostic tools and mentality to around 1880 (1985, p. 75). The reasons for this delay were, first, the reluctance of medical schools to incorporate the new ideas into their curricula and, second, the resistance of older doctors to change their medical outlook, which was grounded in pre-modern medical theories (Shorter 1985, p. 78). Since the modern approach to illness did not show any significant *curative* results until the development of micro-biology in the 1880s (with the possible exception of the benefits of better surgical technology), or indeed until the therapeutical success of antibiotics in the 1930s and 1940s, it is not very hard to understand the scepticism of these old-fashioned doctors.

In order to explicate the significance of the profound change that took place in the history of Western medicine around 1800 in the school of Paris, I will compare two very different historical theories dealing with this event. The first, which I will call 'the progressive view', is propounded by traditional medical historians such as Richard Shryock and Owsei Temkin; the second, which I will call 'the epistemic view', mainly derives its origin from the influential works of Michel Foucault and other historians of medicine working in his wake.

According to the progressive view, the birth of modern medicine was the result of the scientific discoveries and hard practical work of enlightened and brave men who challenged religious tradition, superstition and ignorance. They only placed their trust in evidence, which they could actually see with their own eyes, and did not hesitate to do the dirty work of dissection themselves. Temkin here emphasizes surgery and the influence it had upon medicine in the eighteenth century as decisive (1977, p. 491); whereas Shryock instead stresses the importance of quantitative and instrumental procedures (1948, p. v). The progressive view tends to look upon medical history as a series of discoveries by different individuals, who challenge the theories of pre-modern medicine (humoral pathology and other speculative theories based on sensibility, irritability and similar concepts). The sound empirical knowledge that these men amass finally culminates in a massive body of thought that succeeds in toppling the old system, which was supported by a religious and conservative ideology. This intellectual coup is admittedly not an isolated phenomenon: it would not have been possible without changes in other sciences and in the social structure of society. Still, according to this view, medical history advances progressively and cumulatively, and the role of science in this progression is to provide medicine with increasingly sophisticated theories and techniques, with the help of which medicine can better promote the well-being of mankind.

The epistemic view of Foucault regarding the same events is a totally different one. According to Foucault, historical changes do not come about through the isolated inventions or discoveries of individuals, which then accumulate in a progressive way, but rather depend on epistemological shifts in discourse[27], which make the new inventions and theories of individuals possible:

> I am not concerned, therefore, to describe the progress of knowledge towards an objectivity in which today's science can finally be recognised; what I am attempting to bring to light is the epistemological field, the *episteme* in which knowledge, envisaged apart from all criteria having reference to its rational value or to its objective forms, grounds its positivity and thereby manifests a history which is not that of its growing perfection, but rather that of its conditions of possibility; in this account, what should appear are those configurations within the *space* of knowledge which have given rise to the diverse forms of empirical science. Such an enterprise is not so much a history, in the traditional meaning of that word, as an 'archaeology'. Now, this archaeological inquiry has revealed two great discontinuities in the *episteme* of Western culture: the first inaugurates the Classical age (roughly half-way through the seventeenth century) and the second, at the beginning of the nineteenth century, marks the beginning of the modern age.... Not that reason made any progress: it was simply that the mode of being of things, and the order that divided them up before presenting them to the understanding, was profoundly altered (Foucault 1994b, p. xxii).

The two epistemological 'grids' that predetermine knowledge in the classical versus the modern age can, according to *Les mots et les choses*, be summarized in the terms 'representation' and 'human being'. In the case of the history of medicine – to which Foucault, three years earlier, in 1963, had devoted a whole book, *Naissance de la clinique* – classical medicine as a representational phenomenon is most obvious in the nosological catalogues of different diseases assembled by physicians such as Thomas Sydenham, François de Boissier de Sauvages and William Cullen. They worked according to a botanic principle (1994a, p. 7). Like Linnaeus, they created systems of diseases – taxonomies – which classified ailments according to similarities and differences in the symptoms and clinical signs of the patients. A table in which all diseases were thus described and arranged *represented* the diseases as they actually manifested themselves on the surface of the patients (for example, as spots on the skin, or as irregularities in the excrement, urine or sputum or of the temperature of the skin or of the quality of the pulse). These nosological systems, according to Foucault, left no room for the patients (or the doctors) as human beings; they were reduced to little more than 'disturbances' in the representational system of diseases:

> In the rational space of disease, doctors and patients do not occupy a place as of right; they are tolerated as disturbances that can hardly be avoided: the paradoxical role of medicine consists, above all, in neutralising them, in maintaining the maximum difference between them, so that, in the void that appears between them, the ideal configura-

---

[27] It is hard to give any good account of this famous term, which plays a key role in Foucault's theories. To analyse 'discourse' must of course mean to analyse the structure of language, rather than human experience, but whether this emphasis makes Foucault's project a structuralist one is a disputed issue. Foucault himself explicitly rejects the phenomenological approach in favour of an analysis of 'discursive practice', but also at the same time resists the label 'structuralist' (1994b, p. xiv). For a lucid, critical discussion of his position, see Dreyfus and Rabinow (1982), Part 1.

tion of the disease becomes a concrete, free form, totalized at last in a motionless, simultaneous picture, lacking both density and secrecy, where recognition opens of itself onto the order of essences (1994a, p. 9).

Human beings did not come to occupy the centre of knowledge, the focus of the medical gaze, until the modern clinic was born and the epistemological shift from the classical to the modern age had taken place. But the import of this shift of epistemes can be stated even more dramatically: 'Before the end of the eighteenth century, *man did not exist*', to quote the notorious words from *Les mots et les choses* (1994b, p. 308). In the modern clinic, for the first time, it becomes possible to view the patient as an integrated, functional object with a *depth*, not just as a surface upon which diseases are read and classified. But this is not all: with the arrival of the modern doctor and patient we also witness the birth of the individual human being who is not only the *object* of the medical gaze, but also structures knowledge in the sense of being its true *subject*, its origin.[28] Man as a biological object – a living space of functions – is born contemporaneously with man as an autonomous subject – a modern individual who is the condition of knowledge. Thus, in the preceding classical age there could exist neither physiology, nor any individual, autonomous doctors or patients. The representational grid of diseases in medical discourse would have thwarted any such tendency of the human being to move towards either the origin or the focus of the medical gaze.

Why then, does this epistemological shift between the classical and the modern age take place? Foucault never answers this question in any distinct way. The purpose of his archaeology is obviously not so much to offer historical explanations of changes, as to describe the changes that actually took place and find the epistemic patterns in discourse that made and make different forms of knowledge – before and after the shift – possible. But he gives us some hints. 'An erosion from outside', from the other side of scientific thought – that is, from culture – can result in a discontinuity in the epistemic pattern (1994b [1966], p. 50). When Foucault, a few years later, transforms his archaeological method into a *genealogy*, this emphasis on culture, institutions and practice, and on the interdependence of power and knowledge, will become even more obvious.[29] However, even previously, in his first main work, *Histoire de la folie à l'âge classique*, published originally in 1961, Foucault, in opposition to the traditional view of the modern psychiatrist as liberating humanist, had traced the elements of *control* present in the newly founded field of knowledge concerning insanity. The insane were incarcerated and isolated as a distinct group during the classical age in order afterwards to become the object of modern knowledge. A similar process is obviously in operation in the case of the modern physician, who inspects and keeps notes on his patients in the clinic while they are alive, in order simply to open them up more knowledgeably when they are dead. The medical gaze

---

[28] See Foucault (1994b), especially Chapter 9, 'Man and his Doubles'.

[29] See above all *Surveiller et punir* (1974).

is a controlling, dissecting gaze and it is made possible by an *institution* – the clinic.[30]

Is then the non-progressive, epistemic view of medical history which Foucault provides a tenable one? It indeed seems hard to fit in all the medical inventions and theories of the seventeenth and eighteenth century under the general pattern of a representational matrix. What about the 'little animals' that Leeuwenhoek saw in his microscope, and what about the functional anatomy of Boerhaave, just to mention two obvious examples? In what sense did these belong to a representational mode of knowledge? Foucault would surely answer that we project our own mode of knowledge upon these scientists when we include them in the modern episteme. He would say that Leeuwenhoek, for instance, did not actually see what we today are able to see when we look through the same microscope, because the pattern that organizes our gazes is different from that which organized the gaze of Leeuwenhoek (1994b, p. 133). But though microbiology had to wait another 200 years for its emergence as a distinct discipline, it seems odd to deprive individuals of any possibility of thinking 'against their age', as Foucault does (1994b, p. 63). It has often taken a long time for medical inventions, theories and diagnostic practices to receive general acceptance, and their novelty and excellence are, of course, then often recognized in a 'backward-looking' perspective; but were they not, at the same time, themselves important *steps* towards this recognition?

Even stranger is Foucault's tendency to deprive the patient of any other position in classical medicine than as a 'disturbance' in the ideal configuration of diseases that is spread out for interpretation on the surface of his body (1994a, p. 9). As Foucault notices himself a few pages later in *Naissance de la clinique*, the extremely detailed disease catalogues of Sydenham indeed contain as many diseases as there are patients (1994a, p. 15). Indeed, as we have seen in the preceding section, the patient, as the subject of symptoms known uniquely to him and reported by him to the physician, is hardly a mere disturbance in the disease pattern, occupying, on the contrary, a central position in the process of arriving at a diagnosis. The historian N. D. Jewson, who in many ways has a theoretical outlook similar to that of Foucault, considers the 'medical cosmology' of bedside medicine – which in his conceptual framework precedes the modern cosmologies of hospital and laboratory medicine – to be essentially patient-centred, in the sense that the patient as an individual person and his symptoms and the account of his illness 'were the raw materials from which the pathological entities of medical theory were constructed' (1975, p. 233).[31] What

---

[30] For a well-informed and accurate study of the relation between knowledge and power in Foucault's writings about medicine, see Spitzack (1992). The question whether the modern, controlling, medical gaze is also a *male* gaze, and whether consequently the norms of medicine are male norms and forms of repression are interesting ones, which I will not be able to deal with here. See Moscucci (1990), which provides good arguments for an affirmative answer in the case of gynaecology.

[31] Jewson defines the concept of 'medical cosmology' thus: 'Medical cosmologies are basically metaphysical attempts to circumscribe and define systematically the essential nature of the universe of medical discourse as a whole. They are conceptual structures which constitute the frame of reference within which all questions are posed and all answers are offered. Such intellectual gestalts provide those set of axioms and assumptions which guide the interests, perceptions, and cognitive processes of medical in-

Foucault tends to forget is precisely the *practical* aspect of medical practice – the *meetings* between doctors and patients – an aspect which persists, mainly undisturbed by the theoretical works of scientists:

> The social structure of Bedside Medicine consisted of a network of segmental, unregulated patient-practitioner relationships. Medical investigators were fragmented into numerous local groups, each dedicated to the service of one part of this small but multifaceted medical market and each ranked according to the social standing of their patrons. The various shades and grades of practitioners offered a wide selection of theories and therapies to the sick. In the absence of reliable professional, academic or technical criteria, patients selected their practitioners by means of their own personal assessment of the moral integrity and professional skill of medical personnel. The consultative relationship was thus joined on the basis of personal empathy between the parties (Jewson 1975, p. 233).[32]

Given his theoretical outlook we can easily understand why Foucault so stubbornly denies the possibility of a history of the doctor-patient relationship (1994a, p. xiv), despite the historical evidence for its existence and indeed for the major importance of the meeting in the classical and preceding ages. How could there namely exist such a history if no 'individuals' existed in medicine prior to 1800? How one should understand the absence of suffering and communicating subjects in Foucault's account of the history of medicine is a difficult issue. It can surely not be taken in any absurd, literal sense, since Foucault, in fact, gives many examples of suffering patients and doctors and patients speaking with each other. But his provocative thesis clearly has a theoretical significance: patients and doctors and their ways of coming together are merely *effects* of medical discourse.[33] The emphasis is on language and not on practice; 'discursive practice' hardly means *praxis* of human individuals in the Aristotelian sense. As will become clear later on, the philosophical framework which I will adopt in this work, taken from phenomenology and hermeneutics, places

---

vestigators' (1975, p. 226). Jewson notes the similarity to Foucault's epistemic outlook (and indeed to Kuhn's theory of 'paradigms') himself (p. 241).

[32] There are indeed historical studies which put their major emphasis upon medical practice rather than medical theories in contrast to both the 'progressive' and the 'epistemic' views I have described above. Dorothy and Roy Porter's *Patient's Progress* (1989) and Edward Shorter's *Bedside Manners* (1985) are two such studies which I will make (and already have made) use of in this work. There are also other books which focus upon medical practice around the time of the shift from classical to modern medicine, and which, though lacking the general and explicit outlook of Porters' and Shorter's studies on the clinical encounter in pre-modern and modern times, are nevertheless of great importance for a historical study of the doctor-patient relationship. Michael MacDonald in his *Mystical Bedlam* (1981), explores the medical and popular beliefs of insanity and the therapies for healing it in seventeenth-century England through a reading of the manuscript notebooks of Richard Napier, a clergyman and astrological physician. Another example is Roy Porter's *Doctor of Society* (1992), based on the practice of Thomas Beddoes, a celebrated physician in late eighteenth-century England.

[33] Even when Foucault remarks that the old 'What is the matter with you?' has been replaced by 'Where does it hurt?' in modern medicine, and thereby indirectly acknowledges the importance of the meeting in pre-modern medicine, he adds in brackets concerning this very meeting that it is 'a dialogue possessing its own grammar and style', thus indicating his interest in the spoken discourse, rather than the speaking subjects (1994a, p xviii).

far greater emphasis on subjective experience, intersubjectivity and historical continuity than the (post)structuralism of Foucault.

Despite these problematic issues, there is at least one important thing we can learn from the medical archaeology which Foucault proposes, in opposition to the progressive views of traditional medical history. The birth of modern medicine, as he points out, is not only a liberating success of science which implies the possibility of cure and relief for (future) patients. The patient in modern medicine also runs the risk of being reduced to an object – a body, a case in the records – and of disappearing as a person. The meeting between doctor and patient, which has up to this period of transition in the history of medicine formed the obvious essence of medicine, is replaced by a new image: the scientist examining his object. This is problematic since this object – the patient – of course, never ceases to be, at the same time, a person (indeed as a modern autonomous individual he is more so than ever before), and this will give rise to conflict and distrust in the doctor-patient relationship. Modern medical science and technology will change the nature of the medical meeting, but medical practice will, without doubt, at the same time – and this is important to point out even at this early juncture – remain a meeting between persons.

4. MEDICAL TECHNOLOGY

Technology is essentially a feature of modern medicine. Pre-modern doctors were not armed with stethoscopes, X-ray, sphygmomanometers, lab tests and all the other technical devices and procedures which we have learned to associate with medical activity. Their main technical attribute was the *matula* – a bladder-shaped glass for the inspection of urine (Reiser 1978, p. 122). Uroscopy had ever since Galen been an important part of establishing a diagnosis.

With the rise of modern medicine, an increasing number of instruments were introduced to aid the physician in his work. The lancet is certainly not a new device – surgery had been carried out since ancient times – but before 1800 it was not common that the physician used the knife for anything other than blood-letting. Surgeons formed guilds of their own in pre-modern medicine and most physicians did not operate on their patients. This changed with the arrival of modern medicine. Doctors now ceased to hesitate to use the knife themselves. Operations, however, were very dangerous and painful, since disinfection and anaesthetics were not used until the middle of the nineteenth century, and they were of course not carried out for diagnosis or scientific studies, but only when they seemed the only possible way to prevent an otherwise fatal outcome.[34]

In autopsy dissections the human body could be opened up for studies in normal and abnormal anatomy. To make major advances in physiology and pathophysiology, however, one needed to look into the living body and not only the dead

---

[34] Ether and chloroform were first used in the 1840s and antisepsis in the 1860s (Shorter 1985, pp. 95, 133). Before the era of anaesthesia and antisepsis the operations which were most often carried out were cutting for bladder stone, amputation of limbs, setting of fractures and 'a host of grisly procedures in obstetrics' (Shorter 1985, p. 133).

one. This was certainly the great desire of the nineteenth-century physicians: to be able to see with their own eyes what was actually going on in the diseased bodies of their patients.

The difficulties involved in getting beneath the skin of the patient were manifold and would only gradually be overcome. That which physicians, at first, were unable to *see*, they were, however, able to feel and *hear*. The Viennese physician Leopold Auenbrugger had published a book in 1761 on a new examination method he called 'percussion'. The term meant to strike the body (for example, the chest) with the fingers to produce sounds indicating the vitality of underlying organs. Auenbrugger's work was largely ignored until *On Percussion of the Chest* was published in a new French translation in 1808. The book was read by a young physician, René Laënnec, who, following the example of his colleague Gaspard Bayle, in addition to making use of percussion and palpation began applying his ear to the patients' chests in order to listen to the sounds produced by their diseased bodies. One day in 1816 at the Necker Hospital in Paris an important invention was made:[35]

> Laënnec, then 35, examined a young woman who had a baffling heart disorder. To diagnose her illness he tried to use percussion and palpation: the patient's obesity thwarted both techniques. He then thought of placing his ear to her chest to listen to the heart, but the patient's youth and sex restrained him. Then a fact in acoustics flashed through Laënnec's mind. He remembered that sound travelling through solid bodies becomes augmented. Rolling some sheets of paper into a cylinder, he placed one end on the patient's chest and the other next to his ear. Clear and distinct heart sounds emerged (Reiser 1978, p. 25).

The instrument which Laënnec constructed after this incident was called a 'stethoscope', and it brought about a true revolution in the area of chest-disease diagnosis. Not that one was able to cure any patients, but through listening to their lungs and hearts one could actually predict what would be found at the future autopsy. The different sounds which were produced in different states of disease, such as by the caverns in lungs affected by tuberculosis, or by the liquid in the pleura characteristic of pleurisy, could be recognized and afterwards, by means of dissection, proved to have predicted the correct diagnosis. This procedure was so successful that doctors really felt they were 'looking' into the diseased body:

> One metaphor that recurred regularly in the medical literature between 1820 and 1850 was 'seeing' disease by listening through the stethoscope: 'We anatomise by auscultation (if I may say so), while the patient is yet alive,' proclaimed a doctor for whom the ear became an eye through auscultation (Reiser 1978, p. 30).

The stethoscope also had another important function as we learn from the quotation above recounting Laënnec's flash of genius: it introduced a necessary distance between the doctor and patient which prevented the meeting from taking on an intimacy that would be improper. The doctor could now get close to the patient's body,

---

[35] This scene might actually have taken place in Laënnec's private office and not at the Necker Hospital as the original story goes (Lachmund 1996, p. 65). The private office with its more unofficial atmosphere would have made it even more necessary to abstain from touching the woman's chest with the bare hands or ear.

indeed beneath the skin, without running the risk of being accused of the 'wrong form of intimacy'. The medical meeting is an intimate one, but this medical intimacy has nothing to do with the intimacy of lovers (Zaner 1993, pp. 8-9). The physician does not caress the skin of the patient, although for an outsider (someone coming from another culture than the Western one) it might look so. He feels and listens (palpates and auscultates) in order to detect diseases. Medical technology makes the meeting 'scientific' and prevents it from being confused with other sorts of intimate meetings between people in our society. The stethoscope consequently gradually becomes a sort of attribute of the doctor, something he might wear irrespective of any need to use it in his daily practice, simply as a sign of his scientific profession.

The stethoscope enabled the physician to 'listen' to the patient without making any inquiries about his symptoms, thoughts and feelings. The body spoke a far more objective and exact language about diseases than the voice of the person. Physicians consequently began to regard the detailed symptoms that the patients described as of minor importance and even came to distrust the stories that they presented (Reiser 1978, p. 31). The consultation changed character as the patient was treated more as an object of scientific investigation and less as a suffering person.[36]

But the sounds heard in the stethoscope were not always easy to tell apart or to describe to other physicians. The eye is far more powerful than the ear when it comes to identifying lesions and to comparing different structures irrespective of *who* is investigating. The metaphor for knowledge in the West has always been to *see*, not to listen; the gaze carries objectivity.[37] During the nineteenth century several instruments were designed to look into the living body: the ophthalmoscope, the laryngoscope, the gastroscope, and so on. These different 'scopes' made it possible for the physician to enter into the living body of the patient by way of natural body orifices with the help of speculum and light.[38] The peak of this development is of course the invention of X-ray in 1895 by Wilhelm Röntgen. At last the physician become capable of literally looking through the skin of the patient. The invention was viewed as true magic and was readily adopted in daily medical practice, since it not only provided the physician with new diagnostic capabilities but also inspired respect in patients due to its magical character (Shorter 1985, p. 89).

The microscope had existed at least since the seventeenth century, and we have already discussed the discoveries of Antoni van Leeuwenhoek in the 1680s.[39] Leeuwenhoek saw red blood cells, spermatozoa, protozoa and bacteria through his magnifying lens, but was not able to put these findings into any systematical context. With the rise of modern medical theory the microscope becomes an important tool for research. Xavier Bichat's systematization of different forms of tissues, Rudolf Vir-

---

[36] Or the symptoms and stories of the patient are represented in the medical records, but now in the terms of pathological anatomy (Foucault 1994a, p. 187), a distinct sign of the changed attitude.

[37] See for example Jonas (1966, p. 135 ff.).

[38] Almost every technical 'invention' of modern medicine, seems to have had a forerunner. In the case of scopes, there is evidence that elaborate vaginal speculums were used in ancient medicine (Nutton 1993, p. 7)

[39] See here Bracegirdle (1993).

chow's cellular pathology, and the development of bacteriology by Robert Koch and others, rested heavily on this invention and its successive improvement.

With the rise of bacteriology in the 1870s and its subsequent rapid development, allowing identification of different micro-organisms, the causal link responsible for contagious diseases was established. Although it had been understood earlier that some diseases (and indeed the most feared ones) were contagious, and although the recently-launched public health movement had already resulted in improved sanitation, bacteriology furnished this preventive movement with new arguments.[40] Bacteriology also led to the development of vaccines and sera to be used preventively against several diseases. Inoculation against smallpox had existed for a long time but now one could explain *why* it worked.

The laboratory revolution in medicine with the chemical examination of urine, blood and other substances meant nothing short of a revolution in the procedures of medical practice.[41] Lab tests have, during the twentieth century, become a natural part of most clinical encounters. To find out what is wrong with the patient one now needs both to take a look inside his body (X-ray and, later, various forms of tomography) and to test the bodily fluids for the presence of micro-organisms or other abnormalities. In order to be able to do this, one needs the apparatuses and methods of modern biochemistry. Biochemistry is without doubt the most important scientific field for the development of modern medicine as we know it today.

But modern medicine also developed with the aid of other sciences such as physics and statistics. In the nineteenth century instruments were constructed to *measure* temperature, pulse, blood pressure and lung capacity, and statistical studies were conducted to separate normal values from the abnormal ones of different diseases. Some of these instruments or practices had indeed existed long before modern medicine, such as the thermometer, which can probably be traced back to Galileo (Reiser 1978, p. 110). But although physicians had regarded the pulse and temperature of the patient as important parts of the diagnosis and prognosis since ancient times, they had not attempted to carry out systematic quantifications of these phenomena. To be able to feel the manifold qualities of pulses in different diseases had ever since Galen been a part of the skilled physician's practical knowledge, but it did not occur to these pre-modern doctors that it could be useful to *count* it during a given length of time.

To quantify and to make graphic pictures of temperature, blood pressure, the electrical conductivity of the heart and other phenomena, provided the activities of physicians with a new air of objectivity.[42] Instead of watching, feeling and listening to the patient, the latter can be projected on to a screen by way of medical technology. On this screen the patient's variables can be studied and discussed by a team of

---

[40] See Graninger (1997); Koprowski and Oldstone (1996); and Shryock (1948), Chapter 12.

[41] For the history of the development of the modern clinical laboratory, see Cunningham and Williams (1992).

[42] For an interesting account of the importance of graphic picturing in nineteenth-century and early twentieth-century medicine, see Borell (1993).

physicians. Perhaps the patient is also permitted some comments or at least questions in this conversation, but the attention is not primarily upon *him* anymore, but upon the variables given by medical technology. This has been an obvious tendency in modern medicine from the very beginning:

> Wunderlich's treatise elevated thermometry to a highly regarded diagnostic technique in the 1870's. Many physicians declared that thermometer readings were beyond control of the patient's will, or of extraneous circumstances, and thus were unerringly accurate. The instrument seemed to work by itself: 'While the doctor is chatting with his patient, or interrogating the friends, the thermometer may be silently recording its truthful tale in the patient's axilla' (Reiser 1978, p. 118).

The mathematicalization of nature in modern physics was gradually adopted in medicine which quantified and measured bodily phenomena. The blood pressure cuff, the thermometer and the watch for measuring the pulse are simple instruments which still hold an important place in the clinical encounter. To these and other instruments, such as the X-ray tube, the apparatuses of the clinical chemical laboratory and the electrocardiograph, can be added the rapidly increasing number of 'high-tech' medical devises used today which rely on powerful computers: ultrasound, computed tomography, nuclear magnetic resonance, positron emission scans and DNA tests. Computer-assisted diagnosis – which makes use of programs designed to suggest which disease the patient is suffering from when given clinical data – is yet another of these recent medical tools (Reiser 1993).

Computer-assisted diagnosis highlights a problem which has become ever more pressing in modern medicine and which concerns the topic of this study: the fading focus on the *meeting* in medical practice. If, as we have seen, the voice of the patient is threatened by the loudening hum of medical technology, the computer as a judge in matters of diagnosis and therapy may also gradually replace the voice of the *doctor*. The future scenario of the patient 'meeting' with a computer, instead of with a physician, would mean the end of medical practice as a meeting between two persons. We are certainly not there yet (and, one can hope, will never be faced with this situation); the physician still makes use of the computer as a tool, as an advanced form of technology which *guides* him in the meeting with the patient. In order to see why the meeting is essential to the success of medical practice, and why the emphasis on the patient, not as a person, but as an object investigated by different forms of scientific technologies, not only has lead to a prospering, but also to a crisis of modern medical practice, we need to move on in our historical survey of the development of medicine.

5. THE MODERN MEDICAL MEETING – SUCCESS AND CRISIS

As I remarked earlier, the emergence of modern medicine in Paris around 1800 did not have many immediate effects on medical practice outside the university hospitals. It took some time until the new thoughts and the new technology were taken up and integrated into the doings of the small-town and countryside physicians. Doctors trained in the old style did not see any reason to change their behaviour, since the diagnostic abilities of the emerging science at first did not show any major therapeutic effects. It was indeed a problem for many to understand that, for instance, Laënnec's writings not only concerned pathology, but also diagnostics (Nicolson 1993b, p. 135). As I have showed in Section 3, this was indeed the very step that led to modern medical thinking – to be able to link the findings of pathological anatomy to systematic chart-keeping. Establishing a place for this new thinking in the medical curriculum and replacing the established doctors, who were too old to learn new ways, took some time.

Around 1880 the reputation of physicians began to improve and soon reached impressive heights.[43] Patients began to trust and look up to their doctors in a way that, earlier, had been true only of priests. People, much more than had been the case before, actually started to believe that doctors could really *cure* them when they were ill, and the doctors gained new self-confidence. The heroes in the white coats were on their way:

> The encouraging results attained in medical practice, especially after 1900, were bound to affect the whole spirit of the medical profession. The revolution in surgery, the services of endocrinology and dietics, the value of serum and chemotherapy, the accomplishments of hygienic procedures – these in themselves were sufficient to banish the nihilism of 1850. The negative enthusiasm of that day, which found its chief service in disclosing the uselessness of traditional remedies, was now replaced by positive amelioration and cure. Most of the drugs and procedures abandoned by the first generation of critical physicians were given up for good; their places were now taken by a limited number of remedies of proven value. No longer could one say, with Oliver Wendell Holmes, that if most medicines were thrown into the sea it would be so much better for mankind and so much worse for the fishes. Quinine, morphine, insulin, salvarsan, and diphtheria antitoxin were too precious for that (Shryock 1948, pp. 256-257).

Although these drugs were helpful, the main reason for the disappearance or retreat of terrible infectious killers like smallpox, yellow fever, diphtheria, cholera, typhus and plague was the public-health movement and not medicine itself.[44] Improved living standards with better sanitation and nutritional conditions were chiefly responsible for improved health in the early twentieth-century Western world. But the decline of many infectious diseases did not result in mass unemployment for physicians. On the contrary, new groups of patients began coming to the doctor – including increasing numbers of women and children, two groups which, previously, had rarely sought medical help. In addition, patients began seeing the doctor for colds and for stomach and bowel ailments – conditions which previously had been treated within the family. The modern patient clearly becomes more attentive to symptoms and more often interprets them as caused by a disease. Also, due to the new confidence felt for the doctor, he visits him in cases in which he earlier would have tried to heal himself. The scientific development in itself indeed created entirely new symptoms, such as those associated with hypo- and hypertension; having heard of these phe-

---

[43] The main source for this section is Shorter (1985). The details are taken from this book if no other references are given.

[44] See Porter (1993).

nomena, patients could now believe themselves to be experiencing them and begin reporting them as complaints.

It seems, however, as though the reputation of the early-modern physician and the respect he enjoyed from his patients came largely from his diagnostic and not from his curative skills. His new technical, diagnostic tools separated him from the quacks in the eyes of the patients, and also gave him the possibility of finding out what was physically wrong with the patient and what could possibly be done. According to Shorter (1985) the medical meeting in these early days of modern medical practice (c. 1880-c. 1945), despite the lack of effective cures, *was* successful. It is possible to discern four main reasons for this new success and patient satisfaction. The first we have already mentioned: the modern doctor could carry out a correct differentiated diagnosis and could thus tell the patient what was wrong. The second reason we have also touched upon: new cures or symptomatic treatments for diseases were actually developed and the old useless (and often even dangerous) ones were got rid of. The third reason for the success of the meetings was the new scientific aura surrounding the physician, which led to a feeling of confidence among the patients. This confidence in itself had a therapeutic effect probably comparable to the later proven placebo effect of biologically ineffective drugs. As mentioned before, the modern doctor did not have many effective drugs to offer until the time of the Second World War. But as shown in many scientific investigations the placebo effect is a powerful one and it should not be despised or underestimated.[45] The fourth reason for success was the time and the interest these physicians devoted to their patients and the sympathy they felt for them. According to Shorter, these physicians were not only scientists, but also gentlemen and humanists interested in their patients as unique individuals with engaging life stories (1985, p. 106). The physicians had not only a scientific, but also a moral status as wise men rich in life experience, and they educated and admonished their patients like good fathers. They had what Aristotle termed *phronesis* – practical wisdom – which had been the mark of the good doctor since ancient times. Thus the doctor successfully treated not only physiological disorders but many illnesses which we today would call 'psychosomatic'.[46] This brings us to a subject I have not dealt with at all so far in this work: mental illness.

Modern psychiatry and psychoanalysis are children of the late nineteenth and early twentieth century. True, the Paris clinics, with persons such as Philippe Pinel, witnessed the beginning of a new attitude towards the insane – a more scientific one. The medicalization of madness, as Foucault (1972) and others have shown, takes place around 1800; that is, at the same time as modern medicine is taking form.[47] But psychiatry did not profit from the studies of pathological anatomy; it had to find other ways for development of theories. The gruesome imprisonment and treatment methods the mentally ill were exposed to during the nineteenth and a large part of the twentieth century will not be dealt with here. Most of these psychiatric patients rarely

---

[45] See Harrington (1997).

[46] On the history of psychosomatics, see Shorter (1992).

[47] For a good introduction to the history of psychiatry, see Shorter (1997).

saw a doctor and indeed were seldom part of a doctor-patient relationship. They were diagnosed as chronically ill, kept under surveillance and exposed to cruel 'therapies'. But, aside from these patients, many of whom we today would call 'psychotic', many other people from the late nineteenth century and onwards (almost all of them were women) were treated for milder mental 'diseases' like neurasthenia and hysteria.[48] The dividing line between mental and somatic illness was not at all clear in these days (as it has never been and will for different reasons perhaps never be) and many of these women were treated by gynaecological surgical procedures such as hysterectomy – removal of the uterus. But the doctors did not only operate on these patients; they listened to them and talked to them about their lives in a sort of proto-psychotherapeutic way. These conversations were indeed more authoritarian than the Freudian analysis. The physician had a more active role as a sort of life educator and the therapy was rather one of moral persuasion than a self-liberating analysis. But physicians such as Paul Dubois and Edwin Bramwell were rather successful in their persuasion: many patients actually got better from these cures of moral persuasion and 'positive thinking'. This probably did not have very much to do with the design of the different cures in themselves (since all of them seemed to work), but was rather due to the fact 'that the medical consultation in itself, when conducted in a friendly, leisurely way, can have a curative power' (Shorter 1985, p. 178).

The psychoanalysis of Freud has had a great impact upon theories about the medical meeting and probably also upon the meeting itself, not only in psychiatry, but also in general practice, as we will see later. It is not easy to say exactly in what way this impact has manifested itself; the influence of psychoanalysis has probably been manifold. The first thing one notices is that psychoanalysis seems to have restored the voice of the individual – the voice which the objectification of the patient in modern medicine threatened to silence. But as we have also seen, the doctors in Freud's time actually still had a great deal of interest for their patients as individuals. It is, thus, probably more correct to say that psychoanalysis restored, to some extent, the *influence* of the patient, in a meeting that had come to be increasingly dominated by the physician. But then again, analysis, at least in its original Freudian form, essentially leaves the interpretation to the analyst and not to the client.[49]

Psychoanalysis has undoubtedly meant more than any other field of study when it comes to understanding that psychological problems can have effects on somatic health and illness, and that a conversation about a patient's life situation and his illness can have significant effects not only on his mental, but also on his somatic, health. But in addition to this emphasis on the meeting between two persons as cru-

---

[48]See Johannisson (1994) and Moscucci (1990). The question is of course which implications follow from the obvious 'cultural construction' of these diseases. That they belonged to a social pattern which repressed women, which indeed considered 'the feminine' as an illness *per se*, is fairly obvious. The more controversial question is the status of *contemporary* medical science. To what extent are the diagnoses of our time cultural constructs, instead of value-neutral descriptions? I will return to this question in Section 7 of this part.

[49]This is obviously a disputed point, but I think anybody who devotes some time to Freud's case studies, evolving out of his own practice, would agree with me.

cial to medical practice, psychoanalysis has also had a tendency to *change* this medical meeting into a scene of combat between different desires of unconscious origin. To put it in extreme terms, there are no longer only two parties engaged in the medical meeting, but rather (at least) four: the conscious part of the patient and the conscious part of the physician as well as the *unconscious* parts of their minds. Transference and countertransference change the meeting into an interpretive enterprise of systematic suspicion. The patient does not know what his symptoms mean; their meaning can only be found out through an interpretation, performed by the analyst, of the patient's account. Thus, the *true* significance of the patient's complaints often differs greatly from – or, indeed, is found to be in direct contradiction to – the meaning the patient himself accords them. For example, resistance on the part of the patient towards a given interpretation is to be considered an indication of truth, since the unconscious fights the uncovering of repressed ideas.[50]

So far in this section we have only dealt with the *successes* of modern medicine. We will now approach the reverse side of these successes, a phenomenon which has become increasingly obvious since the Second World War, and which I will call the *crisis* of (late-)modern medicine. It is this crisis that makes the project I am embarking upon in this book particularly urgent, since the crisis seems to stem precisely from a tendency to neglect what I claim to be the essential part of all medical practice: the meeting between two persons – doctor (or other clinical professional) and patient. This tendency towards negligence can be traced back to several different traits in the development of modern medicine, many of which we have already dealt with above. These traits can be summarized by two key features: objectification (the reduction of the patient to a biological-physiological object) and specialization (the partitioning of this object between different medical specialities).

Medical technologies, built on the theory of modern medical science and applied increasingly in modern medical practice, tend to objectify the patient. The physician no longer has direct contact with the patient but examines him as a biological organism, objectifiable in graphical, chemical and numerical illustrations. Why ask the patient if you are not interested in his opinions, but in his patho-physiology? This objectifying tendency escalated after the Second World War when the use of antibiotics was firmly established in medical practice and was quickly followed by other modern drugs for endocrinological, immunological and mental diseases. Biochemistry could now not only be applied as a diagnostic tool; it could also be used to effect real cures for diseases which had earlier been plainly incurable. No wonder the physicians (and patients) were impressed by this development. It lead to a change in medical education in the fifties by which biochemistry, microbiology, pharmacology, immunology and genetics were given much more detailed attention than before. Every doctor should now become a scientist.

---

[50] It is hard to give an adequate reference here without ending up mentioning too many of Freud's works. Paul Ricoeur's *Freud and Philosophy: An Essay on Interpretation* (1970) gives a good survey of Freud's theories and is particularly appropriate in the context of this study given its focus on hermeneutics. See Part 3, Section 4, of the present work for an analysis and comparison of the hermeneutics of psychoanalysis and the hermeneutics of medicine.

Scientists are forced to specialize in their studies, and this has led to a reinforcement of a tendency present since the birth of modern medicine: medical specialization. The general practitioner – the family doctor – has been on the retreat since the 1880s, if one compares the number of generalists to the number of specialists (Reiser 1978, p. 144). This specialization of medicine was firmly established as the only alternative in the 1950s. The patient is thus partitioned between different medical specialists, who take care of different parts and aspects of the organism. During our century, more and more medical activity has been moved from the private clinic or the patient's home into the hospital – a development which has resulted in a tendency to 'divide up' the patient in different parts and then add them together in the diagnosis. But the patient is hardly just the sum of his biological data. Hans-Georg Gadamer has made this point in his book *Über die Verborgenheit der Gesundheit*:

> We have, for example, the disintegration of the person. This happens within medical science when the individual patient is objectified in terms of a multiplicity of data. This means that the patient is assembled as through a card index in the clinical examination of today. If this is done correctly all data (Werte) belong to the individual patient. But the question still remains whether the value of the individual (Eigenwert) is recognized in this process (1993, p. 108).

Gadamer is hardly the first to state this critique of modern medicine.[51] It has been stated many times and worn many different guises. Reductivism and specialization give rise to ethical problems. Patient autonomy movements and bioethical committees did not exist before the Second World War. Still another effect of the scientific turn of medicine is the problem of how to deal with illnesses which do not fit the biological paradigm – such as so-called psychosomatic illnesses. This form of illness – in which the physician cannot find any physiological abnormalities – afflicts many of the patients who seek medical aid today.[52] Still another critical voice against the scientific medical paradigm comes from patients suffering from chronic illness. Chronic diseases have come to be far more common as medical science has developed means to deal with many of the acute diseases. People live longer, are more conscious of somatic symptoms and demand more help for them. A disease which cannot be cured but only relieved demands attention to the person which is suffering from the disease – to his situation in life, to his thoughts, feelings, wishes and possibilities etc. – and such an approach is hard to combine with objectification and specialization.[53]

---

[51] An early acknowledgement of the threat of science on the art of medicine and the care of the patient was Francis Peabody's now classical essay from 1926, *The Care of the Patient* (1987).

[52] It is very hard to give exact statistical data here for obvious reasons. The percentage of patients suffering from symptoms without having any disease varies with time, culture, clinic and physician. One should also be aware of that many diseases are defined symptomatically, rather than etiologically, which renders the distinction fuzzy anyway. The experienced and uncontroversial family physician Ian McWhinney estimates that 'no disease-specific diagnosis is possible in 25 to 50 percent of patient visits to family physicians' (1989, p. 111).

[53] See Toombs et al. (1995).

Yet another kind of critique, that is particularly influential in the United States, and this for obvious reasons, focuses upon the problems of medicine as embraced and controlled by capitalism.[54] According to such a view, doctors are not interested in their patients anymore, but have chosen their profession mainly out of the prospect of making a lot of money. The tendency in health-care economics to think about the clinical encounter in terms of a seller-consumer relationship rests firmly on such an unquestioned capitalist ground.[55] As we have seen, however, the seller-consumer model in medicine is not only a modern phenomenon. Patients have shopped around among different healers since the days of Hippocrates.[56]

In the next section I will try to give a survey of investigations and theories which have dealt with the doctor-patient relationship in our time. As we will see, these approaches, in different ways, can be viewed as emanating out of the historical situation of success and crisis in modern medicine which I have sketched the outlines of above.

6. RESEARCH ON THE CLINICAL ENCOUNTER IN THE TWENTIETH CENTURY

Just as it is beyond the scope of this study to offer a detailed account of the historical development of Western medicine, it is also impossible here to give a complete report of modern research on the doctor-patient relationship. The literature is enormous as well as significantly heterogeneous.[57] What I will try to do in this section is to trace the outlines of some main currents in this literature.

What one notices immediately in reviewing the literature on the clinical encounter is that most of the research has not focused upon the meeting itself, but rather upon the effect that the meeting might have on outcomes such as health, compliance, patient satisfaction and patient autonomy. In order to improve upon these outcomes different 'models' have been developed to help the doctor change his consultant style and approach towards the patient. A dominant part of the literature is significantly 'practical' in its outlook.[58] Rather than asking ontological and epistemological questions such as 'What is a medical meeting?' or 'What is the nature of the knowledge established in and through such a meeting?', the research highlights a preferred outcome of the consultation and tries to find a meeting-model which will achieve this outcome.

Ever since the advent of modern medicine around 1800, and of modern medical practice in the 1880s, which I have described above, there has been a resistance and

---

[54] See Starr (1982).

[55] Although my general approach to the medical meeting in this work is critical towards a seller-consumer model, I do not directly enter into this debate since it would take me too far off target. Such a philosophical critique would have to involve theories evolving out of a Marxist tradition, and especially the school of Critical Theory, which makes a direct connection between science and capitalism.

[56] See Edelstein (1967) and Porter and Porter (1989).

[57] Good recent surveys are given by Ong et al. (1995) and Roter and Hall (1992).

[58] See for instance Myerscough et al. (1992) and Pendleton et al. (1984).

a reluctance to accept the new ideas and techniques. There was, from the beginning, a general fear that the scientific approach would ruin the *art* of medicine, the practical skills and wisdom of the experienced family doctor, who keeps close contact with his patients and knows the history of their personal problems as well as their somatic pathologies. As touched upon above, much of the health problems that a general physician encounters in his practice are not due to any known diseases (states or processes which tend to effect physiological dysfunction) but are rather illnesses (experiences of symptoms). Many of these illnesses without disease, although very 'real' in the sense of suffered and not simulated, probably have something to do with the patient's psychological and social situation.[59] The illness could of course be due to an undetected or perhaps still unknown disease, but diseases as well as illnesses afflict patients in different situations in life and the situation demand attention as such from the physician, whether the disease is caused by this situation or not. We will return to these issues of health, disease and illness in a more systematical way later in this work, but it is important to point out from the beginning that viewpoints which are often referred to as new 'holistic' insights are not new at all, but indeed as old as medicine itself. They were only brought to the surface and demanded new attention as soon as the modern, medical technologies started to affect the doctor-patient relationship (Reiser 1978, p. 174 ff.).

Psychoanalysis provided physicians who were interested in the communicative aspect of the clinical encounter and in psychosomatics with new tools for understanding the 'art' of medicine. Psychoanalysis had an immediate influence on psychiatry – indeed it is in part responsible for the founding of modern psychiatry – but it also had a more gradual impact on general practice. After the Second World War, Michael Balint started to work with his later famous 'Balint groups' in the Tavistock Clinic in London. His idea was that a changed personality and consultant style of the general practitioner, based on psychoanalytical insights, would have significant effects on the health outcomes of patients with illnesses which were essentially 'neurotic', 'functional' and 'psychosomatic'.[60] The doctor's personality and the meeting itself would be the 'drug' that the patient needed to get well. This demanded a changed consultant style. Diagnosis should take place on a 'deeper' level, involving the life history of the patient (Balint 1972, p. 120).

Balint soon understood that the project of letting general practitioners go through personal psychoanalysis – a long and expensive procedure – was quite unrealistic. The short psychiatric, theoretical courses that were given as a part of the medical curriculum were also dissatisfying; what was needed was practical, conversational exercise through which the physicians could develop psychoanalytic skills.[61] For this purpose Balint started to work with small groups of general practitioners who met

---

[59] The standard case of illness is, of course, illness *with* disease. I will deal with these matters in a much more detailed way in the second part of this work, 'The Phenomenology of Health and Illness'. For an introduction to the distinctions between illness and disease, see Sachs and Uddenberg (1984), Chapter 3.

[60] Balint uses all these terms in *The Doctor, His Patient and the Illness* (1972 [1957]).

[61] See Balint (1972), 'Appendix 1. Training'.

once a week for two or three years together with a psychiatrist to discuss their patients. Through this form of 'group analysis' the physicians would learn basic analytic skills. They would develop sensitivity to phenomena like transference and countertransference and become attentive to the unconscious wishes and drives of their patients. These skills would enable them to help many of their 'difficult' patients through bringing them to understand that the 'basic fault' was not a disease but a life situation that needed to be changed (Balint 1972, p. 252 ff.). The self-image and personality of the patient, according to this view, can have a pathological influence on his physiological state and the doctor can help the patient realize this and change this state of affairs.

Psychosomatic medicine has, of course, not been restricted to Balint groups, and I cannot deal with this diverse research tradition here.[62] Nor does it seem motivated, since the medical meeting and its outcomes are generally not the focus of this literature. The research on doctor-patient communication has, however, by no means been limited to its effect on psychosomatic problems, but has also focused upon patient satisfaction and health outcomes which are not thought to have much to do with psychosomatics, but rather depend on the vital effects an improved communication in itself can have upon treatment.[63] To ask the patient about his symptoms, and about his feelings and beliefs about his illness enables the doctor, not only to develop a correct diagnosis, but also to design a treatment which, because it takes into account the special requests of the patient and his situation in life, makes sense to him. Such an approach will also make the patient feel better about the meeting and increases the chances that he will actually follow the advise of the physician; that is, it will increase *compliance*, which is a key concept in modern clinical medicine.

Alvan Feinstein's classic work *Clinical Judgement* (1967) is a good example of the literature that approaches the 'art of medicine' from within the modern medical tradition. While maintaining the scientific point of view of modern medicine, he at the same time wants to emphasize its clinical aspect. This aspect, he claims, is as scientific as any laboratory research and should not be treated as something mystical that cannot be studied systematically in the same way as all other parts of medical science (1967, p. 291 ff.). But clinical medicine is also different from all other parts of medical science in that it focuses precisely upon *clinical* judgment:

---

[62] Some of the investigators who have dealt with the doctor-patient relationship and its effects upon the psycho-somatic health of the patient demand special attention in this work, since they have worked in, or close to, the philosophical tradition I take as my point of departure, phenomenology. I am thinking of philosopher-physicians such as Ludwig Binswanger, Medard Boss, F. J. J. Buytendijk, V. E. von Gebsattel, Karl Jaspers, Herbert Plügge, Erwin Straus and Viktor von Weizsäcker. (For a good introduction to this, mainly German, tradition in psychosomatics see Rattner and Danzer 1997.) I will return to some of these thinkers and their works in the two following parts of this work. The Swedish physician Olle Hellström has developed an approach to the consultation which he calls 'dialogical medicine', which places emphasis upon the patient's life situation and illness as a way of dealing with an un-acceptable situation and self-image (1994). Hellström's main theoretical sources are Martin Buber and system theory, but much of what he says comes quite close to psychoanalytical and phenomenological points of view.

[63] See Stewart (1995).

> All good clinicians use a distinctly clinical type of reasoning, called *clinical judgement*, for making decisions about prognosis and therapy of patients. We often refer to a clinician's judgement as being good or bad according to the wisdom with which he makes those decisions. The reasoning in this type of clinical thinking is quite different from the deductive logic employed to establish diagnosis, aetiology, or pathogenesis of a patient's disease. Clinical judgement depends not on a knowledge of causes, mechanisms, or names for disease, but on a knowledge of patients. The background of clinical judgement is clinical experience: the things clinicians have learned at the bedside in the care of sick people (1967, p. 12).

But this practical knowledge, according to Feinstein, as all other medical activities, can be systematized. Systematization of terminology and detailed, unbiased examination lead to better clinical judgment. The clinical data can then be linked to the establishing of a diagnosis and a possible cure. Clinical medicine, as noted in the above quotation, deals with patients and not with diseases, and Feinstein accordingly stresses the importance of an interest in people among physicians (1967, p. 301). But in the end, for Feinstein, this interest is merely put in the service of the scientific ambition of cultivating one's clinical judgment for the purpose of making medical diagnoses. What the patient says offers clues for scientific investigation. The medical meeting and communication are themselves, however, not essential to medical practice. The important thing is not to find out what the patient thinks, feels and wants. What is important is detailed, standardized clinical *investigation*, which provides the physician with the possibility of making a correct diagnosis in scientific terms, and enables him to design a cure for the particular disease found to be the cause of the patient's complaints.

The type of literature which I have talked about so far in this section, although very heterogeneous in character, shares a focus upon the outcomes of the consultation – health, satisfaction, diagnosis, compliance – as something related to the skills of the physician.[64] These skills may be psychological, social, artistic, or technical in some other sense, but they are all centred on the physician and his style and personality. Most of the models aim at an improvement of the skills of the physician, not a re-evaluation of his *position* in the meeting. The latter goal, however, is the major concern of another main current in the doctor-patient relationship literature: the current centred on patient autonomy.

The movements of patient autonomy in medicine were formed after the Second World War when clients began demanding influence in the medical institutions and began accusing the doctors of a 'paternalistic' behaviour. The physician had, up to this time, in a natural way, acted as the good father without many protests being voiced, and, indeed, as we have seen, had also been generally successful in this role (Shorter 1985). Modern medicine provided the physician with new influence and power – as both a scientist and a father figure. One must not forget, however, that modern medicine arose contemporaneously with the modern 'enlightened', autono-

---

[64] Byrne and Long (1976) is a seminal work in this tradition.

mous human mind; and one found 'newborn', autonomous individuals not only among doctors but also among patients.[65]

In 1956 Thomas Szasz and Marc Hollender published an article which can be considered a sort of archae-text in the patient-autonomy tradition of research on doctor-patient relations. Just as in the case of Balint, the basic influence on the authors is the theory and practice of psychoanalysis, but Szasz and Hollender come to very different conclusions about the optimal format for the encounter. The authors describe three basic models of the physician-patient relationship. The first one is the 'activity-passivity model' which pertains to cases in which the physician simply does something to the patient without asking his permission. This is the case for example when the patient is unconscious. The prototype of this model, according to the authors, is the parent-infant relationship. The second model is called the 'guidance-co-operation model' (sic), and here the physician tells the patient what to do and the patient simply has to obey. This is the case for example in states of acute infection. The prototype for this model is the parent-child (parent-adolescent) relationship. The third model is the 'mutual participation model', in which the physician helps the patient to help himself, as is the case in psychoanalysis. The prototype for this model is of course the adult-adult relationship, and the authors claim that it is all too often absent from medical practice. Szasz and Hollender do not intend to say that the other two models should never be used; they have their rightful place, for instance in the paradigm examples the authors mention (unconsciousness and acute infection, respectively). But, according to the authors, these models are also applied in many other cases, in which the adult-adult relationship model would be more appropriate – for instance in most chronic illnesses.

Szasz and Hollender argue for a new role for the patient as a full-fledged partner in the medical meeting; a partner who takes responsibility for his own health and life situation and who also, accordingly, is allowed to exert influence upon this situation:

> The model of mutual participation, as suggested earlier, is essentially foreign to medicine. This relationship, characterized by a high degree of empathy, has elements often associated with the notions of friendship and partnership and the imparting of expert advice. The physician may be said to help the patient to help himself. The physician's gratification cannot stem from power or from the control over someone else. His satisfactions are derived from more abstract kinds of mastery, which are as yet poorly understood (Szasz and Hollender 1956, p. 588).

The literature which has developed around the doctor-patient relationship and which has focused upon the patient's participation and rights in this process has used many

---

[65] Modern medicine – especially pathological anatomy – was indeed not only contemporaneous with, but also played a vital part in, the birth of the enlightened modern mind. Dualism and materialism are supported by a new attitude towards human corpses: 'It seems clear that the idea that the human body can and must be considered "in itself", as if there were no soul attached to it (the discovery of *anatomy*), has its correlate in the idea that the human soul must therefore also be considered "in and by itself", apart from its own embodying body (the idea of *autonomy*)' (Zaner 1988, p. 287). If, however, the time lag of the modern doctor-individual coming to power in medical practice seems to have been about eighty years (c. 1800-c. 1880), the modern patient-individual apparently had to wait an additional seventy years (until c. 1950) to acquire power and influence.

different tools and has found territories in many different disciplines. Philosophy – mainly ethics – is one of them; others are sociology and language studies.[66] Elliot Mishler combines all three of these approaches in his *The Discourse of Medicine: Dialectics of Medical Interviews* from 1984. His point of departure is discourse-analytical with an investigation of the spoken language of a large number of consultations, but he combines this social linguistic approach with an interest in the struggle for power in the consultation and in the social context in which this struggle is situated. The phenomenological concept of 'lifeworld' – which we will return to later – is used by Mishler in order to discuss the different 'voices' of medicine and everyday life which clash with one another in the encounter between doctor and patient. In this struggle for influence the author does not remain impartial, but rather defends the rights of the patient to have his voice heard in the consultation, not only because of the salutary effect this would have on his health or satisfaction, but also because it is his right as an autonomous individual to make decisions about his own health. This outlook firmly places Mishler in the second current which I have sketched in this section, and as a paradigmatic example from this tradition, his work gives us an idea of the viewpoints which characterize this literature.[67]

7. THE SOCIAL AND CULTURAL BACKGROUND

Medical meetings do not take place in a context-free clinical setting separated from the rest of society, but are part of a social reality and its structure. This social, cultural setting obviously has significant impact upon what the healing relationship of medicine looks like in different times and parts of the world. Despite this I have claimed that there exists a general continuity that enables us to talk about a *Western* tradition of medicine from Hippocrates and onwards. The most important development in this tradition was the dawning of modern medicine around 1800, which gradually changed medical practice the way I have outlined above.

I do not want to argue against the view that factors such as class and gender can have a significant influence on the structure of the medical meeting. They might influence the way doctors and patients talk to each other, what they talk about, how many and what types of clinical investigations are carried out, just as they obviously influence the types of health problems which prevail in different social groups.[68] But recognizing these differences, I still find it possible to talk about *one* tradition of Western medicine. The unity of this tradition makes it possible both to regard modern Western medicine as a distinct entity, and to carry out a philosophical analysis of *medicine* as a distinct human activity. Western medicine, as I will try to make evi-

---

[66]Examples of recent, representative works in these disciplines are, in ethics, Nikku (1997); in sociology, Tuckett et al. (1985); and, in language studies, Larsson (1989).

[67]Good surveys of this multifaceted literature are given in Childress and Siegler (1984) and in Hydén and Mishler (1999).

[68]See Fitzpatrick and Scambler (1984) and Helman (1990).

dent later in this study, is a meeting and a practice which has a certain ontological and epistemological structure – a hermeneutical one.

When it comes to non-Western societies things are different. Healing interactions as they are carried out for instance by the Ndembu people in Zambia, by the Hopi Indians in Arizona, or in classical Tibetan medicine, might not be similar enough to the activities carried out in modern Western clinics to be embraced by my philosophical analysis. Although we also in these cases are dealing with *meetings* between healers and clients and different kinds of interpretations of presented ailments – hermeneutics – the hermeneutical patterns are very different from that of Western medicine. When the medicine man in Zambia blames a sorcerer for being responsible for illness and performs magical rituals to remove the curse, this interpretation and activity might not have enough in common with what is performed in a medical clinic in Stockholm to be called medicine in the sense in which the word is used in this work. The healing practices in Zambia – and the cosmology and beliefs underlying these activities – are significantly different from ours. The medicine man and the physician pose different questions to their respective clients and carry out different activities. Admittedly, the client in Zambia and the patient in Stockholm share the desire to get healthy, and it is this desire that brings them to the medicine man or the physician; but, at the same time, they presumably have quite different thoughts about what being healthy means and different expectations concerning what the healer will be able to do. They also have different ideas about the cause of their illness, and they may very well experience very different symptoms even in cases in which their ailments are pathophysiologically identical.

This last statement – the same disease process can be experienced and interpreted differently by patients from different cultures – is obviously problematic. The reason for this is that the interpretational matrix of modern Western medicine here is taken as a truth about how things in the world *really are* beyond the interpretation of different cultures. But, one may ask oneself, is not science itself an activity which is carried out within a culture? Is not science itself determined by social and cultural circumstances which conditions its claims to truth? We have discussed, earlier in this study, the theories of Foucault and his notion of 'epistemes' which determine the scientific thoughts of different times and cultures. Thinkers such as Ludwik Fleck (1980) or Bruno Latour (1987) would provide us with similar theories concerning the culture-ladenness of science.

The phenomenological starting point which I will adopt and later expand upon in this study views science as a human activity carried out against the background of a pre-scientific meaning-pattern – a lifeworld. Science takes on meaning as a certain attitude towards the world: a specialized, abstract, theoretical way to view and construct the world that relies on the everyday, concrete meaning-patterns of the lifeworld which constitute its foundation.[69] Diseases would no longer be diseases without the persons who suffer from them and experience them as changed meaning-patterns in their everyday life – as, for example, pain, paralysis, nausea, dizziness,

---

[69] See, in particular, Husserl (1976b). This discussion will continue in Part 2 of this work.

weakness, anxiety, memory loss, or impaired speech or thinking. This is the way we identify 'dis-eases' as the word itself indicates. The scientific investigations of biological, functional disorders is carried out against the horizon of an illness-world of symptoms that afflict persons.[70]

On the other hand, science clearly has an impact upon our everyday lifeworld; for instance, a sore throat is thought of as an 'infection' – as an invasion of microorganisms – by most modern people. The success of medical science in the West stems not only from its ability to present explanations for experienced illnesses that make sense (one could say that about many non-Western and pre-modern medical cosmologies as well); modern medicine has also made it possible to develop effective *therapies* against many of the diseases it has identified, and this provides it with a rather special position compared to other medical cosmologies. Science is undoubtedly a human activity which is carried out against the background of everyday life, but it is a rather special activity when it comes to understanding and manipulating the world. This special position is very obvious in the domain of health and disease.

I naturally do not see any possibility of settling the issue of the 'objectivity' of medical science here (whatever that would mean). What I will do in this section is to take a look at some works which deal with healing in cultures other than the modern Western one. These works will offer contrast to the medicine we know in our own culture and make it easier to discriminate the ontological structure of medical practice. The reason for this is mainly that living within a culture tends to make one blind to the meaning structure pervading that culture. The success of modern medical science has made it hard to see that medicine is a healing relationship between two persons and not just a scientific investigation of a biological organism. The dissimilarities between healing in different societies will make us aware of the cultural context belonging to the modern medical enterprise.

Medical anthropology is a rather young discipline. The first decisive steps in its development were taken in the early twentieth century by anthropologists such as Franz Boas and Ruth Benedict, who, in their studies of foreign cultures, among other things, focused upon healing practices and beliefs about illness among 'savages'.[71] The most important works on the healer-patient relationship in other cultures compared to the doctor-patient relationship in our own were, however, not carried out until the seventies in sub-disciplines which are often referred to as 'ethno-medicine' and 'cross-cultural psychiatry'. Psychiatrists and anthropologists such as Arthur Kleinman and Byron Good carried out fieldwork in Asian societies (Taiwan and

---

[70] By this I do not want to say that all diseases (abnormal biological processes or states) must in every case lead to an experienced symptom (illness). Most diseases do sooner or later, but there still exists the possibility of a 'silent' or 'self-abortive' disease – for instance a tumour which stops growing or even regresses before it leads to symptoms of illness. In the standard case, however, a disease will be identified and indeed called a disease because it leads to illness. This is the message of the opening quotation of this part of my work, taken from Georges Canguilhem (1991, p. 226): 'In pathology the first word historically speaking and the last word logically speaking comes back to clinical practice.'

[71] See MacCormack (1993).

Iran), through which they highlighted the differences in various types of healing relationships in these societies, and drew attention to the cultural frameworks that these relationships were situated in. They attempted to study these 'primitive' practices in an unbiased way by leaving behind 'Western prejudices' about illness and its treatment. This was a necessary step in order to focus upon the 'explanatory models' (Kleinman) or 'semantic networks' (Good) of illness in these societies and thus make sense of the structures of the healing relationships.

Kleinman's magnum opus, built on a decade of field research and theoretical attempts published in several articles during the seventies, is *Patients and Healers in the Context of Culture* from 1980. In this book he compares four different types of healing practices in Taiwan: the practice of Western medicine, of classical Chinese medicine, and of shamans (tâng-ki) and ch'ien fortune tellers, who both receive their clients in shrines. These four types of healing relationships are compared on the basis of a large number of empirical studies recording differences in the following categories: institutional setting, characteristics of the interpersonal interaction, idiom of communication, clinical reality, and therapeutic stages and mechanisms (Kleinman 1980, pp. 207-208). Through keeping a record of these variables, one can give a systematic picture of the differences between the four healing relationships. The symbolic and magical care structure of shaman healing can for example be contrasted to the disease-oriented therapy approach of the Western practitioner. But the truly significant result of Kleinman's study is that some variables which differ from the structure of the doctor-patient relationship in the West are constant in all four types of healing relationships in Taiwan (including the Western practice on the island). The two most important of these variables are the focus upon the family and the tendency to present somatic instead of psychological problems.

The *family* is the locus of responsibility and indeed the help-seeking part of the healing relationship in Taiwan, whereas the individual patient occupies this place in the Western world. Illness is considered the business of the whole family in Taiwan, and it is related to family history and conflicts. Family members often accompany the patient to the practitioner and indeed direct the conversation in a manner which would be possible only in the case of children in the West. *Somatization* is also a phenomenon present in all four types of relationships in Taiwan. Mental illness is stigmatized in Chinese culture, and therefore, people tend to experience and present illness through the body instead of feeling depressed or complaining of psychological and social problems. These two general phenomena make the non-Western healing practices in Taiwan far more effective than they would be if imported into our society, since they are designed to give illness a meaningful place in the family structure and to give the patient an opportunity to enact psychologically the problems which burden him in a socially sanctioned way. Through blaming the illness on ghosts or other supernatural phenomena related to the family history and performing rituals which the client takes part in – often involving dancing, screaming and cursing – the shaman actually often heals the patient from his illness:

> Based upon the material presented, I draw the perhaps surprising conclusion that in most cases indigenous practitioners must heal. Why? As we have seen, indigenous

> practitioners primarily treat three types of disorders: (1) acute, self-limited (naturally remitting) diseases; (2) non-life-threatening, chronic diseases in which management of illness (psychosocial and cultural) problems is a larger component of clinical management than biomedical treatment of the disease; and (3) secondary somatic manifestations (somatization) of minor psychological disorders and interpersonal problems. The treatment of disease plays a small role in the care of these disorders. Therapeutic efficacy for these problems is principally a function of the treatment of the psychosocial and cultural aspects of the illness (Kleinman 1980, p. 361).

Interestingly enough, these three types of disorders (at least 2 and 3) seem to be similar to the cases that we, in Section 5, established as constituting the main problems for late-modern Western medicine.[72]

Why do the healing relationships in Taiwan display a general consistency, regarding the variables family-centredness and somatization, that is absent from the medical meeting in the West? Kleinman's answer is that healing practices and explanatory models for illness depend on, and are embedded in, a cultural system, and that the system present in Taiwan is different from the one present in the West. This system which Kleinman calls the 'health-care system' (not to be confused with the physical and administrative organization of health care) determines all health activities — including Western practice — in Taiwan. The health-care system provides the context through which healing and illness in a culture can be understood:

> Put somewhat differently, the health care system, like other cultural systems, integrates the health-related components of society. These include patterns of belief about the causes of illness; norms governing choice and evaluation of treatment; socially-legitimated statuses, roles, power relationships, interaction settings, and institutions. Patients and healers are basic components of such systems and thus are embedded in specific configurations of cultural meanings and social relationships. They cannot be understood apart from this context. Illness and healing also are part of the system of health care. Within that system, they are articulated as culturally constituted experiences and activities, respectively. In the context of culture, the study of patients and healers, and illness and healing, must, therefore, start with an analysis of health care systems (1980, pp. 24-25).

But how does one study such systems? They are indeed abstract entities — 'conceptual models held by the researcher', as Kleinman writes — which are not part of the physical world (1980, p. 25). The only way to study such systems of cultural meanings seems to be through the attitudes and beliefs of, and relations between, the agents of the system themselves. What Kleinman aims at comes close to a phenomenological analysis of the lifeworld(s) of patients and healers. The ambition to adopt a neutral standpoint is similar to what we in Part 2 of this work will term the phenomenological *epoche*:[73]

---

[72]Influential articles developing this point of view are Eisenberg (1977) and Engel (1977).

[73]Kleinman's relation to phenomenology is an ambivalent one. He refers to the works of Alfred Schutz (a Husserl scholar and a sociologist), but does not make use of the phenomenology of Husserl (or of other phenomenologists) in his analysis. In a recent work Kleinman praises phenomenological theory for its possibilities in describing and understanding human suffering, but also criticizes its predilection for an esoteric terminology (1995, p. 118). See also (1988), in which Kleinman deals not only with chronic illness but also with its narrative (hermeneutic) structure.

> What I am describing is the process of medical ethnography through which local health care systems are reconstructed. In order to conduct such an ethnography, the investigator usually needs to step outside of the cultural rules governing his beliefs and behaviours, including his own health care involvement. Otherwise he risks contaminating his analytic model of the health care system with his largely tacit actor's model of his own health care system. . . . If he chooses to study his own culture, however, the researcher must systematically alienate himself from his inner model of the system within which he is an actor, a most difficult task (1980, p. 26).

The anthropologist Byron Good has recently carried out an ethnographic study in his own culture – Harvard Medical School – of the type which Kleinman describes. Through this study Good wants to show that 'medicine formulates the human body and disease in a culturally distinctive fashion' (1994, p. 65). Several interviews with medical students focused upon how students change the way they think about, and look upon, the human body and being, as they pass through different stages of medical education. The preclinical years in the anatomy lab change the way they *look* and *name*:

> Medical education begins by entry into the human body. Viewed through the microscope, entered physically in the gross anatomy lab, seen with astounding clarity via contemporary radiologic imaging, or presented by master scientists, the body is revealed in infinite, hierarchical detail. Students begin a process of gaining intimacy with the body – attempting to understand its gross organization and structure three-dimensionally, examining tissue from gross function to molecular structure; students are as geographers moving from gross topography to the detail of microecology. . . . Within the lifeworld of medicine, the body is newly constituted as a medical body, quite distinct from the bodies with which we interact in everyday life (1994, p. 72).

The following clinical years change the way the students *talk* and *listen*. A student describes his experiences from the hospital:

> You're not there just to talk with people and learn about their lives and nurture them. You're not there for that. You're a professional and you're trained in interpreting phenomenological descriptions of behavior into physiologic and pathophysiologic processes. So there's the sense if you try to tell the people really the story of someone, they'd be angry; they'd be annoyed at you because you're missing the point. That's indulgence, sort of. You can have that if you want that when you're in the room with the patient. But don't present that to me. What you need to present to me is the stuff we're going to work on (1994, p. 78).

Thus the medical school is a cultural framework – a lifeworld – within which the student is shaped by a certain style of perceiving and thinking. The body becomes a hierarchical structure – an organism framed in a special language. The patient becomes a case with a diagnosis and a prognosis, documented in the language of the chart. Becoming a physician is not only about learning a lot of facts that you add to your old knowledge. In medical school you learn what is important and what is not, you learn how to organize knowledge and how to communicate it. But adopting this role, this style of thinking, might mean difficulties when it comes to relating to the everyday experiences and beliefs of patients.

Good himself, like Kleinman, has done a great deal of research on the healer-patient relationship. In this research, mainly carried out in Iran, Good has made use of what he calls a 'meaning-centred' approach to medical anthropology (1994, p. 52 ff.).[74] While Kleinman has invented terms like 'explanatory models' for illnesses and 'cultural systems' of health care, Good has employed the concept 'semantic network' to capture the meaning of illness in a culture.[75] In *The Heart of What's the Matter: The Semantics of Illness in Iran*, from 1977, Good analyses the semantic network surrounding heart distress. The heart occupies a central position in Iranian culture as an idiom for expressing emotion. People who experience stress and anxiety in life situations which are hard to handle complain of their hearts beating too fast or too hard.[76] This is a source of misunderstanding when these patients visit Western practitioners, since the doctor cannot find anything physiologically wrong with the patient's heart. By bringing to light a semantic network between terms associated with heart distress, Good is able to illuminate a field of experiences and beliefs characteristic of the illness. The network in this particular case includes terms such as 'anxiety', 'sorrow', 'death', 'mourning', 'interpersonal problems', 'worry', 'nerves', 'blood problems' and 'madness' (1977, p. 46). Networks are distinctively polysemic tools. They are not hierarchically or systematically organized, but they nonetheless enables the researcher (and physician) to get closer to the meaning a certain illness carries in a culture.

In a more recent article – *The Meaning of Symptoms: A Cultural Hermeneutic Model for Clinical Practice* – Good has focused upon the difficulties which physicians might have interpreting the illness symptoms that patients, especially from foreign cultures, present. For the attentive physician, knowledge of the semantic network makes a cultural, hermeneutic reading of the illness possible in addition to the biomedical investigation of diseases. This integrated approach, according to Good, is crucial if the consultation is to be successful, in terms of diagnosis, compliance and patient satisfaction (1981, p. 181). Knowledge of the cultural framework enables the physician to understand the patient's illness and thus find a possible strategy for treating it.

As we have now seen in our survey of theories on the medical meeting from psychology, sociology and anthropology, the terms 'phenomenology' and 'hermeneutics' have cropped up on several occasions. Most often they have been employed by the author in a rather everyday sense, to mean something like 'giving detailed descriptions of experiences' and 'providing correct interpretations'. Before we take a

---

[74] This tradition for Good includes the works of Kleinman as well as those of Allan Young, Mary-Jo DelVecchio Good and others, who all in different ways make use of an interpretive paradigm.

[75] In (1997), Chapter 5, Karin Johannisson introduces the notion that different 'grammars' are essential to different medical cultures. This is in many ways a more radical approach than the semantic one, since it suggests that what separates modern Western medicine and folk medicine are different types of *logical* structures, for instance regarding the explanation of illness.

[76] This tendency towards what Westerners would call somatization of psychological problems is present in Chinese culture as well, as we saw in Kleinman (1980). Also the central place of the family in health care is true of Iranian as well as of Chinese culture. Are these two phenomena characteristics of Asian culture? Or are they rather characteristics of pre-modern culture generally? As I have pointed out above, the intimacy of the medical meeting – as a meeting between two persons – was not a common thing in the West before the advent of modern medicine.

deeper look at the theories of phenomenology and hermeneutics and their relation to health and medicine – indeed the task of the two following parts of this book – we need to say more about the relationship between philosophy and medicine. Phenomenology and hermeneutics, in the forms in which they will be employed in this work, are philosophical theories, and we need to approach the *philosophy* of medicine in order to see how these theories will provide an opportunity to present an ontological and epistemological theory of medicine as an interpretive practice.

8. PHILOSOPHY OF MEDICINE

The relationship between philosophy and medicine has been a long and intimate. As I pointed out in the first section of this part, the two disciplines in the days of Hippocrates were closely united with analogous duties: philosophy cared for the well-being of the soul – *psyche* – and medicine for the well-being of the body – *soma* – of the free men in the *polis* (Nussbaum 1994). The true physician should also be a philosopher, as Galen is known to have said. But though one finds many medical examples in classical philosophical texts, this relation of apparently mutual influence was decidedly unbalanced: ancient medicine got most of its ideas and theories from philosophy, whereas the practice of medicine did not significantly influence philosophical theories.[77]

In our century the balance of this relation has shifted direction. Medical science left philosophy behind around the year 1800, dedicated itself to empirical studies and shunned the influence of 'speculative' philosophies such as the systems of the German Idealists.[78] The development of modern philosophy of science (biology) in our century has not significantly changed this pattern of medical ignorance of – and even hostility towards – philosophical theories. The development of modern medicine has, however, in our times, and especially during the last three decades, come to have a significant influence upon philosophical disciplines – particularly upon the philosophy of mind and ethics. Neuroscience and genetics raise questions regarding our conception of the essence of man and regarding whether all alterations of human life made possible by the powerful new technology are ethically defensible. These developments have not only built a new bridge between medicine and philosophy, they have also had a vitalizing effect upon philosophy and created an increased interest in the discipline – in fact, cognitive science and bioethics are becoming ways of earning a livelihood for philosophers.

What to a large extent is still missing, despite this development and new contact between the two disciplines, is a philosophy that focuses upon clinical practice and deal not only with the advances in medical science. A theory of medicine as a distinct enterprise cannot only consist in the sum of selected parts of the philosophy of mind, biology and ethics. This insight became widespread in the seventies, as reflected by the founding, during that decade, of new journals – first and foremost,

---

[77]Edelstein, 'The Relation of Ancient Philosophy to Medicine', in (1967, p. 350).

[78]See, for example, Shryock (1948), Chapter 6: 'Science in a Romantic Age, 1800-1850'.

Journal of Medicine and Philosophy, and later, *Theoretical Medicine* – and the appearance of new books – notably the *Philosophy and Medicine* series, published by Reidel since 1975 – which deal with the philosophical aspects of medicine and health care. These new journals and books in no way fostered a consensus upon the possibility of a philosophy of medicine as a distinct discipline,[79] but the need for a philosophy of clinical medicine, a philosophy dealing with medical practice – the activities of doctors and other health-care personnel in the clinic – and not only with medical science as a research activity, was clearly felt.

This need became urgent in the state of crisis of modern medicine I have sketched out above. The reverse side of the success of medical science is, as we have seen, a distrust and lack of understanding between doctor and patient, which has crept into the clinical encounter. A number of recent phenomena, such as the popularity of patient autonomy movements, the renewed relevance of medical ethics, and the increasing attention given to psychosomatic and chronic illnesses – forms of illness that present problems unsolvable in a reductive scientific manner – have made doctors aware of the importance of treating the patient as a person: this historical situation has created a new interest in a philosophy of medical practice.[80]

The first coherent and systematic attempt to fill the gap was Edmund Pellegrino's and David Thomasma's book *A Philosophical Basis of Medical Practice* from 1981.[81] The authors use methods and insights from so disparate philosophical traditions as Aristotle, American pragmatism, phenomenology and language-based conceptual analysis in their attempt to provide an ontological theory of medicine (1981, p. 27 ff.). The definition of medicine they arrive at with this 'pluralistic methodology' reads as follows: '(Medicine is) *a relation of mutual consent to effect individualized well-being by working in, with, and through the body*' (1981, p. 80, italics in original).

The first thing one notices in this definition is of course the insistence upon medicine being a relationship – a meeting – to effect well-being – health. Medicine is consequently first and foremost a practice, an activity of healing, and not a theory.

---

[79] See, for example, the round-table discussion in the first volume of the *Philosophy and Medicine* series edited by Engelhardt and Spicker (1975).

[80] In this context I would especially like to mention the books by Eric Cassell, which in an excellent way analyse and propose solutions for the crisis of modern medicine: *The Healer's Art* (1976), *Talking with Patients* (1985), and *The Nature of Suffering* (1991).

[81] It is always risky and perhaps unwise to make such a categorical statement – that a book is the very *first* to develop such and such a view. By adding 'coherent' and 'systematic' I would like to indicate that, although most of what the authors say indeed is not new, they make an attempt to put old insights into a coherent and systematic pattern with the aim of developing a philosophy (and ethics) of medical practice. Whether the philosophy of medical practice which they develop in this (and later) books really is a systematic, coherent philosophy *of* medicine and not only scattered, theoretical remarks *about* medicine which lack the underpinning of a consistent methodology is a matter that has been discussed by Verwey (1987). I agree with many of the points made in Verwey's competent and elaborate reading, but would still put a greater emphasis on the statement found in the prologue of Pellegrino's and Thomasma's book: 'This book is a *first step* toward what we hope will become a systematic philosophy of medicine' (1981, p. 3, my italics). As such a first step the book has proved very important and has had an impact upon the modern philosophy of medicine which is unparalleled.

As a practice, however, it is not to be though of as merely applied medical theory (applied medical science). The essence of medicine according to Pellegrino and Thomasma *is* clinical practice and not medical science. This is not meant as a denial of the worth of modern medical science, but rather as a reminder that the results of the research and theories of medical science must be put into practice in the clinical encounter between doctor (or some other health-care professional) and patient and thus, as parts of modern medical practice, are situated in the framework of a meeting between persons.[82] Consequently, if medical science and technology are used in other settings than the clinical meeting (as, for instance, when DNA samples are used in courts, or biomedical research is used in the food industry), it is, according to the definition of Pellegrino and Thomasma, not a question of *medicine*, but only of applied medical science. This is an important distinction which I myself will adopt in this study. A philosophy of medicine should be a theory about clinical practice, for this is what medicine essentially is:

> Therefore, the method of philosophy must begin in practice and return thereto for a test of its meaning. In other words, a philosophy of medicine must be an ontology of practice, a search for meaning in the practice of medicine, and specific applications of the results of this search (Pellegrino and Thomasma 1981, p. 50).[83]

The attempts made in the field of the philosophy of medicine, following the publication of *A Philosophical Basis of Medical Practice*, to define medicine as a certain form of practice, have lead to a return to Aristotle's classical distinctions, made in the *Nicomachean Ethics*, between *episteme, techne* and *phronesis*.[84] *Episteme*, in

---

[82] Pellegrino's and Thomasma's theory of medical practice is meant to cover the activities of all health-care personnel: 'All health professionals enter, in some degree, into this nexus of relationships; therefore we include all health professions in our concerns. We use medicine and the physician-patient relationship as our paradigm because of its moral, legal, and historical precedents. What we say of the healing relationship is equally significant for nurses, pharmacists, dentists, clinical psychologists, medical social workers, and allied health workers' (1981, p. 5). This statement by the authors about the different actors in the clinic and their place in medical practice seems to me either too narrow or too wide. It can be read as stating that 'medicine and the physician-patient relationship' is the *paradigm* which is of significance to the activities of all other types of clinical professions without these other paramedical meetings being included in the definition of medicine. This seems too narrow, since health professionals other than doctors (in particular, nurses) obviously take part in *medical* meetings. On the other hand, the lines can be read as including all the cited professions in the practice of medicine, which seems to me too wide a definition, since, for instance, medical social workers do not approach their clients in the same way as doctors do. The theory of medicine that I will develop in this book will have its centre in the activities of the general practitioner, but I will allow for the fact that professionals other than doctors (nurses) may have a significant role in this medical activity. See Part 3, Section 7, of this work for an extended discussion of this issue. See also Nordenfelt (1996).

[83] Siegler (1981) stresses the practical approach for a theory of the doctor-patient relationship. The test of any health theory should be its applicability in clinical practice. Although I share Siegler's focus upon clinical practice as the starting point for a philosophy of medicine, I am not as sceptical as he when it comes to the usefulness of philosophical theory for medicine. To reflect on what kind of activity medicine might be, one needs to step back from it and use philosophical tools, if only in order to return afterwards to the everyday world of clinical practice.

[84] Pellegrino and Thomasma discuss these distinctions in (1981), and, more extensively, in later works such as (1993). The most important articles dealing with Aristotle's different forms of knowledge in re-

that work, signifies theoretical, scientific knowledge. Aristotle's notion of science is, however, tied to the knowledge of eternal things – *a priori* knowledge – in a way that does not apply for modern medical science, but only for disciplines such as mathematics (p. 1140b30 ff.). Regardless of what Aristotle would have thought about modern empirical science, his definition of practical knowledge – *techne* – bears resemblance to the knowledge of clinical medicine. *Techne* is the kind of knowledge involved in making and doing directed towards a certain goal (often the making of an object – *poiesis*), not through the application of a deductive system of theoretical knowledge, but rather through a sort of 'tacit' knowledge learned through practice. This reminds us of the debate surrounding the *art* of medicine in contrast to its theory mentioned above.

In addition to *techne* – which is useful in describing the craft of medicine – a second Aristotelian notion – *phronesis*, or practical wisdom – seems to be applicable to medical knowledge. To have *phronesis* a man must know how to deliberate in difficult situations in life, which can only be learnt through experience, since this knowledge presupposes familarity with the individual, particular situation, which, as unique, cannot be subsumed under general principles. *Phronesis* never gives certain knowledge in the same way as science, since it deals with human beings and matters of life on which choices have to be made without any possibility of grounding these choices in infallible knowledge:

> Practical wisdom on the other hand (in contrast to science) is concerned with things human and things about which it is possible to deliberate; for we say this is above all the work of the man of practical wisdom, to deliberate well, but no one deliberates about things invariable, or about things which have not an end which is a good that can be brought about by action (NE, p. 1141b8).

Rephrased in modern philosophical terms we would say that deliberation in situations dealing with persons always involves normative issues, which cannot be known and settled by scientific research. Medicine is such a value-laden activity since it involves the entire social and psychological dimension of the individual person seeking help and not only his biology. Medicine, as many authors have pointed out, is an inherently value-laden and moral enterprise.[85] This does not, however, make medicine into *only* an art. The central place of science in modern medicine is obvious

---

lation to medical practice are Davis (1997); Gatens-Robinson (1986); and Widdershoven-Heerding (1987).

[85] See above all the detailed and original discussions by Zaner in (1988). If medicine is inherently moral, this means that one cannot separate the two questions 'What is medicine?' and 'What ought medicine be?' in any simple way. If medicine has an inherent goal – the health of the patient – as I, in agreement with Pellegrino and Thomasma, will argue in what follows, it is an activity that cannot be conceptualized separately from that goal. We cannot first ask the question 'What is medical knowledge?' and after having settled this issue go on to ask 'What ought we do with this knowledge?', since the nature of the knowledge can only be understood in the first place by grasping its goal. Clinical medicine cannot be understood merely as medical science, which we choose to apply in different ways, asking ourselves what we ought to do with it. (Whoever 'we' might be.) The measure of what ought to be done in medicine must be sought in medicine itself by analysing its ontological structure. The relation between ontology and ethics in medicine is an urgent issue, to which I will return in Part 3, Section 9, of this work. Regarding this issue, see also Svenaeus (1996).

from the historical survey I have given above. The crucial task for a philosophy of medicine is to explain how art and science are *united* in the encounter and activity that we call medical practice. I will attempt to do this in the third part of this work by making use of hermeneutic theories. We will then be able to explain how science is present in the human encounter by explicating different forms of *understanding*.

One way to single out medicine from other human encounters and activities is to pin-point the *goal* of the clinical event. Different activities have different goals. According to Pellegrino and Thomasma the goal of medicine is 'to effect individualized well-being by working in, with, and through the body'. It is clear from other passages in the book that the authors by well-being mean health and not quality of life, which is an important distinction (1981, p. 32). The emphasis on physical cure in their definition seems, however, to limit the goal of health in medicine to somatic health and to exclude mental aspects of the concept. Consequently, psychiatry, for Pellegrino and Thomasma, is not a part of medicine, since it involves mental therapy (1981, p. 25). This exclusion seems strange given the many non-physical aspects of health and medicine. As I will try to show in Part 2 of this work, an analysis of the concept of health is needed to straighten out the relation between somatic and mental health as goals of medicine.

On the other hand there might indeed be dangers involved in giving too wide a definition of the goal of medicine. This is what Eric Cassell in *The Nature of Suffering* (1991) risks doing when he states that the goal of medicine is to remove or relieve human suffering. A great deal of human suffering is due to other things than illness and is consequently not in any obvious way the business of medicine. As Pedro Lain Entralgo stresses:

> The proper aim of the medical relationship is the health of the patient; nothing could be more obvious than that. All the same, it is as well to emphasise the fact, because present-day medicine, intoxicated by its new and wonderfully effective techniques for controlling human nature, is sometimes led to believe that the doctor's ultimate aim may be man's moral goodness (to make men good) or the happiness of humanity (to make men happy), rather than the physical health of the invalid (1969, p. 154).

The aim of clinical practice, it seems, is to restore health that has been lost (or, in the cases of congenital defects, to bring it about for the first time). I will in this work adopt Pellegrino's and Thomasma's characterization of medicine as a meeting that aims at restoring the lost health of the patient, as a starting point to be further explored and explicated through phenomenology and hermeneutics. There are problems involved, however, even in this initial sketch of health as the goal of medicine. What about diseases which cannot be cured and what about preventive measures taken when the patient is healthy? The treatment of chronic illness and preventive medicine are, however, clearly directed towards health, or at least towards a 'healthier life' for the patient: in the first case, the patient is rendered more able to cope with his illness; in the second case, if preventive measures are successful, the future health of the patient is guaranteed.[86] Parts of medicine that are not in any obvious way aimed at restoring health such as, for instance, obstetrics can thus be understood as having a preventive function.

Those forms of plastic surgery that do not aim at restoring the patient's health or preventing future illness, but rather at increasing his quality of life, are harder to handle. Given our initial characterization of medicine here, face-lifts and silicon breast implants indeed might not be considered parts of medical practice. But this in no way contradicts our theory, it only highlights the fact that the ontological investigation of medicine upon which we are embarking here has a normative as well as descriptive side. The *fact* that modern medicine finds itself in a continuous process of expanding its field – what is usually referred to as the 'medicalization of life'[87] – should not lead us to the immediate conclusion that this is what it *ought* to do. The goals and structures of the activities in question need to be examined. That which is termed medicine might, for instance, turn out to be applied medical science rather than medical practice.[88] We will return to these issues in Part 3, but I find it appropriate to introduce this dual aspect of my analysis already at this early stage.

The next thing we need to do in this work in order to bring light to these issues, is to discuss the concepts of health, illness and disease. Health theory is crucial to the philosophy of medicine. It does not help much to say that the goal of medicine is to restore health or to cure and relieve illness and disease, if we do not know the meaning of these concepts.[89] Pellegrino and Thomasma acknowledge this fact, although they do not carry out very much of the work themselves:

> Intimately related to the philosophical conception of man are the definitions of health and disease, of cure, and of disability. The presuppositions physicians hold about these conceptions shape medical theory and practice. Since health is the end and purpose of medical knowledge, the clearer the definition we can give to that term, the more order and priority we can give to our uses of medical knowledge (1981, p. 32).

---

[86]Some forms of preventive medicine – screening, for instance – seem, nevertheless, to resemble applied medical science *only*, rather than a meeting between persons. Once the patient has given his consent to be screened, no essential dialogue takes place. The dialogue between health-care personnel and patient often starts only when something is found to be *wrong* through the scientific tests.

[87]The sword of medicalization is double-edged, since it not only conquers life territories that were earlier ruled by other thoughts and disciplines than medicine, but does this precisely by *re-designating* something previously regarded as, for example, a moral problem a *disease*. Thus to try to resist the process of medicalization by saying that the proper aim of medicine is health does not help much, if we do not, at the same time, analyse the concepts of disease and health in order to determine how the terms could and should be used in medical practice.

[88]This is not merely an empty terminological issue, but an ontological question, which could guide us in practical-political matters like the design of the health-care system and the financing and control of research. Applied medical science should not be treated like medical practice in cases in which it is not a part of it.

[89]Khushf (1997) shows in a convincing way, not only that ethics is in need of a philosophy of medicine, but also that the philosophy of medicine depends on the elucidation of the concepts of health and disease.

I will aim at giving such a clear and adequate theory of health and illness by focusing not only upon medical theory, but also upon the *experience* of being ill and healthy. Phenomenology will accordingly be our guide in the next part of this book.

PART 2

THE PHENOMENOLOGY OF HEALTH AND ILLNESS

'Oder müssen gar Krankheit und Tod überhaupt – auch medizinisch – primär als existenziale Phänomene begriffen werden?'[90]

What is health? The answer to this question is by no means obvious. And yet in a way most of us know what it is like to be healthy, since this is the state in which we most often find ourselves in our normal life. Illness to most of us is an exception, a contrast to and interruption of our normal way of being in the world. Merely to experience something and to conceptualize it, however, certainly are two different things, although firmly connected. We can trace the theories of this connection at least as far back as Plato's world of ideas explaining and supporting the world of appearance. The nature of the relation between experience and concept has, in the discipline of philosophy, been a constant source of debate and generated many different theories. This part of my work will take its starting point in one of the philosophical attempts to found a theory about the structure or *eidos* of experience – phenomenology.

Before entering the philosophy of phenomenology and trying to trace the outlines of a phenomenological theory of health, it will be useful to take a look at theories of health which have their origin in other schools of philosophy. This will be a rather long detour, but it is motivated since we need to know what we should expect from a theory of health. In what sense will a phenomenological theory be different from other theories of health and in what sense will it be similar? Why, indeed, do we need a phenomenological theory of health (instead of simply contenting ourselves with a biomedical science of diseases) when we develop a theory of medicine based on clinical practice? These are questions which I hope will find answers in this part of my work.

1. THE ANCIENT TRADITION

Health theory is not a new subject in the history of philosophy. Actually, the reverse is the case: in antiquity the philosophies of health (*hygieia*) and medicine (*iatrike*) formed vital subdisciplines to philosophy. This was the case in the philosophies of

---

[90]Heidegger, *Sein und Zeit* (1986, p. 247).

Plato and Aristotle and in many other Greek and Roman philosophical schools as well.[91]

The theories of health in antiquity were built around different thoughts about balance and harmony (*isonomia, taxis, kosmos*); the most famous and influential was the Hippocratic theory about the balance between the four bodily fluids – blood, phlegm, yellow and black bile. This balance between fluids or other elements – such as air, water, fire and earth – in the human body mirrored an order of the entire world in classical Greece. Man was seen as a microcosmos, built according to the same principles as the order of all things – the *kosmos*.

Galen, the Greek physician from the second century A.D., linked the theory of balance between fluids to the theory of the four elements and their qualities. Each fluid had the qualities characteristic of one of the elements: blood was hot and moist like air; phlegm was cold and moist like water; yellow bile was hot and dry like fire; and black bile was cold and dry like earth (Temkin 1977, p. 423). The excess of any of the fluids in relation to the others, according to the Galenic doctrine, could not only result in illness, but was also representative of a certain type of character. The fluids accordingly represented different *humours*; and an excess of blood was thought to produce a sanguine character, an excess of phlegm a phlegmatic character, an excess of yellow bile a choleric character, and an excess of black bile a melancholy character. This theory was to maintain its influence for more than 1500 years. Not until the emergence of modern medicine in late eighteenth-century Europe was it deemed faulty and irrelevant.

This is not the place for a detailed survey of ancient health theories – that would be well beyond my abilities. It might be interesting, however, to lay out some basic features of the most influential theories in order to compare them with the modern health theories I will discuss later on. I have already mentioned the concept of balance as central to the ancient theories. In Plato's works we find the outlines of at least five different health theories, each centred around the idea of balance.[92] Three of these theories propound notions of equilibrium that are similar to Hippocratic-Galenic doctrines: balance between different parts of the body; balance between the four elements of the body; and balance between different pairs of opposites, such as dry-moist, less-more, fast-slow, big-small, cold-warm, and sweet-sour, in the body. All three of these Platonic outlines look upon health as a state of balance in the body (*soma*). In other places Plato also brings in soul (*psyche*) into his discussions concerning health. In the *Timaios* he seems to hold that health consists in a balance and

---

[91] As was made clear in Part 1, this study limits its scope to the Western tradition of medicine and health. I do certainly not, however, argue against the view that ancient Greek culture and philosophy were influenced by or built upon Egyptian and Mesopotamian culture, nor do I want to dispute the importance of Indian and Chinese healing practices and theories of health. The Hippocratic tradition (dating from c. 400 B.C.), however, (just like ancient Greek philosophy in general) seems to provide the starting point for a specifically Western cultural praxis and way of thinking. It also, as we have seen in the first part of this work, forms the starting point for a unique medical relationship with a certain structure of helping and healing.

[92] I rely mainly on Petersson (1995) here. Specific references to all passages in Plato's work in which the philosopher addresses these different concepts of health are found in this paper.

harmony between the abilities of the soul and the abilities of the body; and in the *Charmides* balance is to be established not only between soul and body, but also between the parts of the body and between the parts of the soul (Petersson 1995, pp. 113-114).

Is there accordingly in Plato not only a theory about somatic health, but also a theory of mental health? The question is not easy to answer. One must realize that the 'healthy' soul, not only in Plato, but in other ancient philosophies as well, resembles that which we today rather would call the virtuous soul. One also has to remember that the Greek word *psyche* is not synonymous with 'soul' in the (Christian) sense of spirit and that many of the Greek philosophers were materialists. *Psyche* simply stands for all the 'life-activities' of the organism (Nussbaum 1994, p. 13). Thus *soma* and *psyche* were not divided in ancient Greece in the dualistic manner characteristic to much of later Western thinking.

Excellence of character (*arete*), characterized by temperance (*sophrosyne*) and self-control (*enkrateia*), was, accordingly, for the Greeks, both a moral project *and* a health project. To cultivate oneself, to live a good and flourishing life (*eudaimonia*), was a *life* project, a matter of shaping and creating oneself.[93] This involved all sorts of habits (*ethos*): sexual habits and techniques, company with one's friends, exercise habits, what to eat and when to sleep, what to study, and so on. It was thus a matter of cultivating the body as well as the soul, and, consequently, the cultivation of the *psyche* cannot be thought of as an ethics in the modern, mainstream philosophical sense.[94] To be able to control oneself and choose the right goals in life – that is, to be able to realize the 'life plan' of the good life – was just as much a matter of the *health* as of the virtue of the soul.[95]

The healthy body (*soma*) demands a healthy – virtuous – soul (*psyche*) in ancient Greek thought. It is a significant and interesting fact that the theories of health as a balance between different parts, elements or fluids in the body, in Plato and Aristotle, as well as in other Hellenistic schools of philosophy, have a counterpart in the balance between different parts of the soul that characterizes the virtuous man who leads a flourishing, good life (*eudaimonia*). In the *Nicomachean Ethics* Aristotle (the son of a doctor) refers countless times to the art of medicine and compares it to other activities. The doctor must be able to adapt his judgement to the individual, concrete case and not just apply general rules (pp. 1097a, 1103b-1104a). This approximates the practical wisdom (*phronesis*) of the virtuous man. But there are also some important differences, so the analogy does not hold entirely: the ill man does not have

---

[93] See the last two parts of Michel Foucault's *Histoire de la sexualité* (1984), 'L'usage des plaisirs' and 'Le souci de soi', for an examination of this theme.

[94] Regarding the difference between Greek ethical thought and the non-cognitivist ethics characteristic of modern philosophical thinking, see MacIntyre (1985).

[95] Here we seem to come close to the modern holistic health theories of, for instance, Ingmar Pörn and Lennart Nordenfelt, which I will discuss later on. The main difference, however, is that the good life (*eudaimonia*) in ancient Greece was a normative and *objective* concept. The individual himself had no influence upon what was to be considered as a good life *for him*, as is the case in Pörn's and Nordenfelt's theories.

to learn medicine to get healthy (p. 1143b), but one has to learn philosophy to become virtuous (or at least it helps significantly).

Hygieia is one good (produced by medicine) among many other goods produced by other activities, as is stated on the first page of the *Nicomachean Ethics*. *Soma* and *psyche* in Aristotle, as in other classic philosophers, I repeat, must be thought of as joined together – in the case of Aristotle as the matter and form of the organism – in a union by which the activities of the *psyche* shape the organism. Although it is clear that health for Aristotle is primarily a somatic state and not a mental one, his theories of the virtuous character as a disposition (*diathesis, hexis*) enabling us to realize the good life are very similar in *structure* to the ancient health theories I have discussed above. The balanced state of the body of the healthy man, has its counterpart in the balanced, moderate state of the soul of the virtuous man, a state of temperance. The balance is to be established between what Aristotle in the *Nicomachean Ethics* calls the rational and the irrational elements of the soul; that is, between thinking (*logos*) and the emotions and desires (*pathe*) (p. 1102a). In the *Nicomachean Ethics* this is mainly conceptualized as the *logos* of the *psyche* taking control over the irrational *pathe*.[96]

I will return to the relation between the good life and the healthy life and to the roles played by thoughts and feelings within them later in developing a phenomenological theory of health. Let us now, however, proceed to some health theories of modern time.

2. THE BIOSTATISTICAL THEORY – BOORSE

The ancient health theories, as we have seen in the first part of this work, preserved their influence for a very long time – they were not superseded until the birth of modern medicine. They at last, however, yielded to a modern, scientific approach to medicine, inaugurated after the Renaissance and predominant after the coming together of the modern clinic and pathological anatomy in Paris around 1800; and they

---

[96] As Nussbaum has showed in her study of the second book of Aristotle's *Rhetoric* (dealing with *pathe*), however, Aristotle was not entitled to hold such a view, since he had, in that book, established that emotions are complex *cognitive* dispositions. *Pathe* are thus not irrational, neither in the sense of being non-cognitive, nor in the sense of always being false or inadequate (Nussbaum 1994, p. 81 ff.). Emotions, such as anger or love, are, according to Aristotle, directed towards objects and involve certain beliefs which can be true or false. (The anger of the man who is angry at his wife is directed towards *her* and involves the belief that she has deliberately done him wrong when she was unfaithful.) The reason Aristotle is so hostile toward *pathe* in the *Nicomachean Ethics* is probably because he in that work mainly identifies them with bodily appetites and desires and not with more complex emotions. We must thus think of the balance or harmony of the soul in another way than the cognitive, active elements simply conquering and taking control over the irrational, passive parts. Aristotle held a much more complex and positive view of the emotions as forming a part of the good life. Consider, for instance, Books VIII and IX of the *Nicomachean Ethics* discussing love and friendship – *philia*. As Nussbaum shows in her book (1994) many other ancient schools were more hostile towards *pathe* in their prescriptions for the 'ethical health' of the patient. The Stoics in this sense represented the extreme position of endeavouring an extirpation of all passions, since they considered them to represent false beliefs which caused suffering and led the philosopher astray in his search for the good life.

THE PHENOMENOLOGY OF HEALTH 63

are today viewed as curiosities of the past. As mere metaphysical speculation they did not meet the criteria of scientific, empirical investigation.

Health, though still an important subject for philosophers such as Descartes, Locke, Kant and Schelling, eventually was given up in the modern era as a subject for philosophy and became instead a subject for empirical science. Somatic as well as mental health consequently became the indirect research objects of medical science. I write indirect, because doctors and medical scientists are in most cases not really interested in health, but rather in possible compromisers of health such as diseases, impairments, injuries, and other defects. To identify and classify these different maladies – mainly diseases – to study their aetiology and effect their remedy, palliation and prevention are considered the main tasks of modern medicine.

During the last three decades we have witnessed what might be called a revival of the philosophy of medicine and health. For different reasons – which I have discussed in the preceding part of this work – the insight has become more widespread that the success of medical science by itself will never provide us with answers to all problems of clinical practice. Medical science itself does not provide us with a language in which we can carry out a philosophy of medicine; that is, a language in order to broach such questions as 'What is medicine?' and 'What is medical knowledge?'. As I want to show in this part of my work, the same is true when we discuss health. In formulating a theory of health, philosophical reflection is an indispensable tool. But since medical science is the discipline investigating empirically the diseased and the healthy organism (pathology, physiology), the *philosophy of* medical science (philosophical reflection on the status and meaning of medical scientific results and theories) certainly seems to be a possible starting point for a theory of health. Though not the first philosopher of health to work in the field of the philosophy of science, Christopher Boorse may very well be the most comprehensive and the most interesting.[97] I will in this section give a survey of his theory as an example of what might be called a biological-statistical theory of health.

Boorse's theory – just like the empirical theories of medical science – is based on the notion of disease. Boorse interprets disease in a very wide sense in order to include other maladies, such as congenital defects, injuries, and impairments (end results of diseases) (1977, pp. 550-551).[98] The test for a state (or possibly a process) to be called a disease is whether it prevents a part of the body from functioning in a normal way.[99] If the organism is not afflicted by any diseases it is healthy. Health is

---

[97] The three most important articles by Boorse on health theory were published in the seventies (1975, 1976 and 1977). Boorse has recently defended his theory against the many different forms of critique it has given rise to in *A Rebuttal on Health* (1997).

[98] Boorse writes in *A Rebuttal on Health* that he would today prefer the term 'pathological condition' to 'disease', in order to avoid misunderstandings (1997, p. 41 ff.).

[99] Boorse uses the term 'state' when he discusses diseases, although it would be more appropriate to call many diseases 'processes' (consider, for example, the various forms of cancer). The disease, in Boorse's framework, *causes* an abnormal functioning (or more exactly the inability to function normally) of a part of the body. Sometimes, however, Boorse seems to allow the possibility of identifying the disease with the state of abnormal functioning *itself* (1977, p. 567). This possibility seems to arise from cases in

accordingly the *absence* of disease. Boorse's theory puts a sharp focus upon biological *functions* – or rather upon *normal* biological functions. Normality, as it is used here, is a non-evaluative, descriptive concept, based solely on empirical investigations and statistics. The ancient theories of health were analogically built around normal functioning of the body and mind[100] of the individual; but, in these cases, 'normal' tended to mean 'in accordance with nature', and the 'natural' state was obviously relative to cultural norms.[101] It is interesting, however, that the ancient conceptions of health as different states of balance seem to have survived, in transmogrified form, in the modern, physiological concept of *homeostasis*. Walter Cannon, in his book *The Wisdom of the Body* from 1932, synthesized a huge amount of research and was able to show that the healthy organism is dependent upon the preservation of a stable inner environment. This environment can be described numerically; there is a normal value for the amount of water in the body in relation to other compounds, for the concentration of salts and minerals, for the temperature of the body, the blood pressure, the pH, and so on.[102] This inner environment is preserved – balanced – by different control systems which often work in opposite directions (the sympathetic and parasympathetic nervous systems and different endocrine systems, for instance).

---

which the cause of the abnormal functioning is not known, or in which the cause is known to be an external factor (such as pollution).

[100] I will not discuss Boorse's theory of mental health here separately, since it is in almost every sense similar to his theory of somatic health. The only difference lies in the possibility of the existence of other primary goals for the organism than survival and reproduction when *psychological* functions are taken into consideration in the theory (1976). Everything that the theories of psychology (and sociology) have to say about the normal functions of the individual should, however, in principle, be possible to express in the languages of chemistry and physics; there are no qualitative differences, and hence, the science of (neuro)physiology still seems to be the ultimate ground for Boorse's philosophy of mental health.

[101] As touched upon in Part 1 of this work, I will not consider the question whether science itself is value-laden, in the sense of depending on external constituting factors. It is not necessary for my argument to take a stand on the issue of the objectivity of science; the important thing is that there are other forms of knowledge in medicine than medical science. These other forms of knowledge, which I will try to explicate through the theories of phenomenology and hermeneutics, are based in clinical practice and focus upon the patient as a person and not exclusively as a biological organism. The degree to which science is a social construction or depends upon a preceding historical 'episteme' is consequently an issue that will not be dealt with here. I hope it has become obvious, from the first part of this work, however, that I do not proceed primarily from a theory of social construction, but from a phenomenological theory, based on the concept of lifeworld or being-in-the-world rather than on social relations of political power. The meaning-structures of the Western lifeworld are of course not historically static, but some basic strata are more reluctant to change than others. The caring, medical relationship which is the subject of this book is one example of this. The phenomenological structure of health, which I will try to outline later in this part, is another example. That science is an activity which *proceeds* from the basis of a cultural lifeworld and that it needs to be linked to this everyday world in order not to lose its meaningfulness, is however a phenomenological thesis which follows from my approach (Husserl 1976b). But, on the other hand, it is also obvious that science during the last two centuries has, indeed, in many ways, changed the lifeworld in which we experience and seek help and remedy for illness.

[102] An important forerunner to this modern theory of homeostasis was the work of Claude Bernard, who more than 80 years before Cannon founded the discipline of physiology and conceived of the normal physiological state as the preservation of a stable inner environment, which can be measured and assigned certain values. See Canguilhem (1991, pp. 260-261).

Boorse, however, is not willing to proceed directly from the concept of homeostasis, although he does not reject its importance:

> Homeostasis cannot, however, profitably be viewed as a general model of biological function. Many life functions are not homeostatic unless one stretches the concept to cover every goal-directed process (1977, p. 550).

Biological functions – the starting point for Boorse – are *goal-directed*, they have an aim: the goal of the kidneys is to remove some substances from the blood, while retaining others, in order to preserve its stable composition; the goal of the heart is to pump the blood through the vascular system in order to deliver oxygen and nutrients to the tissues, and so forth. Most parts and systems of the body – cells, tissues, organs, groups of organs – have many different functions with different goals. The kidneys, for example, do not only clear the blood; they also produce a number of hormones. The ultimate goal of every function of the parts of the body, according to Boorse, is, however, to contribute to the survival and reproduction of the organism.

All of the goals Boorse refers to are functional goals; that is, they are the goals of biological processes and are not aimed at in any intentional, *purposive* way. They are, however, indeed *purposeful* in the sense of serving survival and reproduction, but they are not the conscious aims of any person. To explain the function of the heart in terms of it pumping the blood *in order to* deliver oxygen and nutrients to the tissues is thus to give what Georg Henrik von Wright calls a 'quasi-teleological explanation'[103], since the whole set of events could instead be explained in terms of causality and laws of nature. We will return to this issue in the next section when I discuss another way of approaching health and again in Section 1 of Part 3, which deals with explanation and understanding in medicine.

The primary goals of the organism – survival and reproduction – can be achieved if the organism's biological functions, the functions of its parts (organs, tissues, cells), are normal with respect to its species. This analysis is essentially based on the same type of reasoning as in physiology: the body is looked upon as a complicated machine, the functions of which are analysable in terms of the functions of its parts. The biostatistical theory of health has consequently been called the 'machine model' of health.[104] If the parts of the organism have the ability to function in a normal way (the normal being calculated from empirical investigations of a large number of individuals and the biological function of every part being connected to a subgoal ultimately serving the primary goals of survival and reproduction) then the organism is healthy, according to Boorse. If not, the organism is diseased. Health is consequently looked upon as the absence of disease, and diseases are defined as internal states re-

---

[103] See von Wright (1971), especially Chapter 2: 'Causality and Causal Explanation'.

[104] See Jensen (1983). It might today, in the face of the development of recent biomedicine, be more accurate to speak of an informatic model in medicine than a machine model. The computer rather than the automobile seems to be the current model of the human body (Borck 1996). Boorse's theory, in any case, is intended to apply to animals as well as to human beings. This in a way seems to be inevitable, since his concept of health is based on the *organism* and not on the *person*. I will elaborate on this theme in the next section when I discuss a holistic theory of health.

ducing the ability of biological functioning below the normal value.[105] For a person to be ill, it is necessary that some part of his organism function in a subnormal way. If the organism is not afflicted with any diseases it is healthy, since it will have the ability to perform the biological functions of its parts in a normal way.

According to Boorse health is a *theoretical* concept and not a practical one. The question of whether a person is diseased or not is a strictly empirical question and not a matter of evaluation. The terms used to specify normal functions are all terms from science – biology, chemistry and statistics – and so even the functions and goals of the whole organism are analysable in these theoretical terms. The individual's evaluation – his feelings and thoughts – about his state of health is not relevant in any final sense when we try to determine whether he is healthy or not. The evaluation might often be relevant in an instrumental sense, of course – guiding the physician in his search for a disease – but it is not the final word on the issue of health. Many people are indeed diseased and unhealthy (in Boorse's sense) for a long time without having any symptoms or ever requiring any medical treatment.

There are a number of problems associated with the biostatistical theory of health.[106] Boorse's theory is designed to meet and solve some of these difficulties, for example, by allowing for super-normal biological functioning of parts of the organism without the organism being defined as diseased, or by allowing for differences within the population of a species which are related to sex and age. But many other problems remain to be solved. At what level of complexity should the function-goal structure whereby we identify disease be located? Since the aim of the theory is to analyse the health of the organism in terms of its parts, we could choose to look at the functions of organs, tissues or cells. Boorse's theory is an *analytical* theory; that is, he considers the function of the whole organism to be a system determinable from an analysis of the functions of its parts. The problem is that the biological function of an organ can be statistically normal even if parts of it do not work and are in a condition that we would normally refer to as diseased. If on the other hand we choose to focus on smaller parts of the organism such as the cells, we will always find some malfunctioning parts, and, consequently, according to Boorse's theory, all organisms would be diseased. (The malfunctioning would not be statistically species-normal since different types of cells would be functioning on a subnormal level in different organisms.) Another problem is the question of the dividing line between abnormal and normal functioning. Statistics will not provide us with the interval of normal functioning. Boorse himself admits that this issue will have to be settled on conventional grounds 'as in any application of statistical normality to a continuous distribution' (1977, p. 559). But what about statistically *species-normal* subfunctioning due to diseases which are genetically determined or the effect of harmful environmental

---

[105]Boorse does allow for the possibility of supernormal functioning without disease: 'The unusual cardiovascular ability of a long-distance runner is not a disease' (1977, p. 559).

[106]Most of the problems I refer to here have already been highlighted by Nordenfelt in his *On the Nature of Health: An Action Theoretic Approach* (1987) – a work that I will discuss extensively in the next section – and before him by Canguilhem (1991 [1966]). Other important critiques of Boorse are Engelhardt (1984) and Fulford (1989).

factors? Boorse responds to this critique, and to many other objections to his theory, in the recent *A Rebuttal on Health* (1997). He admits, for instance, that one might have to introduce the concept of an *environment* being statistically normal or abnormal to a species to solve the problem of diseases that seem to be present in nearly every individual in a population (1997, p. 83). The most important aspect of Boorse's rebuttal is that it clarifies a point that was not made explicit in the earlier articles and therefore did not occur to many of his critics. What Boorse wants to do is to make the concept of disease as it is used within *pathology* lucid (1997, p. 48). His health theory is therefore not intended to be a theory that guides the clinician, but rather the pathologist. For instance, in reply to the critique that all of us at all times have several cells that are malfunctioning and that we are therefore always diseased, Boorse remarks that this does not amount to an objection to his theory: 'We do all contain some pathology, of which one dead cell is just a trivial example' (1997, p. 85). Naturally Boorse does not intend to say that the physician should treat every such example of pathology, or, for that matter, that he should treat *only* pathologies (diseases). What we need, according to Boorse, in order to make sense of the activities of the clinic are 'disease-plus' concepts (1997, p. 100). These concepts would, in contrast to the empirical-statistical disease concept of pathology, have to be value-laden; but, according to Boorse, they would at the same time rest on the value-free, scientific disease concept as a kind of bedrock.

Indeed, if disease is taken in Boorse's sense, I believe we do, in fact, need a theory based on 'disease-plus' concepts, in order to make sense of the goal of clinical practice. One could however also argue that to base the disease concept on the activities of the pathologist and not on the experiences suffered by the patients of the clinic is a doubtful move.[107] Since I will base my own approach to health in this work on illness rather than on disease, the question of the soundness of this Boorsian move is not, however, essential to my analysis. We will now take a look at another way of conceptualizing health, which in my eyes is more promising when it comes to a theory of health as the goal of clinical practice. This theory will be a positive theory of health; that is, it will try to explicate what health consists in directly and not by way of the concept of disease.

---

[107]Canguilhem (1991 [1966]) refutes in a convincing manner the biostatistical disease concept, which he shows to have been present in medicine ever since Claude Bernard and Auguste Comte. He also develops a view according to which health should be approached as an evaluative concept studied at the level of personal, clinical experience: 'In the final analysis, would it not be appropriate to say that the pathological can be distinguished as such, that is, as an alteration of the normal state, only at the level of organic totality, and when it concerns man, at the level of conscious individual totality, where disease becomes a kind of evil? . . . The situation is such that if the physiological analysis of separated functions is known in the presence of pathological facts, this is due to previous clinical information, for clinical practice puts the physician in contact with complete and concrete individuals and not with organs and their functions' (1991, pp. 87-88).

3. THE HOLISTIC THEORY – NORDENFELT

The main weakness of the biostatistical theory of health is that it looks upon human beings exclusively as organisms – as sophisticated machines – and not as persons. This claim, which I will try to make evident in the following analysis, could be tentatively formulated like this: Organisms have diseases, and these are certainly, in most cases, the cause of ill health; but only human beings living in the world are ill or healthy. Health and illness are consequently not phenomena analysable exclusively in the terms of science, but are evaluative concepts referring to the experiences, ambitions and abilities of human beings situated in certain contexts – lifeworlds. I will now turn to an attempt to formulate a theory of health in *holistic* terms – terms referring to the person as a whole, in constant interaction with his environment.[108]

The biostatistical theory of health does not pay much attention to the surroundings of the organism and their effect on the physiology of the body. This seems to be a factor of vital importance if one wants to study the normal level of activity and goals of biological functions. The temperature of the surroundings of the organism, just to mention one obvious example, affects the activity of many biological functions. It might be possible, although it is complicated, to integrate such environmental factors in the bio-statistical theory by specifying the circumstances for every biological function when one calculates normality.[109]

The environment, however, not only influences biological activity and function; it also influences the activities and goals of the person. What does it mean to be a person? The concept has a long history and has been used in several, different philosophical theories.[110] The notion of person is commonly reserved for human beings[111] and indicates that, in addition to having body and consciousness, one also has a relation to the surrounding world inhabited by other persons – a world in which one acts and realizes one's intentions. To be a person in this sense means to be an individual – a self – with a certain history and personality related to the history of other persons and to social and cultural institutions. I will return to the concepts of person and self later in this part of my work in developing a phenomenological theory of health.

Actions are *intentional*; that is, they are directed towards goals in another sense than the goal-directedness of biological functions, since they are executed by persons who have certain plans and preferences and attempt to achieve certain ends. Organ-

---

[108]Etymological studies provide some support for developing a (w)holistic theory of health. The word 'health' originally seems to have meant 'wholeness' or 'completeness' (Klein 1966, p. 710). The same applies for the German 'Gesundheit' and the French 'santé' (Ritter and Gründer 1974, vol. 3, p. 560; von Wartburg 1964, pp. 184-186).

[109]Boorse writes in *A Rebuttal on Health* that this was what he intended all the time, although he did not make it clear enough in the earlier articles (1997, p. 79).

[110]The Latin word 'persona' originates from the classical theatre where it meant 'mask', 'role' or 'character'. In the Christian tradition the concept of person was associated first with the Trinity and then with the human individual and his relationship to God. For this and later developments of the concept of person, see Horgby (1995) and Theunissen (1966).

[111]There are exceptions, however. See, for instance, Singer (1993, p. 87).

isms do not act; rather they undergo processes that are the causal effects of other processes, and they move in response to stimuli. The functioning of the organism is, of course, *lived* by the person, and it is therefore certainly essential to him; but to describe the life of the person one needs another language than the language of science, namely a language of teleology. Action theory is a field of philosophy providing us with such a language, and the holistic theory of health I will present in this section has its roots in that tradition.

Lennart Nordenfelt's attempt to formulate a holistic theory of health is by no means the first or only such attempt.[112] His theory, however, has some advantages in comparison with many other holistic theories. It is (most often) in conformity with a general understanding of health, and it has been worked out in some detail. According to Nordenfelt, health is 'ability to realize one's vital goals given standard circumstances'. I will in this section try to render this explication of the concept of health lucid, and thereafter, in the remainder of this second part of my work, move on to a phenomenological attempt to formulate a theory of health and illness much in the same spirit, but within another context and with slightly different ambitions and results.

In action theory the teleology of the person is based on the notions of action and goal. The individual acts in order to realize a plan of attaining certain goals. The actions and goals are dependent upon the environment. The individual finds himself in constant interaction with the environment, the environment being the necessary prerequisite for the possibility of action as well as the possible thwarter of our plans. The environment consequently represents the sphere in which our freedom is both realized and limited. It seems clear, however, that the things limiting our freedom are not only to be found outside the body, since the design of our bodies certainly prevents us from doing certain things that we might desire to do, such as flying (without the aid of any mechanical devices). Often, nevertheless, our plans seem to fail on account of some external event or state, such as other people's actions or the physical design of the environment. As long as we do not specify the circumstances, however, it is impossible to establish whether the frustrating factor is located 'within' or 'without'. If I have the goal of jumping ten meters in the air, we might say that this is impossible because the design of my body prevents me from doing so. But still it would, of course, be possible to jump ten meters in the air if the force of gravity were weaker – which is the case, for instance, on the moon. To change sex was definitely not possible one hundred years ago; today it is possible. To fly might be possible in one hundred years from now if we acquire additional knowledge about how to manipulate the human organism.[113] The attainment of a certain goal through se-

---

[112] The books by Nordenfelt I will proceed from in this section are *On the Nature of Health: An Action-Theoretic Approach* (1987, slightly rev. ed. 1995) and *Quality of Life, Health and Happiness* (1993). The most important forerunner to and source of inspiration for Nordenfelt is undoubtedly Canguilhem (1991 [1966]). For other attempts to formulate holistic theories of health, see Fulford (1989, 1993); Kass (1975); Pörn (1984, 1993); Seedhouse (1986); and Whitbeck (1981).

[113] It could, of course, be said that it is, in fact, possible to fly even today given the right circumstances – the absence of gravity. The point of these examples is to highlight the fact that the abilities, actions and

quences of chains of actions (Nordenfelt 1987, pp. 40-41) always seems to depend upon an interaction between the individual person and his environment. In the terminology of action theory we say that the attainment of a goal through sequences of chains of actions requires both the ability and the opportunity – what Nordenfelt refers to as the 'practical possibility' – to perform the actions involved (1987, p. 42).[114]

To be able to do something depends, basically, on the presence of a certain disposition. Since the concept of action is based on intention, to be able to perform a certain action means that you are disposed in such a way that, if you intend to do x (take a pill) and you are given the opportunity to do x, then you will do x. If, given these premises, you do not take the pill, you are not able to do it. To be able to do x presupposes that you are able to form the intention to do x, since all actions – in order to be actions and not simply events – must be intentional. This might be impossible for some persons due to their mental design or ethical character, though they be physically capable of doing x. That is, supposing the pill is a suicide pill, it might be impossible for a person who does not have the courage to commit suicide, or who believes it is wrong to commit suicide, to take it, even though he is physically capable. It might also be impossible for some people to understand that they actually have the possibility of doing x. It is consequently not possible to decide on solely physiological or behavouristic grounds if an individual is able to perform an action. One also needs knowledge about the individual's intentions and beliefs.

In order to know whether a person is able to realize a certain goal through an action – as I mentioned before – one must specify the circumstances. One must specify what opportunities the actor is presented with when one decides whether he is able to perform the action, since the given opportunity forms part of the meaning of every ability. Nordenfelt in his theory of health does this through the notion of 'standard' or 'accepted' circumstances.[115] That the opportunities are 'standard' means that they are not extreme. If the opportunities are extremely favourable we will be able to do almost anything. If, on the other hand, they are extremely unfavourable we will be

---

goals of a person need to be specified in terms of his environment. In the phenomenological context this will lead us to the concept of 'lifeworld' or 'being-in-the-world'.

[114] A sequence of actions is several actions following in succession. The concept action-chain refers to the fact that an action can be thought of as doing x *by* doing y. The variables here do not refer to different actions in the sense of different events causally related, but rather to the same action under different descriptions. For example, I open the window *by* turning the handle *by* turning my hand. Any action, of which it can be said that there exists no description according to which the action is performed by doing something else, is called a basic action. Other actions are called generated actions. The basic action must still be described as an action; that is, it must be intentional – it must be a description of me or somebody else *doing* something, not of processes in my body that merely take place.

[115] The replacement of 'standard' with 'accepted' in *On the Nature of Health* (1995, rev. ed.) merely serves to underscore the fact that the circumstances must be specified by *someone*, and this determination can never be objective in the scientific sense. Someone has to accept the circumstances as standard; whether, in the case of health, it is to be the person whose health is being examined, some general consensus, or an expert team, has to be settled from case to case. There is no final answer on this issue in Nordenfelt's theory (the same applies, as we shall see later, for what he calls 'vital goals'), and, indeed, this is, in his view, the inescapable (but not damning) consequence of the theory being normative.

prevented from doing things we are normally able to do. But it will never be possible to determine the standard or normal circumstances on purely statistical grounds; they will vary with location, time and culture. Since the holistic concept of health in Nordenfelt's version is defined as the ability to realize vital goals given standard circumstances, it will consequently be an evaluative concept not determinable on purely descriptive grounds. This concept of normality is, indeed, as an evaluative, culture-relative concept, similar to the ancient notion of being 'in accordance with nature'.

Health, in Nordenfelt's theory, is characterized as a certain ability – the ability of an individual to realize *vital goals* given standard circumstances.[116] What are these vital goals? Which set of actions is connected to the realization of them? Nordenfelt's answer is that this also is a matter of evaluation; but, in analogy with how we decide upon *standard* circumstances, we cannot treat the vital goals as strictly synonymous with that which the individual himself considers to be vital. The vital goals are not simply the same thing as every individual's conscious (or even conscious and unconscious) high-priority goals and wants. This would leave us with a health concept that is strongly counterintuitive, since the goals of the individual could be highly unrealistic compared with his abilities. Such a concept of health would indeed come closer to a concept of autonomy or quality of life. If, on the other hand, the individual decides to pursue only a few, quite easily-attainable goals, he could, according to such a health concept, be healthy despite serious disease and disability – which also seems to run counter to our intuitive everyday understanding of health.

But though being healthy may seem to depend upon fulfilling basic physiological and psychological needs – such as the need for food, sleep, safety and love; that is, upon a handful of specific goals the individual is incapable of wilfully choosing, rather than upon a broader range of individual wants – we cannot content ourselves with such a health concept based on need. As a matter of fact, it is not possible, on a purely empirical basis, to determine the basic human needs or drives without running into the same problem that we encountered in the biostatistical theory with individual and environmental variation. Only the extremely basic physiological needs, necessary for survival and reproduction, could be said to be statistically normal in all environments and groups. If, however, we were to call all people who are able to fulfil these basic needs healthy, we would include many persons normally referred to as ill and diseased.[117]

---

[116] Or more precisely: the *second-order* ability to realize vital goals given standard circumstances. Second-order ability is the ability to develop another ability given an adequate training program. I do not, for example, speak or understand Chinese, but given a (rather ambitious) training program, I can learn to do so. It is necessary to introduce the notion of second-order ability into the definition of health, since otherwise, people would automatically develop unhealth simply by moving to an unfamiliar culture with very different standard circumstances and vital goals (1987, pp. 49-50). This is not to say that what counts as standard and normal does not matter when we decide upon the matter of health. As we have already seen above, it is indeed crucial, and someone from a foreign culture deemed unhealthy by us might indeed be perfectly healthy given the vital goals and standard circumstances of his own culture

[117] What we obviously cannot do is to define the basic needs in terms of necessary conditions that the individual must be able to fulfil in order to be healthy, since health is precisely that which we are trying to characterize in the explication of basic needs (Nordenfelt 1987, pp. 57-65).

Opinions about what is vital in life are often coloured by individual preferences and culturally-specific values. To have a job may be vital to some people, but not to others. (This does not mean that people with the vital goal of having employment become ill when they lose it; they have to lose the *ability* to work before we, according to Nordenfelt, are ready to consider them unhealthy.) We have to find a compromise between, on the one hand, granting the authority of what is to be considered a vital goal to the individual himself, and, on the other hand, granting this authority to empirical investigators working in terms of universal, basic needs. Nordenfelt's solution consists in linking the notion of vital goal to what he calls 'minimal happiness'. He therefore calls his theory a *welfare* theory of health:

> The general idea is the following: The vital goals of man are those whose fulfilment is necessary and jointly sufficient for a minimal degree of welfare, i.e. happiness. To be healthy, then, is to have the ability to fulfil those goals which are necessary and jointly sufficient for a minimal degree of happiness (1987, p. 78).

What is happiness? This question has been answered in quite different ways in different philosophical traditions. Is happiness an objective or a subjective concept? Is it a feeling, or a cognitive state, or a way of living a good life – the 'eudaimonia' of Aristotle? Nordenfelt discusses these issues, particularly in *Quality of Life, Health and Happiness*, and comes to the following conclusion: 'P is happy with his or her life as a whole, if and only if P wants his or her conditions in life to be just as he or she finds them to be' (1993, p. 45). In *On the Nature of Health*, Nordenfelt had characterized happiness primarily as an emotion: to be happy meant to feel happy about something (1987, pp. 82-86). In the chronologically later work, however, he makes a distinction between being happy and feeling happy. To *be* happy, which is Nordenfelt's prime candidate for happiness, does not necessarily mean to have a feeling about something; it is rather a cognitive state of equilibrium between one's wants and the belief that these are satisfied (1993, p. 52). This state is looked upon as a predisposition for the experience of feeling happy, but does not necessarily, on each occasion, result in this experience. This notion of happiness lies very far from Bentham's identification of happiness with pleasure. Pleasure, in Nordenfelt's model would only be one of the *objects* of happiness (1993, pp. 50-51). Nordenfelt's concept is thus essentially a cognitivist concept of happiness, since it does not necessarily include any *feelings* of well-being or happiness.

Since happiness, according to Nordenfelt, is connected to the realization (or believed realization) of wants, it does not lie very far from his concept of health. Health, we remember, is defined as ability to realize certain goals (wants). To be healthy and to be happy are, however, two very different things, since the ability to realize goals is perfectly compatible with not realizing them.[118] To specify health we

---

[118]Consider, for example, a person under very unfortunate circumstances living, let us say, in Somalia. This person may be able to realize his vital goals, in terms of physical and mental dispositions, but he is not given the opportunity and consequently is very unhappy. On the other hand the unhealthy person may be very happy, according to Nordenfelt's definition, if he is given extremely favourable opportunities (for example mechanical aids and assistants) to attain the goals that, given standard circumstances, he would not be able to realize.

need to know which goals are vital, and this is obviously the reason why vital goals are connected to minimal happiness. The vital goals are, as stated above, those that the individual needs to fulfil (or to believe himself to have fulfilled) in order to be happy in a minimal sense.

Where does this lead us in our attempt to specify vital goals? They will still vary from person to person since the goals which need to be attained in order for the subject to be even minimally happy are individual. But a subclass of vital goals, which Nordenfelt calls 'basic vital goals', would form part of every person's vital goal profile. These are the goals that are absolutely necessary for all happiness (1987, p. 91). These basic goals seem to be similar to basic needs for survival, such as having food, sleep, love (in some form) and security. It might be possible to extend the class of basic vital goals to include things such as having a mission in life, having a sex life, having friends, and so on; but, we might then run the risk of having included goals which, though necessary for *most* people for the achievement of minimal happiness, are not, in fact, necessary for *all* people.

One way of specifying the vital goals is to claim that they are the goals that one must attain (or must believe oneself to have attained) in order to be minimally happy in the *long run*. One would thus exclude goals that, though they give immediate pleasure and thus might form part of a person's want profile, over a longer period of time, will prove to be harmful to him, such as drug abuse. But could not the taking of drugs, nevertheless, be part of some person's vital goal profile? Nordenfelt's view on this issue is that the final authority about a goal being vital cannot be given exclusively either to the subject himself or to the professional observer. In the standard case the individual himself will know which wants constitute his vital goals – he knows what is acceptable or of high priority to him (1987, p. 96; 1993, p. 59). But the person could always be wrong, since there is the possibility that not all vital goals are known to him. Some might, for instance, be unconscious. If not all the vital goals are fulfilled (or the person does not believe them to be so) the person is unhappy. But, of course, the person could also be wrong when we ask him about this. This is particularly obvious when we remind ourselves of the fact that Nordenfelt's concept of happiness is not tied to the feeling of happiness but is rather characterized as a cognitive state. We could *feel* indifferent but still *be* happy according to this theory. But could a happy life (even a minimally happy life) really be a life totally devoid of all feelings of happiness? And can a person be unhealthy without experiencing any feelings of illness? Nordenfelt's solution here is to separate subjective and objective health, the former being defined by the beliefs about, and feelings of, illness (1993, Chapter 6). The concept of objective health is, however, the basic and most important one and accordingly the one which I concentrate upon in this section. I will return to the issue of feelings later in unfolding a phenomenological theory of health.

Health, as defined by the holistic theory above, might be developed as an absolute concept or as a dimensional one (1987, pp. 97-98). The possibility of a dimensional explication lies in giving priority to some vital goals (for instance, the basic ones) before others. One can then develop a scale from minimal health (the ability to realize all basic vital goals) to maximal health (the ability to realize all vital goals).

If, on the other hand, one simply identifes health with ability to realize all of the person's vital goals, then one has instead posited an absolute health concept. One is either able or not able – either healthy or unhealthy; and one is not healthier in virtue of being able to realize additional, non-vital goals. In either case health would be characterized as a state of balance or equilibrium – between abilities and goals – and Nordenfelt in this respect joins the tradition of the health concepts we have discussed in the preceding sections:

> Note again the formal structure of the concept of health introduced in this volume: A is in a bodily and mental state which is such that, given a set of accepted circumstances, A has the second-order ability to realise all his vital goals. According to this characterisation health denotes a relation of equilibrium between a person's ability and his vital goals given a certain set of circumstances (1993, p. 127).

Health is here defined as a state of equilibrium, a balance between abilities and goals.

Now, what about diseases and other maladies? What role do they play in the holistic theory? Although there remains the possibility of being ill (unhealthy) without being diseased in the holistic theory, diseases and other maladies are still the most frequent causes of illness. The reason for this is obvious: diseases always tend to compromise the abilities of their bearer and to cause pain and suffering. This is indeed the reason why we call them 'dis-eases'. According to Nordenfelt's theory, a disease is a *process* that tends to cause inability to realize the vital goals of the bearer (1987, pp. 105-112).[119] A disease *tends* to cause inability; that is, it does so in most cases, but there still remains the possibility of being diseased and, at the same time, healthy, if the process does not affect the bearer – if it does not affect the state of equilibrium.

Disease then, according to Nordenfelt, is a process rather than a state – a process that interferes with our ability to realize vital goals. Other compromisers of health – such as injuries, impairments and defects – are, according to Nordenfelt, *states* of variable duration that tend to cause disability. We can thus see that, although these different kinds of maladies are not the starting point for the development of a holistic theory of health, they certainly play an important role in it. Indeed, the only way to differentiate between mental and somatic illness in Nordenfelt's theory would be via compromisers of health – maladies. If the individual suffers from a mental process or state that tends to cause inability to realize vital goals, then the person would be mentally ill; if he suffers from a physical process or state that tends to cause inability, then he would be physically ill, according to the theory (1987, p. 100).[120] We will return to the relation between somatic and mental illness in our phenomenological analysis later on in this part.

---

[119]This is an important difference compared to the disease concept of Boorse, who identifies disease on purely scientific, and not on clinical grounds.

[120]For a discussion of the relation between the concept of mental health and Nordenfelt's theory, see Tengland (1998).

I have not yet criticized the holistic welfare theory of health in the way I did to the biological-statistical theory. I will save my critique until I have developed a phenomenological alternative to compare Nordenfelt's theory to. By incorporating and developing his theory in a phenomenological context, I will attempt to extract the most advantageous elements of his theory and re-deploy them within the framework that will guide our examination of health and medicine in the remaining parts of this work. As we will see, other dimensions of human existence than action, such as understanding, language, feeling and embodiment, will receive attention when we turn to the theories of phenomenology and hermeneutics.

A pressing and illuminating question remains before we move on to phenomenology. Does Nordenfelt's proposal really represent a *theory* of health? Is it not just a proposal for a *definition* of health, whereas a theory of health would have to proceed from empirical investigations? Yes, but in a way this is exactly the point of this kind of philosophical theory of health. Boorse's theory too was essentially an attempt to *define* the concept of health being used in medical science. The holistic theory of health I have presented in this section is based, not on the analysis of the language of science, but on the analysis of ordinary language use. Nordenfelt's aim, however, is not only to give a description of how people actually use words like 'health', 'illness' and 'disease', but also to propose a use that would be in line with our intuitions and logically consistent. This is what he refers to as the project of 'weak nominalism' (1987, p. 7). His definition is thus not only descriptive but also normative, although the normative element does not derive from a belief in the 'true essence' of any words. The aim of a *philosophical* theory of health can thus be said to lie in the explication of the *meaning* of health, based on the analyses of already existing theories, conceptions and experiences of health. This brings us back to our point of departure in this part of my book: phenomenology.

4. HUSSERL'S PHENOMENOLOGY

Phenomenology represents another attempt at the explication of meaning, but the object of philosophical reflection here is not the theory of science (as in Boorse), or ordinary language use (as in Nordenfelt), but experience itself. It is still an explication, however, since experience is not looked upon as pure formless content – as sense-data for instance – but as a structure of meaning. This structure belongs to experience itself; it is not 'out there' in the world, or 'inside' the subject as a mental pattern organizing sense-data, but rather the structure linking self and world together as parts or modes of the same synthesis. In what terms this synthesis of self and world is to be understood has, as we shall see, been a constant subject of debate in the phenomenological movement.

Phenomenology today is not one but several philosophical, sociological and psychological theories.[121] They all derive their origin, however, from the philosophy of

---

[121] For a comprehensive survey of the phenomenological movement, see the books by Herbert Spiegelberg (1972, 1982).

Edmund Husserl. The common root comes down to Husserl's claim, in the beginning of this century, on the necessity of going back to 'the things themselves' and the way they are presented to us in order to find a solid ground for philosophy. The conceptualization of appearance, the *eidos* or meaning of experience, is to be found in the phenomena themselves by adopting a certain mode of attention. As mentioned above, this project has been taken up and developed in many different ways, and some of them will be addressed in this work.

But let us begin with Husserl.[122] To do phenomenology according to Husserl means to study our experience as *consciousness* of an object. To experience something, according to Husserl, is always to be conscious about it, to be directed towards it in an act. The life of consciousness – which was the starting point for Husserl – unfolds in a series of intentional processes – *acts*. Acts are intentional, they are directed towards objects – states in the world – (or towards other acts of consciousness). Note that intentionality here is a much broader concept than in the action theory of Nordenfelt I presented above. Intentionality as the basic structure of phenomena in Husserl does not necessarily imply that one intends something in the sense of wanting it or bringing it about. It only means that one's consciousness is directed towards, is about, something in the world.

To be conscious is to be *directed* towards the world. We do not pay attention to this in our normal life – a state that Husserl refers to as 'the natural attitude'. The life of consciousness is transparent in the sense that we focus our attention, not upon the act itself, but upon the object of the act. We do not reflect upon the structure of the act itself, but simply live in and through the acts: looking, smelling, touching, talking, reading, thinking, and so on. The phenomenological move consists in a change in the mode of attention referred to as the *epoche*. We shift our mode of attention from the object to the act itself: to the 'directedness' of the act, to the way the object is *constituted* – that is, to the way it obtains meaning for us. The suspension of the existence of the object is not effected in the spirit of scepticism. The phenomenologist does not doubt that there is a world out there; it is not all in our minds as the idealist would hold. As a matter of fact, the phenomenologist abstains from making any ontological claims about what the acts are directed towards, but rather tries to study the acts themselves in order to investigate and classify them. The acts will thus prove to be of very different types. The ways we are directed towards the world in seeing,

---

[122]The authoritative guide to Husserl's phenomenology, examining the genesis of his philosophy and its main themes, is Bernet et al. (1989; translated into English in 1993). Another valuable introduction to Husserl's philosophy is Zaner (1970). My presentation of Husserl's philosophy in this section is mainly built upon his *Ideen zu einer reinen Phänomenologie und phänomenologischen Philosophie. Erstes Buch: Allgemeine Einführung in die reine Phänomenologie* (1976a [1913]). It is, of necessity, a very cursory introduction, omitting many of the main themes of Husserl's philosophy, especially that which is generally referred to as the 'genetic' part of his phenomenology; that is, the constitution of the transcendental ego, which lives in the stream of acts of consciousness through the non-intentional processes of inner-time consciousness. The reason for leaving out this important part of Husserl's philosophy is that I will turn to Heidegger instead of Husserl when it comes to laying out a phenomenological interpretation of health and thus will discuss the status of the self (ego, person) in the terms of Heidegger's and not Husserl's philosophy. I will return briefly to this theme in the next section.

smelling, touching, talking, reading and thinking are certainly very different manners of approaching the world. Husserl would say that the acts – the *noesen* – have different meaning-structures – different *noemata*. The acts, taking place in time and space, are thus, as intentional phenomena, filled with meanings that the phenomenologist tries to excavate.

Every act involves an object. The meaning-structures of these objects vary depending upon the mode of givenness – *Gegebenheitsweise* – of consciousness, and upon the type of object involved. To think of a book and to look at a book represent two different types of acts: the mode of givenness of the book is different in each case, although the acts could be directed towards the same book. To look at a book and to look at a lion are also two different acts – they have different 'noematischen Sinn' in Husserl's terms; that is, the meaning-structures of the objects involved are different. This does not just have to do with colour and shape; it has to do with the fact that we expect very different things from books and lions. Books do not move; they are not frightening (at least not in the same way as lions are); we expect books to contain pages, filled with letters forming words and sentences which can be read, and so on. Lions in general have four legs; they move about, eat, roar and are dangerous. Books and lions have very different meaning-structures as parts of the same meaningful world of experience. But the two acts also have a great deal in common. All things given in perception – books as well as lions – are given in time and space; they have a reverse side, which we cannot see but still believe to be there; they have a specific form and colour, etc. The meaning-structure of objects given in thinking may be different. When we direct ourselves towards the number two, for example, it is not given anywhere in time and space. The object of an act in a dream or a fantasy has yet another mode of existence – but the act still has a meaning-structure, and it is an intentional phenomenon which can be studied.

The claim of phenomenology is that the meaning of every phenomenon – every act – could be studied by the systematical change in our attention – the phenomenological *epoche* – I have described above. The change from the natural to the phenomenological attitude is also referred to by Husserl as the 'phenomenological reduction'. What is 'reduced' (or 'put in brackets') are all preceding scientific theories about the objects of the world, and what is focused upon is the *experience* of the world. This reduction provides us with a *transcendental* analysis in the sense of being an analysis of the *meaning* of experience – an analysis of the structures of consciousness that make the experience and constitution of the objects of the world possible. Transcendental here has the classic Kantian meaning of 'condition of possibility of experience'. Husserl's theory is consequently not a psychological theory about the contents of consciousness – mental entities would also belong to the world – but a philosophical theory about the structure of consciousness and the constitution of the world through the patterns of meaning of intentionality.

The phenomenological reduction is also generally an *eidetical* reduction, since we are interested in the meaning of different *concepts* – the concept of lion and not the individual lion, for instance. The phenomenologist has specific interests and problems that he wants to solve in his phenomenological investigations, and these are tied to conceptual problems: what constitutes a work of art? for example; what features must necessarily belong to an artwork in order for it to be a work of art and not something else? The phenomenological reduction involves what Husserl called 'free fantasy variation'. We do not only consider all artworks we have experienced, but also, by imagining possible artworks that we *could* experience, try to establish what it takes for an act to be an experience of art – that is, an act directed towards an artwork (and not towards a scientific work, for example).

This fantasy variation is, of course, despite its aim of avoiding particularity, nevertheless highly dependent upon our prior experiences (including not only seeing and listening to artworks but also reading and hearing about them). Through the imaginative variation, however, we reach the mode of philosophical reflection and direct ourselves towards the meanings of concepts and not only towards the meanings of individual acts. What is important here is that the attempt to uncover the meanings of concepts aims at generality; that is, it aims to overcome the limits of one's particular experiences and to attain thereby an objective status.

The method of free fantasy variation, picking up examples from life and imagining other possible ones, is not to be confused with induction. The phenomenologist does not gather (add together) empirical evidence in order to make his claims more general. Rather, he uses examples (experienced and imagined) as the bearers of the different necessary features of concepts.[123] The examples of illness and clinical practice that I will use later in this book are construed in this manner of phenomenological reflection – as illustrations of the characteristic, necessary features of health, illness and medicine.[124]

5. THE PHENOMENA OF HEALTH AND ILLNESS

Let us now return to the phenomena I want to focus upon in this part of my work: health and its opposite, illness. How should we proceed when we want to carry out a phenomenological analysis of health? In many ways the phenomenon of illness seems to be far more concrete and easy to get hold of than the phenomenon of health. When we are ill, life is often penetrated by feelings of meaninglessness, helplessness, pain, nausea, fear, dizziness, or disability. Health, in contrast, effaces itself in an enigmatic way. It seems to be the absence of every such feeling of illness, the state or process which we are in when everything is flowing smoothly, running the usual way without hindrance. Is health then only possible to characterize in a

---

[123] See Zaner (1970) for this interpretation of the method of free fantasy variation in Husserl. It is interesting to note that this phenomenological 'method' bears many similarities to the conceptual analysis of Nordenfelt, who also, to a large extent, proceeds from imaginary examples. Perhaps free fantasy variation should really be considered *the* philosophical strategy, generally?

[124] My chief sources of inspiration for these examples come from my study of clinical encounters at Ekholmen Primary Care Centre, and at the University Hospital in Linköping. I have also found information and stories about experiencing and living with illness, as well as meeting with the doctor, in many books. The accounts I have profited from the most are Fisher (1997); Guthrie and Guthrie (1997); Hardy (1978); Kantoff and McConnell (1996); Kleinman (1988); Richt (1992); and Senelick and Rossi (1994).

negative way? Is it only the absence of illness? And should, consequently, the phenomenology of health focus only upon illness?

As we have seen above the distinction between disease as a state or process causing biological malfunction and illness as the lived experience of the person is an important one. It has formed a platform for thinking about medicine as something more than and different from applied biology in psychology, sociology and anthropology, as I showed in Sections 5, 6 and 7 of the previous part of this work; and it is central to the difference between the biostatistical theory of Boorse, which defined health via disease, and the holistic theory of Nordenfelt, which focused directly upon health and illness.[125] Illness, not disease – that is, the lived experience of being ill – will also be my own point of departure when I try to formulate a phenomenological theory of health and illness in what follows.[126] In my attempt to formulate a phenomenological theory of health, however, illness is not meant as a psychological characterization of the life of the person, in contrast to the 'real' diseases of somatics. Phenomenology, as we will see, is not a psychological theory, and it is not some dualistic attempt to overcome materialism. To focus attention on lived experience as a structure of meaning means to bracket both materialism and dualism in order to get at the foundation – the lifeworld-based underpinnings – of the knowledge expressed in philosophical and scientific theories.

But is illness our only possibility for phenomenological analysis? Cannot health itself be explicated phenomenologically? Hans-Georg Gadamer – a philosopher working within the phenomenological tradition – writes, in his book from 1993, *Über die Verborgenheit der Gesundheit*:

> So what possibilities do we really have when it comes to the question of health? Without doubt it is part of our nature as living beings that the conscious awareness of health conceals itself. Despite its hidden character, health nonetheless manifests itself in a kind of feeling of well-being. It shows itself above all where such a feeling of well-being means that we are open to new things, ready to embark on new enterprises and, forgetful of ourselves, scarcely notice the demands and strains which are put upon us. This is what health is (1993, pp. 143-144).

In spite of its character of withdrawal, Gadamer consequently sees a possibility of conceptualizing health. Unfortunately he does not provide us with this phenomenological theory of health in his book. What he does give us are some ingenious, albeit unsystematized, hints concerning how we should look upon the phenomenon of health:

---

[125] As we have seen above, Nordenfelt's primary concept in conceptualizing health is, however, not lived experience, but ability. See Section 9 below for an analysis of the similarities and differences between Nordenfelt's theory and my phenomenological approach to health.

[126] In addition to 'disease' and 'illness' a third term, 'sickness', is often used in talking about health and its opposites. When contrasted to illness it is often used in the sense of a social role, a 'sick-role', ascribed to a person by other people, rather than being something experienced by the person himself. However, the term is also often used interchangeably with 'illness', especially in American English. To avoid confusion I will refrain from using the term 'sickness' in this work. If the term 'sick' is used in any of my examples it means 'ill' and nothing else. For an examination of the different meanings of the three terms, see the articles by Nordenfelt and Twaddle (1993).

> Health is not a condition that one introspectively feels in oneself. Rather it is a condition of being there (Da-Sein), of being in the world (In-der-Welt-Sein), of being together with other people (Mit-den-Menschen-Sein), of being taken in by an active and rewarding engagement with the things that matters in life.... It is the rhythm of life, a permanent process in which equilibrium re-establishes itself. This is something known to us all. Think of the processes of breathing, digesting and sleeping for example (Gadamer 1993, pp. 144-145).

In these suggestions from Gadamer we can find similarities to other health theories we have surveyed. Health described, not as an introspective state, but rather as a pattern of action of being in the world, recalls Nordenfelt's conception of health as an ability to act. On the other hand, the description of health as a process of self re-establishing equilibrium in breathing, digesting and sleeping, is instead reminiscent of homeostatic theories. Yet, what Gadamer is on the verge of is, I think, neither an ability-based nor a function-based theory, but rather a truly phenomenological account of health. As we will see, the terminology he is using is taken from the phenomenology of Martin Heidegger, which is also where I will begin my search for such a theory in the following sections. First, however, some general and systematical problems of approaching health phenomenologically need to be addressed.

There are not many examples of phenomenologists who have attempted to work out a general theory of health.[127] In spite of this I think that the approach of phenomenology, which focuses upon the *meaning* of phenomena, opens up promising possibilities for the conceptualization of health. But the phenomenon of health does not quite seem to fit the structure of intentionality that we have found in Husserl. The terms that Gadamer uses to characterize health in the last quotation – being there, being in the world, being with people, to be busy with projects in life – indicate that health is something we live *through* rather than *towards*. Let me, in order to illuminate this, give an example of a very common episode of illness: having a bad cold.

When Peter woke up that Monday morning he felt really bad. The few hours of sleep he had been able to get had not done him much good. His throat was sore and aching, it hurt just to swallow, and his head felt like it had been stuffed with cotton. As he tried to rise from bed he noticed how heavy his legs were, his whole body seemed to refuse doing proper service, it obviously wanted to stay in bed. But Peter could not do that, today the big sale was starting in the bookstore and he needed to be there in order to help out. They would not be able to do it without him. He dragged himself out of bed, had a shower and swallowed some aspirins, which by the way was really painful because of the throat. Feeling a little bit better he went to the kitchen for some breakfast even though he was not very hungry. But the coffee did not taste nearly as good as usual and every bite of his sandwich was a pain of

---

[127] See Drew Leder (1995) for a survey of the fragmentary but interesting attempts that have been made, mainly by Kay Toombs, Richard Zaner and Leder himself. I will return to these attempts later in this work. Psychiatrists and psychoanalysts inspired by the philosophy of Martin Heidegger have in a (at least partly) phenomenological manner developed theories of *mental* health and illness. Three well-known and influential examples are the theories of Ludwig Binswanger, Medard Boss, and Jacques Lacan. See Richardson (1993) and Spiegelberg (1972).

tasteless resistance in his mouth. Peter felt dizzy and shivered with cold, he could not take any interest in the morning paper which he usually read, but instead closed his eyes and tried to summon some strength to last through the long day. On the bus to work he felt isolated from the other passengers. He was standing as in a soap-bubble of dizzy shivering and still he felt like the noise from the traffic and the rolling movements of the bus were about to burst the bubble at any time and expose him to a world of threatening, stinging stimuli. The day at work in the shop was hellish. The customers, looking for a fine haul on the first day of the big sale, were in a hurry, irritated and aggressive, asking for books he did not have in or complaining about the prices. Normally he could handle these types of situations with a smile, but today they were really aggravating him and he had to use maximum effort to not snub the customers, or just leave the shop and go home. During his lunch break he did not feel any inclination to talk to his colleagues. He kept to himself in the lunchroom, trying at least to drink a hot cup of tea – he could not even think of food – and swallowed some more aspirins. His head was killing him – through the throbbing pain the world around him had a strange quality of unrealness, as if hidden behind a veil. Even the sympathetic comments he got from his friends did not mean much encouragement to him. He did not want to be there, he only wanted to get away, get away from the bookstore, get away from himself in this transformed condition which was still him but yet so different. He could only think of one thing: getting home and going to bed to sleep. But time passed so slowly that day, as if dragged along by pain and dizziness.

Illness is obviously an obstruction to health and its transparency; everything that goes on without us paying explicit attention to it when we are healthy – walking, thinking, talking – now offers resistance. The body, our thinking, the world, everything is now 'out of tune', coloured by feelings of pain, weakness and helplessness. I will later in this part of my work suggest that this way of being in the world in illness is best understood as a form of homelessness. But to understand this claim fully, we first need to learn more about phenomenological analysis and its vocabulary.

We can see clearly from this simple example that, in order to understand what has changed for Peter in falling ill, it is not enough to study what type of acts he lives through that day in contrast to a healthy day; that is, the simple fact that he does not approach many objects or subjects that day is not the crucial issue, though it is important. What is crucial is the very character of the acts he *does* perform: they acquire a different texture (dizziness, pain, resistance), and as the subject of these acts, he experiences himself differently. Were we, in this work, to stay within the confines of Husserl's philosophy, we would now have had to turn to his theory of selfhood – that is, to the genetic rather than the static level of his phenomenology (Bernet et al. 1989, p. 181 ff.). At the genetic level Husserl investigates the genesis and status of the transcendental subject which lives in the flow of successive acts. But even acknowledging this part of Husserl's philosophy, which I have not introduced here, I think we would have difficulties finding a vocabulary suitable for the development of a theory of health in proceeding from his philosophy. One obvious shortcoming in

Husserl's philosophy is the absence of a phenomenology of feelings for describing the structures of acts and of self. The *attunement* of the self in its being in the world is vital for understanding illness, as we can see from the example above, and as I will try to explicate in more detail below.

Another problem with Husserl's phenomenology in approaching health and illness – which is related to the absence of a phenomenology of feelings – is the focus upon consciousness instead of upon embodiment in his philosophy. As we saw in the example of having a cold above, the character of Peter's embodiment was crucial in describing his illness – pain, resistance, shivers, etc. The Husserlian theory of transcendental consciousness must certainly be grounded in a structure of incarnation if it is going to stay true to lived experience.[128] This embodiment in Husserl's phenomenology – *Leiblichkeit* – means essentially, not only that consciousness is able to move about in the world and view objects from different angles, but also that perception itself is a form of 'kinaesthesis' – it has an embodied structure dependent upon the moving body. This kinaesthesis in Husserl, however, does not really affect the structure of intentionality itself as the directedness of *consciousness*. The lived body does not in itself texture and structure the acts, by, for example, offering resistance.

Health and illness as phenomena one lives through and not towards in one's daily activities evokes domains that are hard to grasp adequately through Husserl's theories. Yet another feature of human existence – aside from feeling and body – seems to be neglected by the model of intentionality of consciousness: action. The holistic theory of Nordenfelt makes this lucid by focusing upon abilities, activities and goals, rather than upon acts and objects. An action need not to be directed towards an object, though it be intended (in the sense of having a goal aimed at by the person). If I drive my car in order to get to work, my consciousness is not directed towards the car; the car-driving is rather something I am absorbed in without paying explicit attention to the car. Husserl will apparently have problems incorporating this type of example in the structure of intentionality expounded in his phenomenology.[129] Some phenomena – and health and illness obviously belong to this domain – seem to demand a different approach than his – a phenomenological approach which does not start with the scaffoldings of consciousness, intentionality and object, but rather investigates the meaning of human experience situated in the world as acting, attuned and embodied.[130] Let us therefore now turn to another version of phenomenology

---

[128] This is particularly obvious in some of the manuscripts which were not published until years after Husserl's death. For a careful examination of this theme, see Zahavi (1994). The first and most important philosopher who developed a phenomenological theory *based* on the intentionality of the body was Maurice Merleau-Ponty. I will return to his work later in this part of my work. See also Zaner (1964) on the problems of the phenomenology of embodiment.

[129] See Dreyfus (1991, p. 46 ff.).

[130] Despite the difficulties indicated above, I do not want to claim here that it would be impossible to work out a theory of health working within the scaffold of Husserl's phenomenology. Two interesting recent attempts to approach questions of normality and medicine on the basis of Husserlian phenomenology are Steinbock (1995) and Waldenfels (1998).

which I think provides a promising place to start looking for a theory of health – the philosophy of Martin Heidegger. I will in the next section try to give an introduction to the most basic themes of his philosophy and then, in the subsequent sections, attempt to deploy them in developing a phenomenological theory of health.

6. HEIDEGGER'S PHENOMENOLOGY

Heidegger, in his first main work *Sein und Zeit* from 1927, widened the domains of phenomenology.[131] Husserl was mainly concerned with epistemology – the theory of knowledge, with an emphasis on the theory of science; whereas Heidegger rather focused the everyday world of being and understanding. His phenomenology is accordingly what he calls a 'fundamental ontology' – investigating different modes of what it means to be, rather than what it means to know.

As his starting point, Heidegger takes, instead of the subject of knowledge, what he calls 'Dasein', the 'being-there' of human existence. This being-there means that we are situated or 'thrown' (*geworfen*) into the world that we live in. We are always already *there* (*da*), involved in daily activities. But the term 'Da-sein' also signifies that we have a relation to our own existence in asking what it means to *be* there at all (rather than not to exist). *Dasein* is the only being that asks the fundamental ontological question of what it means to be (*die Frage nach dem Sein*). Therefore philosophy has to start with an analysis of the understanding human being – *Dasein*. This – as we shall see – is the only way to start, since every other being in the world attains its meaning through the understanding of *Dasein*. Human understanding as a 'being-there' in the world is accordingly the starting point for philosophy as a phenomenology of 'everydayness' – an investigation of the everyday forms of understanding carried out by human beings. This phenomenology of the everyday world is also called a *hermeneutics* of everydayness, since the phenomena Heidegger analyses are precisely the self-understanding activities of *Dasein* – that is, its self-interpretation. We will return to the differences and similarities between phenomenology and hermeneutics later in this section.

According to Heidegger, when we study our relationship to the world, we should not view the world as a collection of objects outside of consciousness, towards which we are directed by way of the latter. We should instead study the 'worldliness' of the world, the way we are *in* the world, giving it meaning through our actions; the world indeed being nothing other than a cultural, intersubjective *meaning-structure*, lived in by us and, ultimately, a mode of ourselves. Human understanding is, consequently, for Heidegger, always a being-there in the sense of being-in-the-world (*in-der-Welt-sein*). The hyphens indicate that *Dasein* and world are thought as a unity and not as subject and object. The world is not something external, but is constitutive for the being of *Dasein*.

---

[131] This presentation limits its scope to Heidegger's early philosophy and first main work, *Sein und Zeit* from 1927: (1986, 16th ed.) The excellent new translation by Joan Stambaugh from 1996 has been a great help in transferring Heidegger's vocabulary into English.

The concept of 'being-in-the-world' resembles in many ways the concept of 'lifeworld' which Husserl (inspired by *Sein und Zeit*) developed in his late philosophy (Husserl 1976b). Heidegger considered the meaning-structure of the world to be more primordial than the qualities of objects in the world explored by science (1986, pp. 356-364). (Medical) science investigates parts of the world and tries to find connections by way of observation and measurements. Every science is, however, also a human activity which is situated in a context – a lifeworld – that will determine what to look for and why.[132] Even though Heidegger in *Sein und Zeit* resists using the terms 'life' and 'living' when he refers to the structure of *Dasein* – since he wants to stay clear of every empirical investigation and also of the successful 'life-philosophies' of his time (such as that of Oswald Spengler, for instance) – he is undoubtedly aiming in the same direction as Husserl would later do with the concept of 'lifeworld'.

It is important to note that the discipline generally thought of as investigating life – biology – belongs to what Heidegger calls the *ontic* disciplines, and not to his fundamental *ontology* which questions the *meaning* of being. Biology does not attain its results through investigating the way life is *lived* – given meaning – by *Dasein*, but through measuring the life-activities of objects in the world (1986, p. 45 ff.). The human body investigated as a living object (*Körper*), and not as a lived, experienced body (*Leib*), is thus a part of the world just as other objects. There is, however, an ambivalence in this ambition to stay clear of the empirical disciplines, since the philosophy that Heidegger develops during the twenties – up to *Sein und Zeit* – strives to practise phenomenology as a discipline investigating not the static, transcendental meaning-structures of consciousness, but the phenomena of nature and culture.[133]

The concept 'worldliness' (*Weltlichkeit*) in *Sein und Zeit* indicates that the structure of the world is built up by the understanding actions, thoughts and feelings of human beings situated in the world and not by any properties that belong to the world in itself as a collection of objects (things, molecules, atoms). Heidegger can therefore write that worldliness essentially is an *existential* – that is, something belonging to *Dasein*, to understanding human beings, and not to the world in itself:

---

[132] As indicated above, I (with Husserl and Heidegger) do not think that this gives rise to any sort of total cultural relativism; see Guignon (1991) for a good survey and formulation of the problem. To start with there will probably exist some meaning-strata that are common to all lifeworlds, and the objectivity of science as a certain activity striving towards the possibility of inter-subjective verification through empirical experiments might be such a stratum inherent in every current (Western) lifeworld. But that science is rooted in the lifeworld certainly means that, if science is left in a limbo, if it loses all connections to the lifeworld it was born in, it will lose its meaning for human beings. Science could then also become dangerous in its tendency to technologize the lifeworld; that is, not only cut its links to the lifeworld but also turn back on it and destroy its structures. Western medicine, to mention just one relevant example, would thus lose its character of a human meeting and end up as merely scientific investigation. This technologization of the world is a main theme of Heidegger's late philosophy (1954b), and of many other German philosophers in this tradition such as Hans-Georg Gadamer and Jürgen Habermas.

[133] In the lecture series from the twenties (see especially 1988) Heidegger does not hesitate to use the word 'Leben' in his philosophical analysis. See Krell (1992), especially Chapter 1 and 2, on this theme. The most powerful influence for Heidegger's own 'life philosophy' was without doubt Wilhelm Dilthey. See Kisiel (1986-87).

> 'Worldliness' is an ontological concept and designates the structure of a constitutive factor of being-in-the-world. But we have come to know being-in-the-world as an existential determination of Dasein. Accordingly, worldliness is itself an existential. When we inquire ontologically about the 'world', we by no means abandon the thematic field of the analytic of Dasein. 'World' is ontologically not a determination of those beings which Dasein essentially is not, but a characteristic of Dasein itself (1986, p. 64).

The meaning-structures of the world are made up of relations, not between things, but between tools (*Zeuge*). That is, the meaning of phenomena, according to Heidegger, is not primarily dependent upon how things look, but upon how they are being used. This makes the connection between the structure of the world and *Dasein* more lucid. For how could the world itself as something independent of human beings lead us to an understanding of the function of any tool? A tool always refers to its user. We will only learn what a hammer is by using it, never by staring at it (1986, p. 69). It is important to stress that the concept of tool or availableness (*Zuhandenheit*) in *Sein und Zeit* is meant to cover *all* phenomena, not only human artifacts in the common sense. The sun, for example, would be a tool for time measurement (1986, p. 71). When we study our being-in-the-world at the level of meaning – the phenomenological level – it is, according to Heidegger, to be understood as nothing but a basic openness (*Erschlossenheit*) to the world which is structured as a 'totality of relevance' (*Bewandnisganzheit*). And the totality of relevance is a totality of tools: a *Werkstatt*.

The relations between the different tools are explicated as an 'in order to' (*um zu*) (1986, p. 68). The tools in this way relate to each other; their meanings are determined by their places within the totality of relevance. One uses a hammer in order to nail the palings, in order to raise the walls, in order to build the house, in order to find shelter from the rain, etc.[134] One need not pay attention to these different levels of subgoals at all times. Indeed, some of the subgoals are never explicitly attended to, but are only revealed in a theoretical analysis of the activity.

The final meaning of every tool is the existence of human being – *Dasein*. The understanding of *Dasein* is the activity in relation to which every phenomenon (tool) takes on meaning. In this activity, as pointed out, we most often do not pay explicit attention to any of the tools. We are absorbed in the activity – as in the example of driving in the preceding section. Heidegger's analysis of the worldliness of *Dasein* stays true to this phenomenological fact by focusing upon the practical relations between tools in the world, instead of upon the intentionality of consciousness, which he holds to be a special form of theoretical activity (1986, p. 69).

The being-in-the-world, the 'worldliness' of human existence, is conceptualized by Heidegger by stressing several different aspects of this existence. Since these aspects belong to the only being that truly exists – *Dasein* – and not to things, they are called 'existentials' (*Existenzialien*). Human beings *exist*: that is, they have a relation to their own being, and they are open to the world as a possibility for themselves. This openness to the totality of tools is a pattern not only of action, but also of thinking, feeling and talking. These three modes of being must, however, not be con-

---

[134]This is Heidegger's own famous example (1986, p. 84); one could think of countless others.

ceived of as attributes of a subject – qualities of a thing – but as a meaning pattern that binds human being and the being of the world together. They must likewise articulate a being that is not merely contemplative but *acts* in the world, as the tool pattern makes obvious. The three main existentials which Heidegger chooses in *Sein und Zeit* in order to make sense of our being-in-the-world are understanding (*Verstehen*), attunement (*Befindlichkeit*) and discourse (*Rede*). These three existentials are thought of as intertwined; they always work together, inseparably, as an attuned, articulated understanding situated in the world. The choice of understanding instead of cognition makes a relation to action possible. Understanding can include the active and incarnated sides of life; and, as we will see, so can the concepts of attunement and discourse.

The phenomenology of being-in-the-world, in the form of different existentials – Heidegger calls it an 'existential analytic' – is developed in order to leave the subject-object model behind. The philosophical tradition, according to Heidegger, has remained enslaved to a metaphysics of sight; that is, it has favoured the gaze, to the exclusion of other ways of encountering phenomena in the world. This has resulted in the positing of a human subject facing a world of objects, in Husserl's case a consciousness directed by means of acts. Husserl's phenomenology of transcendental consciousness is unable to explain *transcendence* – the way human existence is always already *outside* itself, *in* the world, acting and understanding itself from the supra-individual structures of the world. To transcend in Heidegger's phenomenology does not mean to go beyond the world. This is the way the concept has usually been employed in philosophy (or religion), sometimes to indicate a mystical relationship – a relationship to something outside the world (God). In contrast to this, transcendence in *Sein und Zeit* means the way human beings (*Dasein*) are thrown *into* the world (1986, pp. 363-364). This transcendence, which belongs to the being-in-the-world of all human understanding, means that we always find ourselves already in the world, given over to some meaning-structures that we have not chosen. These meaning-structures (*Bewandnisganzheiten*) are intersubjective, historical and cultural; that is, they change gradually between different times and places, but they are nevertheless always there in some form, as a necessary 'facticity' (*Faktizität*) which one must make one's own in order to develop a human understanding and self (1986, p. 135).

To the facticity of human beings also belongs something meaning*less*, or rather something that has not yet reached, and perhaps never will reach, an *articulated* understanding. This is the territory of feeling. With the aid of Heidegger it is possible to see how feelings are one aspect of our way of giving meaning to phenomena as a being-in-the-world. Our grasping of a phenomenon is a part of the ongoing, living activity in the world that Heidegger refers to as understanding. But the understanding must always be *attuned* in order to be meaningful: 'Every understanding has its mood. Every attunement understands' (1986, p. 335). Heidegger thus shuns a cognitivist perspective and gives feelings, primarily in the form of moods (*Stimmungen*), an important position in his philosophy.[135] Moods open up the world to human beings in a precognitive way: '*Mood has always already disclosed being-in-the-world as a whole and first makes possible directing oneself toward something*' (1986, p. 137, italics in original). We find ourselves thrown into the world (*geworfen*) as attuned (joyful, bored, sad), and these moods are the primary and unarticulated form of transcendence through which we can take our place in the meaning-structures of the world.[136]

Attunement cannot simply be equated with different feelings as they are studied by the psychologist. Psychology is what Heidegger refers to as an *ontic* science; it studies the mental states of subjects. Heidegger's fundamental ontology – like Husserl's phenomenology – is developed in order to provide a ground for every such ontic science – psychology as well as biology. Moods form the way we understand and articulate the phenomena in the world, and also, ultimately, the way we understand ourselves and others. The attunement of every situation explains why things matter to human beings. They matter because they are part of a totality of relevance – a cultural tradition – and this 'mattering to' is attuned (1986, p. 137).

Certain moods are indeed the prerequisite for reaching what Heidegger calls *authentic* understanding (*Eigentlichkeit*). Authentic understanding is the philosophical mode of understanding that asks for the meaning of being and develops it as the hermeneutics of being-in-the-world – indeed the project of the book *Sein und Zeit* itself. The famous example of an authentic mood from *Sein und Zeit* is anxiety, but later in Heidegger's philosophy other *Grundstimmungen* – basic moods – such as boredom, joy, awe and sorrow are also highlighted as presenting possibilities for authentic understanding.[137] I will return to Heidegger's concept of authenticity later in discussing health.

If the being-in-the-world of human being is opened up by a mood it is also appropriated and projected towards a more or less articulated understanding (*Entwurf*)

---

[135]This model reminds us of the Aristotelian relation between *logos* and *pathe*, the two elements of the *psyche* which must be balanced in an adequate way in the virtuous (healthy) man. The book by Kisiel (1993) has shown the immense importance of Aristotle's philosophy for Heidegger in the lecturing period of the twenties leading up to *Sein und Zeit*. Volpi (1996) has, in addition to this, shown how Heidegger's philosophy is indeed pragmatic – that is, based in the active and not in the theoretical life (something that I stress in my own interpretation of *Sein und Zeit*) – but in a Greek rather than American sense.

[136]The translation of the term 'Befindlichkeit' into English presents real difficulties. The choice of 'state of mind' in the first translation of *Sein und Zeit* by Macquarrie and Robinson was obviously faulty, since Heidegger's aim is precisely to not get stuck in any psychology or philosophy of mind as opposed to body and world. Stambaugh's 'attunement', in the more recent translation, however, is also problematic, since it identifies 'Befindlichkeit' with 'Stimmung' and 'gestimmt sein', which are also translated as 'attunement' and 'being attuned', respectively, in her idiom. 'Sich befinden' literally means 'to find oneself', and through tying this notion to (but not identifying it with) feeling and mood – 'gestimmt sein' – Heidegger wants to indicate that the way in which we find ourselves in the world, as thrown into a situation together with others, is fundamentally to be thought of as a precognitive phenomenon. *Befindlichkeit* is therefore the link between *Geworfenheit* and *Stimmung* – to find oneself in the world is to find onself as being thrown into a mood.

[137]See Held (1993); Pocai (1996); and Svenaeus (1997).

by the accordingly attuned manner of understanding. We are not only thrown into a world of given necessities, but also transform the possibilities that the meaning-structures offer into our own projects. I organize the things (tools) in the world to reveal new uses and to seek to achieve new goals. These activities are usually not explicitly planned; that is, there are not always 'mental' processes which precede and direct the 'physical' actions, but rather the actions in themselves represent a form of non-articulated understanding (1986, p. 145). The understanding actions thus always remain dependent upon a supraindividual meaning-structure, but they also project this structure in an appropriating way.

To understand, in Heidegger's phenomenology, is to find one's place in the meaning-structure of the world and project oneself towards possible goals (1986, p. 142 ff.). We could say, in analogy with Husserl's explication of the meaning of phenomena as *noemata*, that the meaning of actions is the pattern of understanding – the totality of relevance – in which they are exercised. To be able to act on the phenomenological level of meaning is equivalent to having understanding, to having found one's place in a lifeworld of intersubjective meaning-patterns, where actions can attain meaning, be given goals, and thereby constitute *actions* and not just the movements of an organism.

Discourse (*Rede*), the third main existential I mentioned above, is thematized as yet another aspect of the attuned, understanding being-in-the-world of *Dasein*. Language is the *articulation* of the meaning-structures of the world (1986, p. 161). In language the projection (*Entwurf*) of human understanding reaches its uttermost level of transparency. Through language we can think and talk about the world and make its meaningfulness lucid to ourselves and others.

The term Heidegger chooses in *Sein und Zeit* to thematize the *whole* being-in-the-world of *Dasein*, in the form of the three existentials understanding, attunement and discourse, is 'care' – 'Sorge'. Care designates the transcendence of human understanding as a *coming back* to itself. *Dasein* is always ahead of itself, being thrown into the meaning-structures of the world in an everyday doing; but it is also picking up the possibilities of this thrownness and transforming them into an individualized understanding.[138] Although the possibilities of understanding are not invented by the individual self, they are taken up by him and made his own. Existence – human life –

---

[138] The final meaning of this transcending-returning structure in *Sein und Zeit* is attained through an analysis of time. *Dasein* 'zeitigt sich' – projects itself towards the future in a coming back to the possibilities which have been given to it through the past. In this way Heidegger tries to overcome a philosophy that is narrowed down to focusing upon the present as the mode through which the past and future acquire their meaning. *Dasein's* way of being in time (or rather its way of being as time itself) is 'outstanding' (*ek-statikon*) in the past and future, which are therefore called 'Ekstasen'. It is through this time-structure that Heidegger's famous 'being-towards-death' should be understood. *Dasein* is not only a projecting and coming back of itself through and towards its possibilities, but also a finite project. The certainty of death indeed belongs to the meaning of every human existence. But this certainty not only means that the future will not be forever, but also that *Dasein is dying* at every moment in the sense of a constant uncertainty of what the future will hold – every moment could be the last one (1986, p. 245).

is not only a matter of transcending into the collective world but also a matter of doing it as an individualized self – as a person.[139]

Why does Heidegger primarily use the term 'hermeneutics' in *Sein und Zeit* when he refers to his philosophy? And to what extent does this hermeneutics remain a phenomenology when it is developed as an analysis of everyday being-in-the-world? Human being is chosen as the point of departure since it has *understanding*. It understands the world in the activities of everydayness; but, through this transcendence, it also has the potentiality of self-understanding. It has the possibility of focusing upon the meaning-structures of the world as related to its *own* transcendence into the world – this is the move to what Heidegger refers to as *authentic* understanding. This type of understanding in *Sein und Zeit* turns into *interpretation* (hermeneutics), in the sense that phenomena must be uncovered, freed from a state of disguise (*Verborgenheit*). This disguise primarily comes from the tendency of human beings to view the world as a collection of objects independent of human understanding and to include human beings in this collection of things. Human being has an inherent tendency to fall to the world (*Verfallensein*), as Heidegger writes (1986, p. 175). He thereby emphasizes both the transcendence of all human being as an understanding being-in-the-world, *and* the difficulty of taking a step back and exploring the world as a meaning-structure related to *Dasein*.

The form of authentic understanding which manages to take this step back is equivalent to Husserl's phenomenological reduction as a turn to meaning, although it attains different results and has other prerequisites. In the same way as Husserl performed the phenomenological reduction in order to escape the 'natural attitude' and focus upon intentionality itself as a constitution of objects, Heidegger tries to excavate the meaning-structures of being-in-the-world as the fore-structures of human understanding making the everyday understanding activities in the world possible. I write 'excavate', since these meaning-structures are usually hidden by our everyday doings and 'ontic' theories, and therefore demand systematic, 'authentic' interpretation. Thus, in this work, when referring to Heidegger's philosophy, I (like Heidegger himself) will use either the term 'phenomenology' or 'hermeneutics' without any purpose of making a systematical distinction; the central concept, in both cases, is *understanding*.

---

[139]Heidegger generally shuns the notion of 'person' and uses 'self'. The reason for this is that he thinks that the concept of person is caught up in an 'ontic' tradition, tied to theology, anthropology and psychology (1986, pp. 46-50). This, however, does not seem to be a convincing argument, since almost every concept which Heidegger uses in his fundamental ontology has an 'ontic' pre-history. This is certainly true of *Selbst*, see Taylor (1989). I will therefore in this study not follow Heidegger's advice, but will rather use the term 'person' in a similar way to the phenomenological outline of 'self'. For an illuminating study of the phenomenological concept of self, which uses medicine and illness as clues, see Zaner (1981). See also Chapter 3 of a later work by him (1988) for a phenomenological approach to illness.

7. HEALTH AS HOMELIKE BEING-IN-THE-WORLD

Let us now return to health. Heidegger never wrote anything substantial about the subject. There is no analysis of the structures of the healthy versus the ill existence in *Sein und Zeit*. Although a whole chapter in the second division of *Sein und Zeit* is devoted to an analysis of the meaning of death, Heidegger never links the ontological interpretation of death as the finitude of human existence to an analysis of the meaning of illness and health. He makes clear that the existential interpretation of death is prior to any biology or ontology of life, but he also mentions that the medical and biological inquiry into life and dying could be of importance in the analysis of the meaning-structure of human existence (1986, p. 247). The relation between biology and phenomenology is not further discussed, however, nor is a phenomenology of health and illness developed.

It is tempting to interpret the famous opposition of authenticity and inauthenticity as a difference between health and illness, at least when one considers mental health or the 'health' of a culture; and, as we will see, some interpreters have indeed done so.[140] But I do not think this is an attractive approach, at least not if one intends to preserve the normal, everyday meanings of the terms 'healthy' and 'ill'. Authenticity and inauthenticity in Heidegger's phenomenology, as indicated in the preceding section, are two different modes of understanding. These are the counterparts to Husserl's two different modes of attention: philosophical reflection through the phenomenological reduction, investigating the *meaning* of phenomena; and 'natural attention', which lives *through* phenomena by concentrating on the objects of the world.

This authentic, philosophical understanding (which in *Sein und Zeit* is reached in the moment of anxiety) would obviously not always be identical with a healthy being-in-the-world, however. The phenomenologist could be temporarily ill, but still have an authentic understanding, or he could indeed reach it while (or even through) being ill. Also, the phenomenologist would indeed always have to return to the inauthentic understanding of his daily life, since it provides the necessary background for authentic understanding, by being precisely that which is thereby explored as a pattern of meaning (as the existentials and as the totality of relevance of the world). It would therefore certainly be absurd to regard every human being living in an inauthentic mood of understanding as ill. In *Sein und Zeit* Heidegger associates the term 'das Man' with a certain form of everyday existence lacking genuine selfhood and reflection; but though there is certainly some contempt in his description of

---

[140]Nietzsche's notion of a 'große Gesundheit' seems to be a forerunner to such interpretations (1973, pp. 15-17, 317-319). That is, 'the great health' of Nietzsche could be understood as a form of authenticity – the mode of existence of the 'fitter', stronger, braver individual or culture, which can endure and learn from pain and illness – rather than as health in the usual sense. On this subject see Krell (1996), Chapter 10, and Raymond (1999). The remarks by Nietzsche on *Gesundheit der Seele* in *Die fröhliche Wissenschaft* could also, however, be interpreted as promoting an individualistic, holistic health-concept: 'Es kommt auf dein Ziel, deinen Horizont, deine Kräfte, deine Antriebe, deine Irrthümer und namentlich auf die Ideale und Phantasmen deiner Seele an, um zu bestimmen, *was* selbst für deinen *Leib* Gesundheit zu bedeuten habe' (1973, p. 105).

modern public life, he did not mean to suggest that all human beings who never reach authentic understanding are ill.[141]

The only place where Heidegger comes close to saying something substantial about health and medicine is the *Zollikoner Seminare*, lectures and seminars conducted together with the colleagues and students of the psychiatrist Medard Boss during the sixties.[142] Later, Boss himself, in *Grundriss der Medizin und der Psychologie* (1975), worked out a theory of health, based on what he calls 'Daseinsanalyse' – a form of psychotherapy, which he developed with the aid of Heidegger's philosophy. This theory, just like the one I myself will attempt to formulate below, proceeds from Heidegger's existential analytic. Boss's discussions of health and illness certainly are full of insights and his theory has much to offer for medicine. Despite its general ambitions however, Boss's theory is exclusively concerned with mental health and psychosomatics and lacks a general outlook, which would include somatics and which is my aim in this book.[143] Boss's reading of Heidegger, in my opinion, in addition to this shortcoming, tends to fall into the existentialist trap of focusing upon freedom instead of hermeneutic understanding: authentic understanding is *identified* with the freedom to choose one's own way in life, with the freedom to choose oneself as an autonomous being.[144] This is then also the precondition for health in Boss's theory: lack of health is lack of freedom, and the ultimate illness is consequently a lack of identity and autonomy (Boss 1975, pp. 444, 483).[145]

---

[141]My phenomenological analysis of health does not strive towards changing the everyday meaning of the terms 'health' and 'illness'. One alternative would of course be simply to accept the consequences of these imperfect homologies – between, on the one hand, authentic understanding and health and, on the other hand, inauthentic understanding and illness – and say that people we normally refer to as healthy are not 'really healthy', and that people we refer to as ill are sometimes indeed 'very healthy'. This alternative is in line with the Nietzschean proposal I remarked upon above. My aim is rather to explicate by way of phenomenological analysis what we mean in everyday life by 'healthy' and 'ill'. Of course, however, this analysis could also lead to a change in our view on individual cases.

[142]*Zollikoner Seminare* (1994 [1987]). These seminars appear to be one of the very few places where Heidegger addresses not only health and illness, but also embodiment (*Leiblichkeit*). Heidegger, otherwise reluctant to discuss the *specific* activities of everydayness, is here forced to address these themes in the presentation of his philosophy. The encounter between the famous philosopher and the doctors offers very stimulating reading since Heidegger (even more than in his lecture courses) has to mobilize all his pedagogical skills in the face of the questions of the philosophically untrained audience. Boss writes in his introduction that: 'diese Seminar-Situationen riefen die Phantasien wach, es würde erstmal ein Marsmensch einer Gruppe von Erdbewohnern begegnen und sich mit ihnen verständigen wollen' (1994, p. xiv).

[143]However, the two terms 'mental' and 'psycho-somatic' are rejected by Boss, who employs a Heideggerian vocabulary.

[144]It is a widespread misunderstanding that Heidegger was an 'existentialist' like Sartre, who clearly built his theories on *Sein und Zeit*, but also changed Heidegger's phenomenological hermeneutics into an ethics of authentic freedom. It is ironic that Boss, who wants to be a true Heidegger scholar and who often reproaches others for an anthropological reading of Heidegger's philosophy, falls into the trap of existentialism himself when it comes to health.

[145]It seems to me that the existential psychoanalysis of Ludwig Binswanger, despite its originality and fruitfulness for psychiatry, tends to make the same mistake; that is, health is understood as freedom, and illness is identified with the lack of such freedom. See Binswanger (1962, pp. 118-119). Guignon (1993)

My objections to Boss's valuable book here are not due to the fact that he in the end performs an 'anthropological' reading of Heidegger. Indeed, my own introduction above, stresses the pragmatic, concrete sides of Heidegger's philosophy. As I see it, the problem lies elsewhere: it consists in regarding the perspective on the world and self reached in authentic understanding as constitutive of health. That authentic understanding in Heidegger's sense could be of great help in matters of health is one thing, but to say that it is necessary for health or identical with health is in my view far too strong a claim.

My own alternative for a phenomenological theory of health will not be based upon authenticity, freedom or autonomy, but upon *homelikeness*.[146] The remainder of this part of my work will be devoted to developing and explaining this theory. I want to make clear from the start that what I will present below is not an orthodox reading of Heidegger, which merely explicates a hidden theory of health in his work, but rather a theory inspired by his thinking, which makes use of parts of his vocabulary and many of his insights. The theory is also inspired, however, by other phenomenologists – in particular F. J. J. Buytendijk, Hans-Georg Gadamer, Maurice Merleau-Ponty and Erwin Straus.

In analysing the biostatistical, analytical theory of health above, we already established that the relation between the organism and its environment is crucial if we want to find an adequate concept of health. The holistic welfare-theory of health is built around the ability of the individual – the person – to realize his vital goals by acting in the world. We can now, in the context of the phenomenology of Heidegger, understand this interaction between individual and environment as placement of the individual within a meaning-structure – a totality of relevance, or that which we earlier referred to as *Dasein*'s *Geworfenheit*, its being *thrown* into the world. The thrownness of human existence is characterized by the existential of *Befindlichkeit* – attunement. To be delivered to the world of intersubjective meaning – language, culture, history, etc. – is to *find* oneself in the world (*sich befinden*), and this finding oneself appears in the form of an attuned understanding, in the form of finding oneself in a mood. Our attunement colours and determines our understanding of the world. Every understanding consequently has a mood; this certainly applies for the ill forms of understanding. Heidegger says in the *Zollikoner Seminare*:

> We in all the different cases of experiencing a broken arm, buzzing in the ears, stomach pains, or anxiety find ourselves in a different way. In every case our attunement (Befindlichkeit) is different . . . (1994, p. 81).

Despite the shortcomings of the attempts to identify health with authentic existence, it will be instructive here to go back to the account Heidegger gives of existential anxiety in *Sein und Zeit*:

---

is a good analysis of the role of authenticity in psychotherapy, which is the activity central to both Boss and Binswanger.

[146] *Wohnen* – 'to dwell' – is an important theme, particularly in Heidegger's later works, although he never links the thoughts about being at home in the world to health; see, for instance, (1954a). See also Lévinas (1961) for a phenomenological analysis of the home.

> In anxiety one has an 'uncanny' feeling. (In der Angst ist einem 'unheimlich'.) Here the peculiar indefiniteness of that which Dasein finds itself involved in with anxiety initially finds expression: the nothing and nowhere. But uncanniness means at the same time not-being-at-home. In our first phenomenal indication of the fundamental constitution of Dasein and the clarification of the existential meaning of being-in in contradistinction to the categorical signification of 'insideness', being-in was defined as dwelling with . . . , being familiar with . . . (1986, p. 188).

What authentic anxiety makes evident is essentially the same phenomenon that is brought to attention, not in healthy, but in *ill* forms of life – the *not* being at home in the world. Unhomelikeness – (*Unheimlichkeit*)[147] – which is taken to an extreme in the authentic mood, is, even in our everyday modes of being-in-the-world, a basic aspect of our existence; but there it is hidden by a dominating being *at home* in the world and is therefore covered up (*Verborgen*) (1986, p. 277).

The being-at-home of human being-there (*Da-sein*) – 'dwelling with, being familiar with' – is consequently, at the same time, a being not quite at home in this world. The familiarity of our lifeworld – the world of human actions, projects and communication – is always also pervaded by a homelessness: this is my world but it is also at the same time not entirely mine, I do not fully know it or control it. This is not a deficit, but a necessary phenomenon: I am delivered to the world (*geworfen*) with other people, and being together with them (*Mitdasein*) is a part of my own being (1986, p. 117 ff.). Thus the world I live in is certainly first and foremost *my* world (and not the 'objective' world of atoms and molecules), but to this very 'mineness' also belongs otherness in the sense of the meaning of the world belonging to other people. The otherness of the world, however, is not only due to my sharing it with other people, but also to *nature* (as opposed to culture) as something resisting my understanding.[148] We will return to this alien nature of the world later, in discussing illness and the body.

Health is to be understood as a being at home that keeps the not being at home in the world from becoming apparent. The not being at home, which is a basic and necessary condition of human existence, related to our finitude and dependence upon others and otherness, is, in illness, brought to attention and transformed into a pervasive homelessness. One of two *a priori* structures of existence – not being at home and being at home – wins out over the other: unhomelikeness takes control of our being-in-the-world. The basic alienness of my being-in-the-world, which in health is always in the process of receding into the background, breaks forth in illness to pervade existence. This unhomelikeness will be the central theme in our following interpretation of illness.

---

[147] The double meaning of the German word 'unheimlich' – it means both 'uncanny' and 'not at home' or 'unhomelike' ('unheimisch') – cannot be translated directly into English. For the etymology of the word 'unheimlich' and the relation between the phenomenon of *Unheimlichkeit* and mental illness, see Freud (1919). See also Binswanger (1963), 'The Case of Lola Voss'.

[148] Erwin Straus's idea of an *I-Allon* (I-other) relation as the basis of our being-in-the-world has been very helpful here in my reading of Heidegger. See Straus (1966a, 1969).

8. HOMELIKENESS AS THE RHYTHM OF LIFE

The *attunement* of our being-in-the-world seems to be the phenomenon to focus upon, when we try to get hold of the difference between healthy and ill ways of being-in-the-world. To be healthy or ill is, however, certainly not identical with just having a good or a bad feeling. Attunement is not the quality of a thing – of an isolated human subject – but rather, as stated before, a being delivered to the world, a finding oneself in the meaning-structure of the world as an understanding existence. Recall the quotation from Gadamer I gave in Section 5:

> Health is not a condition that one introspectively feels in oneself. Rather it is a condition of being there (Da-Sein), of being in the world (In-der-Welt-Sein), of being together with other people (Mit-den-Menschen-Sein), of being taken in by an active and rewarding engagement with the things that matter in life. . . . It is the rhythm of life, a permanent process in which equilibrium re-establishes itself (Gadamer 1993, pp. 144-145).

We now recognize Gadamer's terms as derived from the phenomenology of *Sein und Zeit*, and we are able to understand this healthy, rhythmic being-in-the-world as a form of attunement, which is certainly not a state that one feels in oneself, but which nevertheless has a 'tune', a feeling component to it.

Citing another passage from Gadamer's book in the same section, I concluded that the phenomenon of illness seems to be easier to get hold of than the phenomenon of health. When we are healthy everything 'flows', the mood we find ourselves in does not make itself heard or seen. It could possibly be felt as a certain form of rhythm in our being-in-the-world connected to time and to the way we are incarnated – to our breathing and to the beating of our hearts (Gadamer 1993, p. 166). It should not, however, be confused with other *positive* moods like well-being or happiness. Such moods also colour our understanding, but in a much more obvious and manifest way than health. Health is a non-apparent attunement, a rhythmic, balancing mood that supports our understanding in a homelike way without calling for our attention.

In what sense then are we to understand this homelike mood as *balanced*? Gadamer's proposal is indeed in line with the ancient health theories, as well as with the physiological concept of homeostasis and the holistic theory of Nordenfelt, which are all based on conceptualizations of balance; but does the word 'balance' carry more than a metaphorical meaning in the case of phenomenology?[149] Is not balance always something obtaining between different *entities*, such as bile and blood? What does it *mean* to talk about balance on the phenomenological level of meaning? Meaning patterns can hardly be weighed, or measured in any other way, since they do not belong to the things of the world. They are rather world-opening structures,

---

[149] One also finds some support for balance being an important aspect of health in sociological studies focusing upon the everyday experience and understanding of being ill and healthy. The notion of being in a state of balance is often mentioned when one asks people about their thoughts on health. In addition to this, absence of diseases, well-being, and strength, are common denominators of health. Health is considered a sort of imperceptible harmony which is rarely explicitly noticed and thought about except when it is replaced by a feeling of disharmony – illness. See Tegern (1994).

which make the appearance of different things as meaningful phenomena in the world possible.

The homelikeness of health can thus obviously not be a balance between two (or several) entities. The 'balance of health' must phenomenologically refer to the way human being finds its place in the world as a meaning pattern – a being-*in*-the-world. Health is thus not a question of a passive state but rather of an active process – a *balancing*.[150] As an illuminating comparative example in exploring balance and its relation to health, we will therefore choose a human activity, namely the everyday activity of riding a bicycle.

The healthy mood – the healthy attuned understanding – we said in the previous section, is always in the process of receding, since it is a mood of homelikeness. In the same way as you do not think of your homelike being-in-the-world when you are healthy, you do not think of your physical balance when you are riding a bicycle. These moods are similar in this respect, though the first one is more complex, since it is not only an attunement of one activity (bicycling), but of one's entire being-in-the-world. Both are, however, unobtrusive *attunements*, supporting our action and understanding. But are they really moods? Can health be *felt*? As developed above, health is obviously not only a feeling in the normal sense, but as a background attunement it does offer the possibility of a kind of direct attention.[151] You could seek this out for yourself phenomenologically by trying to neutralize every mood that is colouring your understanding and focus the attention upon the way you are *in* the world as a taking place in a meaningful context. You will not manage to extirpate all attunement, but rather will reach a basic form of balanced, homelike attunement that *supports* your understanding in transcending to the world. Heidegger is indeed right when he states that human beings are always in *some* mood (1986, p. 134). The health-mood could be seen as a sort of borderline case of the transparency of attunement. It is there all the time in the alternation between different more intrusive moods, sometimes left alone as the pure background mood of homelike understanding.

If you fall off the bicycle or get ill, however, you will notice. When your balance is challenged – when you ride over a stone, for example – you will make efforts to regain your balance in order not to fall down, but eventually will not succeed and will fall over. The moods of illness, in contrast to healthy attunement, seem to manifest themselves in obtrusive ways, colouring our whole existence and understanding. This is not always an immediate experience – like falling down from a bicycle – but sometimes a gradual process, during which, however, in the same way as in the example of riding a bicycle, one strives constantly to 'stay upright', to keep one's balance, but finally has to give in to illness. Let me try to illustrate how the healthy, homelike attunement gradually can be transformed into the unhomelike attunement

---

[150]This thought is inspired by Straus's essay *The Upright Posture* (1966b), in which, however, the author also tries to give this phenomenon a moral significance which is absent in my analysis.

[151]See Plügge (1962, p. 97).

of illness through giving an example. Jane is telling us about the onset of her diabetes:

I guess I was sick for a year before I knew I had diabetes. It came on when I was about 55, five years ago and I had a classic case but it was a long time before I knew what was happening to me. I would get terrifically thirsty and was not able to satisfy my thirst. I could be watching television, get up and drink a glass of water and be thirsty again before I sat down. And, of course, this meant that I had to go to the bathroom all the time, which was embarrassing, but what was worse was that I could not hold it back. When the urge hit me I knew I had about a minute to get to the bathroom. This was not too bad at home or at work but it could be a problem when I was downtown. I bet I have been in every bathroom in every store downtown. Then I began to have blurred vision. One time when I was driving to work – I work as a lawyer in an office downtown – my eyes began to blur and I could not read the billboards along the way. This prompted me to see an ophthalmologist but because this condition of blurred vision came and went, and I could see all right when I was in the doctor's office, he could not find anything wrong and, for some reason or other, he did not think of the possibility that I might have diabetes and, of course, I did not either. Well, I kept getting worse. I lost weight and my legs felt stiff and painful just from walking around at home and in the office. I have never been much for exercise, but now just the thought of my weekly Sunday walk was too much. I felt tired and irritated most of my waking time – at work and at home with my husband. Did not feel like being with people, did not have the energy. Also, my memory started failing me, I forgot things at work, I forgot what people had told me the day before. I suspected something was wrong of course, but at the same time I kept reassuring myself that all I really needed was a long holiday. I was working really hard at this time and I thought maybe I was simply getting too old to carry on like this. But to change your way of life is not an easy thing, you are caught up in old habits and it is hard to tell your boss that you are getting old and weak. Finally one evening my husband managed to persuade me to go out with him and have dinner with an old friend of ours. As I mentioned I had not felt like going out and seeing people the last year – too tired after work. Well our friend is a doctor and at dinner I started telling him about these strange things that had happened to me lately. He just took one look at me and said: 'You be in my office Monday morning.' I could tell by the way he said it that he suspected what was wrong with me. He did. He told me later that he felt he knew already then, but he wanted to run some tests before he said I had diabetes.[152]

Jane's life – her being-in-the-world – is gradually transformed in a way that bothers and worries her. The taken-for-grantedness, the transparency of her normal activities is changed into an effortful striving just to get done that which she used to perform easily; life now offers severe resistance. She feels transformed: Is this still me? Why

---

[152] The example is taken from Hardy (1978, pp. 232-233). It has however been slightly altered.

do my mind and body no longer work as they used to do? Why have they got out of my control? Life is gradually getting 'out of tune' – she feels dizzy, tired, irritated, painstricken[153] – but these 'feelings' are, in fact, part of her pattern of understanding and are not only isolated states of mind. Jane's being-in-the-world is gradually becoming unhomelike; where there was earlier a homelike attunement, there is now the growing despair of uncanniness.

Being-in-the-world, as we laid out in the introductory section on Heidegger's phenomenology, consists in being thrown into the world as attuned and in projecting oneself into an individualized understanding. We have called this act of going outside of itself and into the world, performed by human being-there (*Da-sein*), transcendence. The unhomelike attunement of illness colours and determines our transcendence into the world. In choosing attunement instead of understanding, thrownness (*Geworfenheit*) instead of projection (*Entwurf*), as our starting point for explicating health phenomenologically, we did not mean to develop a theory of health based in feelings as opposed to thinking and acting. To be attuned is always also to be understanding and this understanding is, in the case of illness, 'out of tune' – that is, unhomelike. The dizziness and weakness experienced by Jane, suffering from incipient diabetes, is an example of this. It is an attunement of unhomelike being-in-the-world, by which the understanding transcendence – taking part in meaningful activities in the world like getting up in the morning, going to work, talking with others, thinking about what to do at the weekend, and so on – is gradually diminished and emptied. The dizziness, pain and annoyance colour and determine the understanding of the ill person, who is thrown back on himself as an obtrusive burden, rather than thrown into the world of the others. The openness of the self towards the world is gradually eclipsed in illness.

It is not simply the case that ill being-in-the-world possesses *less* transcendence than its healthy counterpart. Indeed transcendence cannot be quantified or measured. Rather, ill being-in-the-world is characterized by *defective* transcendence, in the sense of the transcendence not being *coherent* – that is, not offering comprehensibility, sense of order and meaningfulness.[154] The transcendence of the person with incipient diabetes is in the process of losing its transparency and ease; it is obstructed in a mood of fatigue and worry – What is happening to me? Why am I so tired? The being-in thus has taken on a specific quality of unhomelikeness characteristic of illness.

---

[153]Pain would here not be restricted to a sensation in the body, but would consist in an atmosphere, a 'pain-mood' disrupting understanding. See Leder (1984-85). See also Heidegger (1989, pp. 118-119): 'Eine Magen "verstimmung" kann eine Verdüsterung über alle Dinge legen.'

[154]This formulation might remind the reader of Aaron Antonovsky's book *Unravelling the Mystery of Health* (1987). 'Sense of coherence' in Antonovsky's theory is not, however, an attempt to characterize health, but a factor contributing to health. Antonovsky's health concept seems to be similar to the biomedical one – that is, absence of disease. Antonovsky, a medical sociologist by profession, discovered that sense of coherence in one's life seemed to be the most important factor for enduring (and surviving) situations of heavy stress without getting depressed or ill in some other sense.

How is it possible in principle to separate such an attunement of illness from the tiredness some of us always experience getting up in the morning? The answer would generally be given by the lasting unhomelike character of the illness mood. A lasting fatigue is indeed called 'chronic fatigue syndrome' and considered an illness, even though one cannot find any disease responsible for it. If Peter, whom we encountered in a previous section, went on having the same symptoms described during his day in the bookstore for weeks and months, without the doctors being able to find anything biomedically wrong with him, we would indeed have a very ill man, but without any disease. I will return to this possibility of 'illness without disease' in the third part of my work, but would at this point like to stress that a phenomenological theory of health offers new possibilities for understanding illness precisely because it takes as its starting point, not disease, but lived experience.[155]

The lasting character of Jane's tiredness amplifies the unhomelikeness of her attunement. As Gadamer pointed out in one of the quotations above, health seems to be a rhythmic phenomenon. Sleepiness belongs to healthy life as a phenomenon occuring daily that frames our being-in-the-world. The unhomelikeness of illness in the example above, however, means a lasting, never-ending tiredness, transformed into an alien attunement, which has gone out of rhythm. It is important to stress here that the metaphorical reference to 'balanced' being-in-the-world as a phenomenological way to approach health and illness, ultimately means an emphasis on the *balancing*, homelike, attuned understanding. The healthy as well as the ill life has a time-structure built into it. To be-in-the-world means to be open to the future as a possibility of the past (Heidegger, 1986, p. 325). Being-in is a being-towards the future in relation to the past in the moment of presence. Balancing is thus to be understood as a *dynamis* rather than as a *stasis*; or, in the terminology of *Sein und Zeit*, as an *ek-stasis* – a standing-out of the self towards the future and the past in the moment of presence. Openness of the self towards the future in developing given possibilities of the past is that which is maintained in balancing and gradually lost in illness.

Drew Leder, in his book *The Absent Body*, has pointed out that health is not an unchanging state but a process:

> Phenomena such as ageing, puberty, menstruation and pregnancy are a normal and necessary part of the life cycle. They are not in themselves dysfunctional and alienating. As such they should not be associated with the notions of 'bad' or 'ill' that comprise part of the Greek meaning of dys (1990a, p. 89).

As Leder makes clear, referring to studies of menstruation, pregnancy and menopause, this rhythmic character of health seems to be specially prevalent for women, given their form of embodiment (1990a, p. 89).[156] As long as these changes have a

---

[155] For an interesting study of normal and pathological physiology from a phenomenological perspective, see Buytendijk (1974). The following remark by Buytendijk fits in nicely with my attempt at a phenomenological theory of illness: '*Being ill is above all alienation from the world*' (p. 62, italics in original).

[156] It is tempting here to extend this interpretation of health as a rhythmic balancing being-in-the-world to include the regular suffering of mild diseases – such as having a cold once or twice a year, from which one recovers without seeing the doctor or taking any drugs. The homelikeness of health would thus be viewed as a balancing which is sometimes lost, but which constantly seeks to re-establish itself. Recent

rhythmic, balancing character they will not mean unhomelike being-in-the-world, not eclipse the openness towards the future and the world, but merely indicate different tempos, different rhythms.

To the rhythm of a healthy being-in-the-world during a life span normally belongs temporary sadness and despair. Very much analogous to the difference I have explicated between different forms of tiredness is the difference between the grief one experiences after the death of a loved one and and an endemic depression. Indeed, an attunement of sadness need not at all be an unhealthy mood, if it merely *colours*, but does not prevent one's understanding in transcending in a coherent way. The border between grief and depression can only be drawn by studying the attunement of the person in question and its temporal dimension. If the future is permanently lost, for instance, this unhomelikeness would surely involve illness.

In approaching health and illness through attuned understanding and its temporal dimension, we must also be attentive to changes which have to do with ageing. People's thoughts often change character when they get older by becoming much more centred around the past and the present than around the future. This does not mean that the elderly are no longer open to the future, but rather that they approach the future *through* the past in a more obvious sense. The 'pulse of their life' indeed beats more slowly and their moods of understanding are different. Their transcendence is accordingly different than that of younger people, but it might nonetheless be just as (or even more) *coherent*. The attunement of older persons' being-in-the-world is therefore sometimes more at home than it has ever been before, although their physical abilities are diminished and their openness has been gradually transformed and has come to centre more upon the past than the future.

As we grow older we gradually start having problems performing activities which we earlier performed with ease, like running or jumping. The presence of several mild and severe diseases seems to be connected to nearly every process of ageing. According to the biostatistical theory of health nearly all old people would indeed be chronically unhealthy.[157] But should elderly people really be considered unhealthy just because their way of being-in-the-world changes character in a way characteristic for ageing? By focusing upon being-in-the-world as rhythmic transcendence, and by separating the healthy from the ill through paying attention to the homelike and the unhomelike, we can give a more adequate description of elderly people's situation and find out what medicine is supposed to do for them. This is an illustration of

---

studies on the functioning of the immune system could be invoked to support such a theory. Canguilhem's view upon health as a capacity to institute new biological norms in changing circumstances also seems to point in this direction (1991, pp. 196-197).

[157] Even if one, like Boorse, tries to solve this problem by specifying different levels of normal functioning for different ages, one cannot deny that some of the causes of these lower levels of functioning would indeed normally be called diseases. Nordenfelt would try to solve the problem of a decreased ability to realize vital goals in life by saying that the vital goals change throughout life (1987, p. 113). This is indeed true, but many other things in addition to abilities and vital goals change throughout life, and the phenomenological theory is meant to be better suited to give an explication of these changing circumstances, which are of importance for a discussion of health.

why we need a phenomenological theory of health – in contrast and in addition to medical science – in working out a philosophy of medical practice.

Transcendence and coherence are an ongoing process of mutual support. They are so to say two sides of the same coin. Through coherent transcendence one develops a coherent self.[158] Lack in transcendence always implies some lack in coherence, but in most cases of illness the transcendence preserves the kind of coherence necessary for being the transcendence of *one* coherent self. Some mental illnesses would however provide us with the extreme case of a transcendence that is so incoherent that it no longer represents the being-in-the-world of one coherent self. The most obvious example would be multiple-personality disorder. The being-in-the-world of the psychotic person lacks homelikeness and this manifests itself primarily in a lack of coherence, which is so strong that it threatens the constancy of the self. The lack of true communication in the behaviour of the psychotic person is an illustration of this.

The homelike attunement of the healthy person indicates that he is experiencing wholeness in his being-in-the-world. He inhabits a world that is his world *and* the world of other people – it is a meaningful world. The person need not be happy – he might well be sad; but, in the mood, we find an attuned understanding that transcends in a coherent way – the homelike balancing is there. This homelikeness of the healthy being-in-the-world is – as I will try to show – the goal of clinical practice. What we have done in this section, and what we will do in the two following sections, should be seen as ways of further explicating the phenomenological concept of health as *homelike being-in-the-world* – by linking homelikeness to other concepts, by using illustrative examples, and by making comparisons with other theories of health.

9. ABILITY TO ACT AND ATTUNED UNDERSTANDING

A clear advantage of viewing health as a homelike way of being-in-the-world is that it is possible to find a phenomenological – and indeed conceptual – *connection* between that which, on a physiological and psychological level, one would call 'disability' and 'feeling' of illness respectively. Ability – the basic concept of Nordenfelt's holistic theory of health – would in the phenomenological theory find a counterpart in the existential of attunement. To be attuned provides admission to the meaning-structure of the world where understanding actions can be exercised, just as mental and physical abilities make it possible for the subject to act. But the conceptualization of illness in terms of unhomelike attunement also makes it obvious that illness has a feeling, in addition to an ability, component to it. As two existentials attunement and understanding are always connected, always linked to one another as two aspects of the same phenomenon – the being-in-the-world of the person. Unhomelike attunement would, therefore, in the phenomenological theory, always im-

---

[158]For a phenomenological study of the genesis of the self, see Part 2 of Zaner (1981). I have not found it necessary to include such an analysis in this work, although I think Heidegger's phenomenology in combination with the theories of other phenomenologists such as Richard Zaner and Paul Ricoeur – in the case of the latter see especially *Oneself as Another* (1992) – offer great possibilities.

ply unhomelike understanding and vice versa. In Nordenfelt's theory disability is only causally related to the feeling of illness; that is, according to him, disability (to realize vital goals) often causes a feeling of illness, but not necessarily so. This was indeed the reason why Nordenfelt chose to develop his theory from the concept of ability, leaving the analysis of the feeling of illness hanging in the air:

> In most such characterisations (of health) two kinds of phenomena are mentioned: first, the subjective phenomenon of a certain kind of feeling, of ease or well-being in the case of health, and of pain or suffering in the case of illness; second, the phenomenon of ability or disability, the former an indication of health, the latter of illness. These two kinds of phenomena are in many ways interconnected. There is first an empirical, causal connection. A feeling of ease or well-being contributes causally to the ability of its bearer. A feeling of pain or suffering may directly cause some degree of disability. Conversely, a subject's perception of his ability or disability greatly influences his emotional state. . . . The assumption of a conceptual relation between pain and disability will be accepted in the present analysis: a man cannot experience great pain or suffering without evincing some degree of disability. But a man may have a disability, and even be generally disabled, without experiencing pain or suffering. There are some paradigm cases of illness where pain and suffering are absent. One obvious case is that of coma. Another is present in certain mental disabilities and illnesses. When a patient cannot reflect over his own situation, then his disabilities need not have suffering as a consequence. In short, wherever there is great pain or suffering there is disability, but the converse is not true (1987, pp. 35-36).

In the phenomenological theory we cannot talk about causal connections in the same way as Nordenfelt does, since causality belongs to the world of objects. Heidegger's philosophy is not a psychological theory; that is, it is not primarily about entities, mental or somatic. We cannot say that the attunement of boredom *causes* our understanding to change its patterns, at least not in the strong sense of causality; that is, a necessary empirical connection between two separate events. Attunement and understanding are not separable in this sense although they are distinguishable.

Adopting Nordenfelt's view, as I see it, one has two possibilities: either one can talk about the objects of the world and the causal connections that hold between them established on an empirical basis; or one can talk about the meaning of words used in talking about the world. The latter is always the case when Nordenfelt talks about conceptual relations: it belongs to the *meaning* of the words 'pain' and 'suffering' that the person referred to is disabled. In the phenomenological theory, however, the meaning-analysis extends to cover not only language use, but the entire worldliness of the person. That the ill way of being-in-the-world is attuned in an unhomelike way *and* is played out in the form of a defective understanding are consequently not two related facts, but two aspects of the same meaning-pattern. The analysis of this meaning-pattern – as I have attempted it above – is not carried out via an analysis of language use (how people use and should use terms relating to illness and health), but via the experience of illness itself. There is certainly a first-person perspective in this approach, but the phenomenological reduction, through which our attention is directed towards the meaning of phenomena, in Heidegger's case the meaning-patterns of being-in-the-world, strives toward arriving at the intersubjective perspective – at a description of the basic structures of not only my but everybody's experiences.

That the different aspects of the meaning patterns of being-in-the-world are not causally related to each other in the sense of separated events, of course, does not mean that a somatic process or state – a malady – could not be responsible for a change in the meaning-patterns. When virus invades the organism the meaning-patterns of the person's being-in-the-world certainly change. But only the virus and the organism – and not the meaning-patterns of being-in-the-world – can be analysed in terms of causes and effects of *objects*. It might be appropriate here to talk about different forms of causality; for a more basic form of causality than the physical form is applicable on the phenomenological level of the person. This basic, everyday, causality means that, although one cannot predict or strictly explain the effect with the help of the cause, the cause is *responsible* for a situation which is lived and interpreted in a different way than the preceding one by the person.[159]

Now, how shall we deal with Nordenfelt's two examples of disability (in his sense of illness) without pain or suffering. A person in a coma – say, after having a stroke – and a deluded psychotic, unaware of his illness, says Nordenfelt in the quotation above, do not *suffer* from their illnesses. These two cases seem to be counter-instances to my phenomenological reworking, in terms of attuned understanding, of Nordenfelt's concept of ability, since the moods typifying illness are here absent, although the ability to act is disturbed. Let us begin with the first example and do so in the form of an illuminating concrete case:

Mary was sorting her mail at her desk when the headache began. It was a dull ache, similar to the ones she had had lately almost every day. She rubbed her forehead and gave it no notice. But Mary's mind soon began to wander; she felt light and unfocused. She looked out her office window. She noticed the men and women in the windows across the way, the men without jackets, their ties flying as they walked from office to office. She could almost hear the women's high heels clicking on the floor. They looked like miniature, mechanical figures, like a music box. 'Like a music box', Mary thought, before she lost her breath, before the headache blinded her, before she fell unconscious, scattering her just-sorted mail on her polished desk.[160]

The woman in a coma – we will encounter her later in more detail – would after falling down unconscious on her desk not be living in the meaning-patterns of the world

---

[159] In the *Zollikoner Seminare* Heidegger talks about the possibility of releasing (*auslösen*) moods through electric shocks (1994, p. 244). The method, however, does not produce (*bewirken*) moods – this is impossible since moods are not objects or states that can be produced, but meaning-patterns of existence. The mood is only *correlated* to a brain state: 'Die Gestimmtheit wird nur *ausgelöst*. Je einer Gestimmtheit ist ein bestimmter Gehirnzustand zugeordnet. Der Gehirnvorgang ist jedoch nie hin-reichend für das Verstehen einer Gestimmtheit, nicht hin- und zu-reichend sogar im wörtlichsten Sinne, weil er nie in die Stimmung als solche hineinreichen kann.' We will return to these issues in the first section of Part 3, which discusses explanation and understanding in medicine.

[160] The example is taken from Senelick and Rossi (1994, p. 70) and is continued in the next part of this work.

at all. Therefore, it is true, one might say that Mary has lost all attunement and understanding.[161] It makes sense to refer to her as diseased or not diseased in a physiological sense, but not as ill or healthy in the phenomenological sense. She is currently just a body – a living and not a dead body, it is true – but still not for the moment a *lived* body; that is, not an incarnated, phenomenal body forming a vector of existence, a 'corps propre' as it is put in the philosophy of Maurice Merleau-Ponty.[162] To refer to her as disabled and ill is therefore correct if ability means 'internal – bodily or mental – resources for performing . . . actions' (Nordenfelt 1987, p. 46), but not if it means attuned understanding in Heidegger's sense. This is obviously a difference between Nordenfelt's theory and my Heideggerian outline. What is important here is that Nordenfelt's ability concept is applicable on the same level as disease processes – that is, it can be used to describe not only lived experience (as mental states), but also the presence or absence of physiological functions. With understanding we do not have this double possibility: the physiological functions must be *experienced* in some way in order to affect and involve understanding, and this does not seem to be the case when one is in a coma.[163]

Although the woman in the coma currently lacks all transcendence, she is nonetheless a part of *other people's* being-in-the-world. Her appearance will immediately give rise to efforts to help her. We do not treat unconscious persons as things – we do not even treat corpses as things – but rather as a part of the world-structure that

---

[161] This of course presupposes that the comatose person is really *unconscious* and not merely sleeping. Dreams are clearly examples of a form of existence having attunement and understanding.

[162] We will soon return to Merleau-Ponty in discussing the lived body. This, however, might be the proper place for an urgent question that might already have entered the reader's mind in my presentation of Nordenfelt's theory: What about children (infants) and animals? Are they all deemed unhealthy by the holistic and the phenomenological theories? Nordenfelt tries to solve the dilemma that infants are not able to realize vital goals by introducing the notion of 'standard adult support' (1987, p. 104). The phenomenological answer would be similar, since infants are not immediately but only gradually thrown into the intersubjective meaning-patterns of being-in-the-world. This process certainly demands support and teaching – consider language use, for instance. The transcendence and coherence one demands for a child to be healthy would therefore gradually increase. It is important to remember that I do not identify illness with a *total lack* of transcendence. This indeed would only be the case when a human being is dead or in a coma. Illness is a *defective* transcendence, a partial breakdown in the meaning-patterns of worldliness of *Dasein*. Now, what about animals? Do they have vital goals? Do they have worldliness? Heidegger's answer would be something like, no, or, if so, only in a reduced sense. In the lecture course from 1929-30, *Grundbegriffe der Metaphysik: Welt – Endlichkeit – Einsamkeit* (1983), he compares the being-in-the-world of human beings and animals. Do they both have *Dasein* – that is, openness to the world as a meaning-pattern? Heidegger writes that human beings are at the same time part of the world – as bodies – and *have* world – they are *weltbildend*. Animals are part of the world and *weltarm* – 'world-poor'. They are not, however, in the manner of a stone, *weltlos* (1983, pp. 261-264). Does this 'world-poorness' indicate that we could ascribe health in the phenomenological sense to higher animals in the same way as to infants? I do not have any definite answer to this question. The main reason for Heidegger to deny animals worldliness in any full sense is their lack of language. But do not some animals speak (dolphins, chimpanzees)? And do not many animals live in intersubjective moods as well as individualized suffering (illness)? See Krell (1992) for an interesting discussion of many of these themes. See also Buytendijk (1958).

[163] See here again the excellent book by Leder (1990a), which particularly tries to investigate the forgotten field of lived somatic functions.

we relate to as a being-with (Heidegger 1986, pp. 117 ff., 237 ff.). We care for our fellow beings even if they are not currently conscious; this is true of many paradigm situations in medicine. And these efforts to help are indeed geared towards the comatose person *regaining* attunement, ultimately a healthy one. This, as we shall see in the next part of this work, was what happened to Mary. Her colleagues, who found her comatose on the desk, called for an ambulance, and Mary, having after a while regained consciousness, then experienced a very different being-in-the-world than before the stroke, an unhomelike one indeed.

What about Nordenfelt's second example – mental illnesses in which the subject cannot reflect on his own situation and consequently does not feel pain or suffering? The lack of what I have referred to as a 'pain-mood' is certainly possible. Not all illnesses involve pain. But does that mean that these patients do not live in illness moods – that is, moods of continuous unhomelikeness? Not necessarily. They could very well live in moods of unhomelikeness, though unable to reflect upon the fact that they are ill. Mental illness seems to be a typical case of different forms of deviant attunements. The moods in which the mentally ill live need not always be powerful, in the sense of anxiety or the boredom of depression, but there nevertheless seems to be a strong case for claiming that all people who are mentally ill have their patterns of understanding coloured by an unhomelike attunement.[164]

In this section I have tried to approach questions regarding the relationship between a theory about the mental and the somatic, on the one hand, and a phenomenological theory, operating at the level of meaning, on the other hand. I attempted to reinterpret Nordenfelt's holistic theory in terms of my Heideggerian proposal for a theory of health and noted important similarities and differences. Both theories stress the importance of the environment of the individual and his plans and actions. In the end, however, Nordenfelt's theory stays true to a third-person, rather than a first-person perspective. Abilities in the form of mental and somatic states are chosen, rather than interpretation and feeling as the lived experiences *of* these states, as the basis for a theory of health. As we shall see in the concluding Section 11 of this part, the two approaches have different advantages in defining and understanding health, respectively.

It is important to point out that although phenomenology is situated at the level of the *meaning* of experience, it is certainly an attempt to explicate the meaning of the very world that surrounds and permeates us. How meaning is lived by the person in his being-in-the-world is therefore in every way *connected* to the things that surround the person and to the 'thing' that he lives through (body-mind). The theories about these 'things' are not, however, taken as the *starting point* for the analysis; rather, it is lived experience that performs this role. To develop a phenomenological theory of health is therefore not meant as an attempt to replace biomedical research. In light of

---

[164]Interesting borderline cases here are the types of mental illnesses which seem to lack attunement altogether: persons suffering from alexithymia and some psychopaths, for instance. If one does not have any feelings at all, how can one then suffer from an attunement of homelessness? But in many such cases, what the subject lacks is *empathy* rather than feelings, and this does not mean a total lack of attunement, although it certainly means a very defective one. See Svenaeus (1999a).

the successful history of modern medicine we have surveyed in the first part of this work this would certainly be an absurd project. Phenomenology is meant to enrich our understanding of health in adding to the disease-level analysis a level that addresses the questions of how the physiological states are lived as meaningful in an environment. As mentioned earlier, we cannot talk about a strict causal relationship between these two levels. The way diseases are taken up and lived is not only dependent upon physiology, but on the place they come to inhabit in a meaning-pattern, a being-in-the-world of attuned understanding.

This level of meaning forms a very significant part of medicine. It is a telling fact in itself that the doctor's telling a patient about a disease that he did not know of before the clinical encounter sometimes seems to be able to 'cause' illness just as much (or more) than the disease itself:

Ted a few weeks after his 55th birthday went to a routine medical examination. These examinations were offered by the company where he worked and he used to go to them every year. Ted was feeling fine. He was in good physical shape, exercised several times a week and had never experienced any problems with his weight or blood pressure. He had a job that he was satisfied with. As a caretaker, he was not very well paid, but he liked the job, he had many good friends at his work place and the job was not too stressful. He had plenty of time for his family and hobbies. The medical examination went as usual – everything was normal – until the doctor asked Ted if he could take a PSA test. He explained to Ted that this blood test – prostate specific antigen – was newly developed and was used to screen for prostate cancer. Since Ted was approaching an age where prostate cancer was a common disease, the doctor thought it might be a good idea to have the test. If we detect prostate cancer in time, he said, we can do something about it before it has spread to other parts of the body. Anyway the risks were of course not very high that Ted had cancer in the first place, but would it not feel good to be certain? Ted did not at first understand how it was possible to have cancer without knowing it, without feeling any symptoms. The doctor said that the symptoms of prostate cancer, such as having problems with urinating, often did not develop until the tumour had grown so big and metastatic that the disease would be hard to treat. Ted agreed to have the test. He came back three days later to get the results and they were positive. He had an elevated PSA level of 4.0 nanograms per millilitre. Ted was terrified, was he going to die or become impotent from treatment as he had heard about? The doctor told him that it still was not certain that Ted really had cancer. The elevated level was not extreme and could be due to a so-called benign prostatic hyperplasia (BPH) which was not malignant. To find out they had to run some more tests – a digital rectal examination and a biopsy. He tried to calm Ted down and made an appointment for him the same day with an urologist at the same hospital, who was to carry out the tests. The urologist received Ted the same afternoon and after reading his chart and asking him a couple of questions about possible symptoms of prostate pathology, such as trouble urinating, carried out a digital rectal examination – he inserted his rubber-gloved finger into Ted's rectum to feel the posterior portion of the prostate, checking for swelling and hardness. He told Ted that he was not able to detect any malignancy this way, but that he wanted to do a biopsy as well just to be sure. In the biopsy the doctor took six small cell samples from Ted's prostate using a so called spring-loaded biopsy gun. Ultrasonic waves are used to scan the prostate looking for suspicious areas to stick the needle into. These procedures were of course rather unpleasant in themselves, but the fear for the results Ted felt was much worse. The following days waiting for the results from the biopsy Ted lived as in a black hole. The contents and prospects of his life had very suddenly changed in a horrible manner. He thought he could feel his prostate ticking in him like a time-bomb. He began thinking back. Had he not had troubles with having to urinate several times during the night lately? Did he not feel a slight resistance when he tried to empty his bladder?[165]

We will return to Ted in the next part of this work, but at this point I want to underline the importance of the patient's interpretation of his situation. This interpretation – an attuned understanding – is not only formed from things we experience directly, but also from things we are *told*. To be told by the doctor that you have cancer almost certainly will 'produce' a feeling of illness in you even if the disease in itself produces no symptoms. The being-in-the-world of the patient seems to change its structure to an attunement of illness as the patient is informed of the disease. This is certainly not a new discovery, but references to 'psychological factors' in medicine are not sufficient for an understanding of how the entire existence of the patient actually changes its structure through the patient being told he has a disease. Ted, in the example, actually starts to reinterpret his past, present and future in the face of the possible diagnosis. Did I not in fact have symptoms before although I did not notice? Do I not really feel something now? What will happen to me and my life in the future?

10. THE LIVED BODY AND THE BROKEN TOOL

Let us return to Heidegger's analysis of the person's being-in-the-world as an attuned understanding played out in the meaning-patterns formed between different tools. How is it possible to get explicit, philosophical hold of these meaning-patterns if we are always absorbed in pre-intentional activity? What in other words is Heidegger's counterpart to Husserl's phenomenological reduction? I have already given a preliminary answer to this question by emphasizing the role of anxiety in *Sein und Zeit* as the prerequisite for reaching authentic understanding. The moment of anxiety signifies a certain form of interruption of all activity in which the world loses its meaning as a totality of relevance for human existence and stands out as perfectly irrelevant – that is, as lacking sense. The focus of understanding thereby changes from the things and goals *in* the world to the *world itself* as a meaning-structure of *Dasein* (being-there-in-the-world):

---

[165]The example has been constructed mainly with the help of Kantoff and McConnell (1996).

> What anxiety is about is completely indefinite. This indefiniteness not only leaves factically undecided which innerworldly beings are threatening to us, but also means that innerworldly beings in general are not 'relevant'. . . . The totality of relevance discovered within the world of things available and objectively present is completely without importance. It collapses. The world has the character of complete insignificance (1986, p. 186).

In authentic understanding the senselessness makes it possible to explicate the world-structure, not as a collection of things, but as a meaning-structure of the phenomenologist's being-in-the-world. In this attitude (the phenomenological attitude) the irrelevant senselessness can be developed into a positive theoretical understanding.

I do not think that anxiety is the only mood that offers the possibility of phenomenological analysis. Heidegger himself in his later works emphasizes other moods, such as the Aristotelian wonder, or the sorrow and joy present in Hölderlin's poetry (Svenaeus 1997). As I made clear in my presentation of Husserl's way to the phenomenological reduction through free fantasy variation, the interests and situation of the philosopher himself seem to be of vital importance. What evokes your wonder and curiosity? This is where to begin (Zaner 1970, p. 75). One of the points with Heidegger's focus upon anxiety in *Sein und Zeit* is, however, that the possibility of phenomenological analysis is not entirely up to oneself, but also depends upon the world that one has been thrown into and lives in. One's attunement, which is where every analysis starts, does not arise in one on account of one having chosen it, but as a result of one's being-in-the-world.

As I have pointed out earlier, authentic anxiety as Heidegger envisages it in *Sein und Zeit* bears resemblance to the unhomelike attunement of illness, which we have focused on above. Authentic anxiety seems to mean a breakdown of all ordinary understanding and activity. Is this not equivalent to the defective transcendence of the ill way of being-in-the-world? Is it not in a way similar to a total lack of transcendence (death, coma)? This would indeed be true if the authentic anxiety lasted for a long time, but according to Heidegger it does not. The total withdrawal from the activities of the world only lasts for a moment (*Augenblick*) (1986, p. 344). After this rewarding experience the phenomenologist has to return to everyday doings – but with new insights, of course, which could change his everyday life. The unhomelike attunement of the ill existence would, in contrast to the attunement of authenticity, be lasting. It could, however, in a similar way, in some cases, offer new perspectives on the worldliness of human being.[166]

Certainly not every breakdown in the ongoing activity of being-in-the-world is equivalent to the anxiety of authentic understanding. First of all, far from all moments of anxiety result in authentic understanding. The reason for this is that the person tends to identify the source of anxiety with a thing in the world and not with the world-structure itself. But in addition to this, very few breakdowns are total, in the sense of making our *entire* existence senseless. Most are merely partial, interrupting

---

[166]Merleau-Ponty (1962) offers an analysis of the meaning-structures of perception performed mainly with the aid of different defects. It is also noteworthy here that to return to health from severe illness generally seems to provide people with new ideas and feelings about the structure and meaning of life.

our ongoing activity on account of the failure, malfunctioning or obtrusiveness of a certain tool in the world.

Heidegger's famous example in *Sein und Zeit* is the hammer (1986, pp. 69, 84). While engaged in building a house, we do not, in the act of hammering, explicitly focus our attention upon the hammer in an intentional way. We are absorbed in the activity. Suddenly, the head of the hammer flies off, and the tool can no longer be used for striking nails. The activity is now interrupted, and we are forced to focus upon the hammer, to become conscious of it as a broken tool which must be repaired or replaced, if we are to be able to go on building the house. Heidegger's point here is that through breakdowns in the activity, it becomes possible to grasp the hammer as a piece of equipment – a tool – and not just as a thing (1986, p. 73 ff.). Similar to authentic understanding, certain breakdowns of activity (which, of course, must also be attuned but not necessarily in the mood of anxiety) make it possible to explicate *parts* of the world-structure as tools. The hammer is seen as a broken hammer and this 'brokenness' of the hammer exists only if the hammer is seen as a part in a totality of relevance – if its function and use in goal-related understanding activity is focused upon. That is, the meaning of the hammer is not revealed if we study it separately as a physical thing with certain qualities – blackness, heaviness, a certain shape and so on – but rather it must be placed in the context of the world as a meaning-structure for human beings. The hammer and its context are difficult to analyse directly in the activity of hammering since this activity is pre-intentional. It can be studied indirectly, however, in different forms of breakdowns and withdrawals from activity, during which the 'sense-lessness', the understanding peculiar to malfunctioning, leads our attention to the meaning-relations between tools – that is, to the meaning-structure of the world.

Heidegger in *Sein und Zeit* neglects to highlight the part played by the body in activity and understanding. The lived body (*Leib*) is merely a part of Dasein's spatiality (1986, p. 108). He never extensively discusses the body as a set of tools or part of the meaning-structure of the world.[167] There is no valid argument, however, for restricting the concept of tool (*Zeug*) as it is used in *Sein und Zeit* to things outside the human body.[168] To place the limit of the meaning-patterns of the world at the surface of the biological organism would be to proceed from a materialist perspective,

---

[167] Many philosophers, like Sartre for instance, reproached him for this exclusion. To deem Heidegger an idealist on these grounds would, however, clearly be wrong, since his phenomenology is intended to transcend both naive realism and idealism (1986, pp. 207-208). Merleau-Ponty's *Phénoménologie de la perception* from 1945, a work highly dependent not only upon Husserl's phenomenology, but also upon the analysis of worldliness in *Sein und Zeit,* makes up for this shortcoming of Heidegger by focusing upon the role of the lived, phenomenal body in perceptual activity. Interestingly enough, the *Zollikoner Seminare* provides evidence that Heidegger was aware of this shortcoming already when he wrote *Sein und Zeit* and that the body as lived – *Leib* – forms a more important part of *Dasein's* being-in-the-world than is evident from the book: 'Sartres Vorwurf kann ich nur mit der Feststellung begegnen, daß das Leibliche das Schwierigste ist und daß ich damals eben noch nicht mehr zu sagen wußte' (1994, p. 292). It is highly likely that Heidegger's analysis of the body in the *Zollikoner Seminare* was inspired by a reading of Merleau-Ponty, though he is never mentioned there.

[168] As Straus has pointed out the original meaning of the Greek *organon* is indeed tool (1966b, p. 150).

and not from the phenomenological point of view which Heidegger adopts in this work. Once the positions of dualism and reductionism have been given up in the phenomenological attitude they cannot be brought in again in order to draw a line between the hammer and the hand in the phenomenological analysis. If the hammer and not the hand can be said to constitute a tool in the phenomenological sense, this line of demarcation must be drawn from the phenomenological position. I will now try to show how this line can be drawn – not at the surface of the biological organism, however, and not by denying the hand the position of a certain type of equipment – but rather by stressing the distinction between *self* and *world* in drawing on the phenomenological analysis of health and illness which I have developed so far.[169]

If the hand instead of the hammer breaks, the activity will likewise come to an end. The hand consequently is also a sort of tool for activity and understanding constituting a nodal point in the meaning-pattern of the world. The hand, like the hammer, can be repaired or maybe even replaced by a prosthesis that would adequately perform the functions of a hand. But the situation of the broken hand is also different from the situation of the broken hammer since it is very differently attuned. The confusion and annoyance of the broken hammer can hardly be compared to the pain we experience having broken a wrist. This pain, if continuous, is typically an attunement of illness.[170] The attunement of illness is linked to a defective understanding, since the meaning-patterns of the world are disturbed as a result – in this case – of the body-tools breaking down. The understanding is limited since a vital part of the totality of relevance has been removed. Still, in a way, it would be wrong to call the body parts tools since they are also part of *Dasein* as a self. They are not only a part of the totality of tools, but also, as lived (*leibliche*), they belong to the projective power of the self. The hand and the hammer are thus rightly regarded as *different* forms of tools; but the line of demarcation is not drawn with reference to the surface of the biological organism. It is rather determined through an appeal to the importance the tool plays in the totality of relevance for the human being in question. If the tool belongs to the region we would identify with the self rather than the world in the person's being-in-the-world, then it would consequently be more likely to result in illness if broken.

The self must, however, always be understood as acquiring its meaning and identity by way of its being-in-the-world. The loss of a beloved could lead to an attunement of illness if he formed an irreplaceable part of the person's self as a being-in-the-world; whereas the loss of some body parts – such as the appendix – could take place without us afterwards experiencing any pain or illness, and in this case it could actually mean a recovery from illness. The loss of all hair, or the loss of an irreplace-

---

[169] Some philosophers before me have suggested the broken tool example in Heidegger as a promising way to a phenomenology of illness. They have, however, never actually carried out the analysis. See Leder (1990a, pp. 19, 33, 83-84), Rawlinson (1982, p. 75), and Toombs (1992b, p. 136 ff.).

[170] The phenomenology of pain is without doubt the best explored area of the phenomenology of illness. A classic case is Buytendijk (1962). I would also like to mention the excellent book by Elaine Scarry, *The Body in Pain* (1985), which explores the effects of torture as severe damage to the person's being-in-the-world. Language, for example, as a way of inhabiting the world, is destroyed through pain.

able toupee that had made one's being-in-the-world homelike again after one had gone bald, would be interesting borderline examples. Could the loss of either of these two 'tools' constitute illness? The question would have to be answered through a careful analysis of the person in question and his being-in-the-world.

The body as lived (*Leib*) would, in any case, just like language, form a vital part of our transcendence into the world. It would indeed seem appropriate to accord the lived body the status of a fourth existential of our being-in-the-world, alongside the other existentials of understanding, attunement and language.[171] Heidegger says to Medard Boss in 1972:

> Everything that we refer to as our lived body (unsere Leiblichkeit), including the most minute muscle fibre and the most imperceptible hormone molecule, belongs essentially to our mode of existence. This body is consequently not to be understood as lifeless matter, but is part of that domain that cannot be objectified or seen, a being able to encounter significance (Vernehmen-könnens von Bedeutsamkeiten), which our entire being-there (Da-sein) consists in. This lived body (dieses Leibliche) forms itself in a way appropriate for using the lifeless and living material objects that it encounters. In contrast to a tool (Werkzeug) the living domains of existence cannot, however, be released from the human being. They cannot be stored separately in a tool-box. Rather they remain pervaded by human being, kept in a human being, belonging to a human being, as long as he lives (1994, p. 293).[172]

That the body is pervaded (*durchwaltet*) by human being (*Mensch-sein*) must certainly mean that it is attuned and transcending. As Merleau-Ponty writes, the body 'understands' and 'inhabits' the world (1962, p. 139). Heidegger expresses this notion through the neologism 'Das Leiben des Leibes' (1994, p. 113). Existence is a 'bodying forth' in the meaning-structures of the world. These meaning-structures are consequently not confined to language or consciousness. Indeed, as early as in *Sein und Zeit*, Heidegger had given priority to everyday *actions* in his analysis.

Interestingly enough Heidegger in the *Zollikoner Seminare* refers to the 'bodying forth' of human being as 'Gebärde' – gestures – a term connected to language, the language of the body:

> In philosophy we must not confine the meaning of the term gesture to 'expression' ('Ausdruck'). This term we should instead use to characterize all behaviour of human being (alles Sich-Betragen des Menschen) as a being-in-the-world determined by the life of the lived body (Leiben des Leibes). Every movement of my body (Leib) as a gesture and behaviour enables me not only to take place in physical space. Rather the

---

[171] This fourfold structure of worldliness would be a parallel (and indeed an alternative) to Heidegger's later notion of *das Geviert* of gods, human beings, sky and earth, constituting the 'dwelling' (*Wohnen*) in the world, see (1954a). The fourfold existential structure would, in the same way as *das Geviert*, include *nature* (the earth meaning nature – animals and plants) in the form of *Leib*, an aspect of existence which is all too absent in *Sein und Zeit*. It would also, however, be centred around *Da-sein*, rather than *Sein*. Human beings would accordingly occupy the centre of the structure and not just one of its nodes.

[172] This quotation inevitably provokes thoughts about the era of organ transplantation which was still in its infancy when Heidegger said this in 1972. There still remain important limits, however, regarding which organs it is possible to store in the 'tool-box' and for how long. Nevertheless, given the emergence of cyberspace and artificial organs, the difference between hand and hammer certainly seems even more diffuse today than in Heidegger's time.

behaviour is always already situated in a region (Gegend) that has been opened up by the thing that I am occupied with, as for instance when I take something in my hand (1994, p. 118).

Body and language are inter-nested just like attunement and understanding. To reach out with the hand and to speak both belong to the transcendence (*Entwurf*) of human being. They are not identical, but rather, just as attunement and understanding, different aspects of our being-in-the-world. The four existentials all permeate and support each other. Illness would mean an unhomelikeness of this structure of being-in, which can be thematized as a peculiar kind of attunement, as a failure in transcendence, or as a breakdown in the tool-structure related to the self.

In many cases of illness the basic experience of being ill is tied to the body. Richard Zaner in *The Context of Self* investigates different ways in which the body announces itself as uncanny in illness (1981, pp. 48-55). My body is not just a tool that I use or a dwelling I live in (this is the basic mistake of dualism) – it is *me* (failing to recognize the significance of this 'mineness' is the basic mistake of reductionism). I *am* my own body. Yet this body, as Zaner remarks, also has a life of its own. As we have come to realize through our reading of Heidegger, I belong to the world just as much as the world belongs to me. In the same way I also belong to my body:

> If there is a sense in which my own-body is 'intimately mine', there is furthermore, an equally decisive sense in which I belong to it – in which I am at its disposal or mercy, if you will. My body, like the world in which I live, has its own nature, functions, structures, and biological conditions; since it embodies me, I thus experience myself as implicated by my body and these various conditions, functions, etc. I am exposed to whatever can influence, threaten, inhibit, alter, or benefit my biological organism. Under certain conditions, it can fail me (more or less), not be capable of fulfilling my wants or desires, or even thoughts, forcing me to turn away from what I may want to do and attend to my own body: because of fatigue, hunger, thirst, disease, injury, pain, or even itches, I am forced at times to tend and attend to it, regardless, it may be, of what may well seem more urgent at the moment. Hence despite its evident 'intimacy', my own-body is as well the experiential ground for frustration, anguish, pain, fear, dread, as well as joy, satiation, pleasure, well-being ('health' as Kass says), and ultimately of death, my own ceasing-to-be (1981, p. 52).

The body is alien, yet, at the same time, myself. It involves biological processes beyond my control, but these processes still belong to me as lived by me. The body seems to be the very form of finitude, in the sense of referring to our being born as well as our having to die. Our finitude is so to say incarnated in the being of the body as our form of existence. Illness is an uncanny (unhomelike) experience since the otherness of the body then presents itself in an obtrusive, merciless way.[173] In illness the body often has to be surveyed – as we shall see later in the case of Jane's diabetes – as something other than oneself, something that has its own ways and must be regulated if one shall be able to survive. The behaviour of the body in illness is often no longer under control; the emptying of bowel and bladder, for instance, takes place

---

[173] As I remarked above the meaning of the German *unheimlich* – 'uncanny' – is related to *unheimisch* – 'unhomelike'. See Freud (1919), and Svenaeus (1999b).

without the ill person being able to regulate it. Of course the body has a life of its own even in health – certain needs must be satisfied; but the inconvenience, experienced in health, of urgently having to heed the call of nature, is very different from the inconvenience of urinating or defecating without noticing it until it is too late. The change in outer appearance and the loss of mastery over one's own body, which take place in many cases of illness, can in themselves be stigmatizing and lead to problems in the relationship with other people.[174]

The unhomelikeness of illness would never consist in one or several of the existentials being totally absent. This is indeed not even a possibility, since the existentials are not merely added to each other as things in the world but permeate each other in an unravellable way, forming the necessary structure that makes being-in-the-world possible at all. The *entire* being-in-the-world of the ill person is always involved in illness. Even if one cannot speak (dumbness) or indeed possesses no 'language' in the usual sense (severe disturbance in mental development) one's body would still 'express' things in its bodying forth in the world. Analogously the tetraplegics who are able to speak or express themselves through writing (perhaps through some sort of computerized device) would still in some restricted sense be present in their own bodies.[175] Consequently, no transcendence and no illness is entirely somatic or entirely mental. On the contrary, these terms are applicable only on the psychological and physiological level – to diseases – not on the meaning-level of health and illness.

None of the cases I mentioned above (dumbness, mental retardation, lameness) would normally be referred to as illnesses, but rather as handicaps. The general difference between ill and handicapped persons on the biomedical level would be that the latter are currently not suffering from any diseases, but rather from defects, injuries or impairments. The handicapped as well as the diseased would, however, be considered unhealthy according to a biostatistical health concept; that is, both groups would have maladies that were responsible for subnormal ability to carry out biological functions.[176] On the phenomenological level handicap would generally be separated from illness by the fact that the handicapped have a reduced or transferred transcendence, but that this transcendence nevertheless has reached a coherence that makes the being-in-the-world of the person homelike although *different* from other people's being-in-the-world. The handicapped are in most cases not in unhomelike attunements of illness, since they have reached a transcendence that undoubtably is different from that of most other people (consider the way the blind use their sense of touch, for instance), but that still enables them to perform their activities in a way that makes sense to them in their life. The being-in-the-world of the handicapped

---

[174]For a study of the stigmatizing effects of illness and handicap, see the classic book by Goffman (1974). See also Toombs (1992a, 1992b).

[175]On the phenomenology of the lived brain see Leder (1990a, p. 111 ff.).

[176]Nordenfelt too must in his theory come to the conclusion that the handicapped person is unhealthy since he does not have the ability to realize vital goals given standard circumstances (1987, p. 128). The handicapped need the assistance of aids, which make the circumstances nonstandard. This might seem counterintuitive since most handicapped people would consider themselves healthy.

person would therefore generally be a healthy, homelike one. Some handicaps might, however, be so severe that a homelike being-in-the-world is not possible. This would probably be the case for most tetraplegics, for instance.

The difference between handicap and chronic illness is not easy to pin-point. Indeed the difference as it is defined on the biomedical level as a difference between impairment, injury, or defect and disease does not make sense on the level of experience. If one is chronically ill (e.g., with diabetes), one generally needs medicine and surveillance (by oneself and professionals); and if one is handicapped (e.g., blind) one is in need of the assistance of aids such as a walking stick. But what is really the difference between insulin and a walking stick? Suppose that we in the future manage to fine-tune the treatment for diabetes in a way that makes it possible for the person with diabetes to live without *paying attention* to his disease, without planning every meal, without monitoring blood glucose levels, without taking any insulin injections, and so on. This may not be a utopia if we consider the rapid development of treatment methods for diabetes during the last few decades.[177] My future scenario is not that we will be able to cure the disease – the pancreas (or the cell receptors) will still function defectively – but rather that it may become possible to compensate for this in a way that makes it possible for the patient to live a totally normal life. In this case we would have a disease, but the person would not be ill in the sense of having an unhomelike attunement in his being-in-the-world.

If one does not have any troubles with a disease, if it does not affect one's being-in-the-world, does it then really make one ill? The answer must indeed be no, and the reason for calling a person with diabetes ill in the phenomenological theory is exactly the 'troubles' that attune the whole being-in-the-world of this person. The blind person has, after a while – supposing his blindness comes from a disease or an injury – adjusted to a new form of being-in-the-world and regained homelikeness. The threat of the chronic illness getting worse is a factor which generally differentiates chronic illness from handicaps. This very threat brings unhomelikeness with it as a constant eclipse of the future, something that is not present for most handicapped. This difference is to be conceptualized on the phenomenological level of being-in-the-world; the threat of ceasing to be or of getting worse is experienced in *lived* time.

To regain homelikeness, to be rehabilitated, for the handicapped might be a long and hard process. It is a process that often requires medical advice and devices. It is also, however, a process in which other professionals and non-professionals than doctors could be of help. And it is first of all a matter of the person himself actively adjusting to a new way of being-in-the-world. The goal for medicine in encountering the handicapped and the chronically ill must indeed be the same: to bring the patient back to homelikeness – that is, to health – or, if this is not possible, as far in the direction of homelike being-in-the-world as possible. 'Back' here does not mean 'backwards'. As we will see in Part 3, to return to a homelike being-in-the-world through the help of medicine often essentially means to go *forward*, to a new and different form of being-in-the-world than the one present before the onset of illness.

---

[177] For future possibilities see Guthrie and Guthrie (1997), Chapter 15.

11. HEALTH AND PHENOMENOLOGY – MEDICINE AND HERMENEUTICS

In closing this second part of my work and moving on to medicine and hermeneutics it might be important to point out once more that the focus upon health and illness as aspects of our being-in-the-world is intended to form, not an alternative, but rather a complement to a biomedical science of diseases. Doctors are indeed very interested in diseases in attempting to heal patients and for very good reasons as we have seen in the first part of this study. What I have criticized here is a too narrow approach to the goal of clinical practice – exemplified by the biostatistical theory of health – and not biomedical science itself. Such a theory tries to define health proceeding exclusively from biomedical science. Given that the goal of the clinical encounter is to restore lost health, this image of health – absence of diseases – would tend to make medicine identical with applied biology.[178] But this is neither what medicine is or what it ought to be. Medicine, as I will develop in the next part, is a meeting between two persons and an interpretation of the ill person's being-in-the-world, with the aim of restoring a life that has turned unhomelike. To find diseases and to cure or mitigate them form significant *parts* of this activity, but the activity includes much more than that.

I have proposed that we should look upon health and illness as, respectively, homelike and unhomelike ways of being-in-the-world. Homelikeness here refers to the patterns of meaning of the existentials (attuned, bodily and articulated understanding) which make coherent transcendence of a self (person) into the world possible. The importance of paying attention to the environment of the person found a first expression in the ancient health theories, which focused upon the individual as situated in a cosmos that mirrored the make-up of his own balanced or unbalanced constitution. Balance in the phenomenological theory of course means something radically different than this, since the balanc*ing* is here thought of as a mode of the person's being-in-the-world and not something present simultaneously *in* the world and *in* the individual analogically or allegorically. The very *being-in* of the individual in the environment as a meaning-pattern is that which is balanced or imbalanced – in the sense of homelike or unhomelike – according to the phenomenological theory. We encountered a first step on the way to such a conception in Aristotle's image of the virtuous, healthy man of temperance, who balances appropriate opinion (*logos*) and feelings (*pathe*) in his habits (*ethos*). Actions, opinions, feelings and even the cultivation of the body can here be seen as different modes of a being-in-the-world, rather than as qualities of an isolated subject. Such a reading of Aristotle – which is indeed a Heideggerian reading – is helpful in working out a phenomenological theory of health.[179]

---

[178] As I pointed out in Section 2, however, Boorse himself, particularly in his latest work (1997), considers such a goal and image of clinical practice far too narrow.

[179] See here again the works by Kisiel (1993) and Volpi (1996) regarding Heidegger's readings of Aristotle.

My Heideggerian outline for a theory of health could also be viewed as trying to give ability to act – which in Nordenfelt's theory refers to mental and somatic dispositions (states) – a phenomenological expression. There would, however, still be important differences between Nordenfelt's theory and mine. As you remember, health in Nordenfelt's theory is defined as ability to realize vital goals given standard circumstances. I have said nothing about *vital* goals and *standard* circumstances. The 'nodal goal points' aimed for and reached in the handling of tools, and the meaning-structure of the world, are indeed intersubjective phenomena, but I have not attempted a 'standardization' of lifeworlds. Is this to be looked upon as a defect or lack in the phenomenological theory? I do not think so, since the holistic and the phenomenological theories have slightly different ambitions. The main point for Nordenfelt's theory is to be able to *define* health, to propose a credible and coherent use for the word 'health' in most contexts. With the aid of this definition it should be possible to draw a clear boundary between people who are healthy and people who are ill.

The point of the phenomenological theory would be rather to give a general *characteristic* of health and illness and provide a vocabulary with the aid of which one can talk about different illnesses and different ill persons and, in each case, be able to understand why and how *this* person is ill.[180] I think that the general scheme that I (through the philosophy of Heidegger) give, with four existentials (understanding, attunement, language, lived body) structuring our being-in-the-world in a homelike or unhomelike way, provides a promising ground for adequate descriptions of different illnesses with different forms of breakdowns of meaning-structures and failing transcendence.

I am not saying, however, that all phenomenology can give us is good descriptions of what different individuals experience. As I have stressed before, phenomenology is not a part of descriptive psychology. The phenomenological description aims at uncovering necessary features of the meaning-patterns structuring our life. The explication of phenomena – in this case, ill persons' experiences – can therefore also help us understand in which sense they are *ill* (and not, for example, merely unhappy). *Unhomelike being-in-the-world* is the feature I have suggested to fill this illuminating role in my analysis. What breaks down in illness are the meaning-patterns of being-*in*-the-world, the way we inhabit the tool-structures we transcend through in our homelike being-in-the-world. The unhomelikeness of illness is consequently a certain form of senselessness, an attunement of, for instance, disorientedness, helplessness, resistance, and despair.

The ill unhomelikeness of being-in-the-world would take on different forms for different people with different illnesses at different times. Different existentials would be primarily involved in different cases and they would relate to each other in different ways. This would often be due to the presence of different diseases, of

---

[180] The books of Oliver Sacks, for instance (1984, 1985), give (without providing any phenomenological theory of health) a fascinating account of the insights phenomenological descriptions of ill persons can provide for medicine.

course; but the diagnosis of disease is not always the *only* explanation of why a person is ill, and it is definitely not the only illuminating thing we can say about ill persons. We will in the next part of this work expand on this theme, in trying to make evident the hermeneutic structure of medicine.

My claim here has been that all forms of attunements of illness are best understood as unhomelike ways of being-in-the-world. But is not unhomelikeness a more general aspect of human existence that is experienced in many different types of situations, and not exclusively in illness? What about the unhomelikeness one experiences in getting lost in the woods, for instance? This attunement is surely unhomelike and uncanny and yet the lost person can hardly be referred to as ill. Just as in the case, explored above, of tiredness upon rising from bed in the morning, I think this counterexample can be met with a reference to the lasting character of an illness mood. Feeling disoriented in one's being-in-the-world happens regularly in exploring new territories (geographical as well as thematic) and is indeed a part of a *healthy* being-in-the-world, the person being interested in learning new things which he does not initially control.

As I wrote above, referring to Erwin Straus, the being-in-the-world of the person can best be understood as characterized by encounters with both familiar and unfamiliar phenomena: the world does not only belong to me, it also has a sense of alienness and is thus basically both homelike *and* unhomelike for me, even when the former phenomenon is predominant. To be permanently lost 'in the woods' – that is, in-the-world – would, however, in most cases, mean illness. We can hardly specify a precise time-lag necessary for the unhomelikeness of being-in-the-world to become ill, in contrast to other types of homelessness. Time in phenomenology always means lived and meaningful time – a structure of human existence – not the objective time of physics.[181]

Stressing the time aspects of illness, while contrasting it to other forms of unhomelikeness, is indeed a start, but it hardly answers all our questions. Existential crisis (after losing a loved one, or losing one's faith in God, man or life in general) is clearly a paradigm example of unhomelikeness, but it is not always synonymous with depression – that is, with illness. Interestingly enough, we here seem to have a kind of mixture of Heidegger's authentic unhomelikeness and the unhomelikeness of illness. The moment of authentic unhomelikeness is mitigated enough to be extended and allow a process of lasting attunement which does not mean total paralysis. Thus life goes on, but is still fundamentally questioned as a foundation for meaning. Existential crisis can be transformed into an illness mood, like in depression, and in this form it is no exception to my analysis. I admit, though, that the permanent unhomelikeness, in which a person questions his place in life, but is not looked upon as ill either by himself or others, seems to be a possible scenario. This situation, however, always borders on illness if it goes on for a long time. The reason for this seems to be that the unhomelikeness in the latter case is tied to a permanent deformation of the meaning-structure of the self, which the person is unable to change. To

---

[181] On the subject of lived time and the illness experience, see Toombs (1990).

see this more clearly let us turn to yet another possibility of unhomelike being-in-the-world without illness.

To be locked up in prison for years and be exposed to horrible conditions is another example of unhomelikeness without illness. First, what is important to stress here is that it is the being-*in*-the-world of the person that counts as homelike or unhomelike in the phenomenological theory. To live in an environment means to interpret it and assign it meaning through feelings, thoughts and actions. Thus the lifeworld of phenomenology is not identical to *physical* surroundings, but is a meaning-pattern partly created by the person himself. Whether being locked up in prison results in unhomelike being-in-the-world depends partly on the world that the person is thrown into (its factical and cultural characteristics) and partly on the way he projects this given world of necessities and possibilities in his life. The prisoner might in some cases be able to adjust to a homelike existence behind the bars, although the conditions of imprisonment in most cases would offer too much resistance to allow this homelike reinterpretation of the subject's life project.

Second, as I stressed in the last section, the unhomelike being-in-the-world of illness is characterized by a fatal change in the meaning-structures, not only of the world, but of the *self*. Although self and world are always interconnected in a synthetic way through the being-*in*-the-world of the self, it is still possible to make a distinction between the person and the world he inhabits. In this way it is possible to distinguish between a more general homelessness of being-in-the-world, which is merely due to breakdowns in the 'external' tool-pattern, and the unhomelikeness of illness, which is always accompanied by a fatal change in the meaning-structure of the self. As we have seen, the parts of the meaning-pattern that are hardest to replace or reinterpret are the ones tied to our own embodiment. The lived body forms the centre of the self. The 'body-tools' are most fundamental for our transcendence, while the surrounding ones often are replaceable to a greater extent. The self, however, is not identical with the lived body, but also has other 'mental' characteristics, which are made lucid by the existentials of understanding and language. My distinction between breakdowns in the meaning-patterns of self versus world should be sufficient to counter the argument that the characterization of illness as unhomelike being-in-the-world threatens to encompass too many conditions that we would normally refer to as unhappiness rather than illness.

On the other hand, however, we have some examples that seem to be cases of illness, which do not readily fit into the pattern of unhomelikeness. I have dealt with the possible counterexamples of coma and mental illness without insight above. Another possible exception is trivial illness. Very mild illness – which does not necessitate a visit to the doctor or demand any medication or major rest – might not bear any clearly apparent character of unhomelikeness. One merely feels a little bit tired and might stay home from work a day or two in order to rest and recover. In this case the unhomelikeness stays in the background and is not striking to the subject – indeed, much as is the case in health, in which, as I have stressed above, a basic alienness of the body and the world is always present in a non-apparent way. This basic alienness is increased even in mild illness compared to in health, but perhaps not always enough to reach direct attention. As I wrote above it is tempting to include such kinds of illnesses in the normal rhythm of the healthy life if they do not occur too often.

In is obvious that my analysis of health is far from complete and calls for further investigation, reflection and development. But, in dealing with possible critiques of my musings on health, I would also like to stress the *kind* of analysis I am pursuing – a *phenomenological* analysis. Such an analysis endeavours to find and explicate the *meaning-structures* of phenomena. It is thus not strictly a matter of defining concepts through an analysis of language – drawing a border *between* the healthy and the ill as in the holistic theory – but rather a way of explicating and understanding two phenomena at the opposite ends of a spectrum through investigating their experienced characteristics. Health and illness, on the phenomenological level, must be seen as graded phenomena, since both homelikeness and unhomelikeness are always present to some degree in our being-in-the-world. The basic alienness of the homelikeness of health has its counterpart in a basic homelikeness in illness. No illness is severe enough to eradicate *all* sense of being-at-home in one's body and world. It indeed always remains *my* body and *my* world, no matter how unhomelike the being-in becomes.

The holistic and the phenomenological theories of health could thus be seen as two different formulations of a similar health theory on two different levels: the ontic level of states *in* the world (physical and mental dispositions to act and understand) and the ontological level of the *meaning* of these states. The lives of human beings, including the dimension of health and illness, are indeed permeated by meaning. Illness is thus always to be understood in terms of a certain form of *lack* of meaning, a breakdown of meaning in the ill person's being-in-the-world. The different existentials, as projective, inter-nested powers of the self and the tool-structures of the world guiding transcendence, help us conceptualize what this lack of meaning as unhomelikeness consists in.

We will carry on our analysis of different types of illnesses in the next part of this work, taking the step over to the medical clinic. The phenomenological outline we have developed will there prove to be of importance. The doctor's obvious focus upon diseases (maladies) as compromisers of health can be filled in and broadened through a theory that makes the positive perspective on health in medicine evident. To be ill means to be unhomelike and the doctor's task will be to *restore* health, to bring the patient back home, or as close to home as possible. As Heidegger told the doctors in Zollikon:

> The strange thing is that your whole profession operates in a negative area in the sense of being privative. You deal with illness. The physician asks the person who comes to him: What is amiss with you? (Wo fehlt es?) The ill person is not healthy. Health (Das Gesundsein, das Wohlbefinden) and attunement (das Sichbefinden) are not simply gone, but rather interfered with. Illness is not the pure negation of the healthy psychosomatic state. Illness is a privative phenomenon. In every privation lies the essential belonging to that which something is missing from. This looks like a triviality but it is incredibly important because your profession is operating in this very area. To the extent that you are dealing with illness you are really dealing with health in the sense of failing health and health to be recovered (1994, pp. 58-59).

PART 3

THE HERMENEUTICS OF MEDICINE

'Das Leben selbst legt sich aus. Es hat selbst hermeneutische Struktur.'[182]

We have now reached the third and last step on our journey towards a philosophy of medical practice. The first two parts of this work could to a large extent be read as self-sufficient studies dealing with the history of medical practice, on the one hand, and the theory of health, on the other. Nevertheless, they have, of course, also been intended to prepare the ground for this third part, dealing with medicine and hermeneutics. In what follows I will consequently draw upon discussions carried out and conclusions reached in Parts 1 and 2, as I attempt to sketch the outlines of a plausible philosophical theory of medical practice.

The questions I aim to answer in this book – namely, 'What is medicine?' and 'What is medical knowledge?' – will in the discussions to follow, be approached through the theory of hermeneutics. I have found it strategically, if not logically, necessary to proceed in the manner I have done in this work in order to make these questions, and the answers I will provide to them, more relevant and understandable. Thus the history of medical practice surveyed in Part 1 is needed in order to provide a framework for the activity in the clinic I will be explicating here. Philosophical questions are indeed always raised at specific moments in history, and in answering them we must pay close attention to our own historical situation and to the past history out of which it has evolved. As I have tried to show, the philosophical questions themselves have a history. Philosophers have since antiquity addressed the questions of medicine and health with variable intensity and ambitions. Although the clinical examples I make use of in this and the preceding part are contemporary, it is therefore nevertheless part of the argument I am developing here that medicine attains its meaning through its own history – through the permanence and changes that have characterized medical practice and the theories of medicine in the past. We will return to the issue of the relevance of a history of human practice later in discussing the relation between descriptive and normative aspects of our analysis.

My clinical examples are employed in an illustrative manner which serves to make a meaning-structure evident that I claim is present in Western medicine generally. This generality, as noted, carries a historical as well as a geographical extension. Not only is the way Western medicine is practised today relatively similar in

---

[182]Gadamer, *Wahrheit und Methode: Grundzüge einer philosophischen Hermeneutik* (1990, p. 230).

Sweden and in the United States (although there obviously also exist important differences depending mainly upon the economic organisation of health care), but the structure of medical practice has preserved certain features which were present from the beginning in ancient Greece. This permanence is exemplified, for instance, by the preservation of the Hippocratic oath. With this I obviously do not want to say that medicine of today is more or less the same as that carried out by the Asclepiads. My claim is only that a certain *basic structure* is present from the beginning and that this structure is expressed differently in different historical epochs. The kind of basic structure I am referring to is indeed the feature which leads us to use the same word for a certain phenomenon appearing at different times and at different places. In the case of medicine we have found this basic structure to be the attempt to help the ill in an interpretive meeting geared towards healing actions. Illness is as old as human beings and man has always tried to understand and fight it. This pattern of interpretation and action, as we have seen, took on a distinct structure in the practice of medicine in the West.

Although I understand my questions here to be historical in the sense that I have indicated above, my analysis not *only* is restricted to the very basic structure present through the entire history of Western medicine, but also aims at explicating the meaning-structure of medicine that is peculiar to the clinic today. Modern medical practice is thus what will be analysed in this part of my work, and the foregoing attempt to increase our understanding of this practice through mapping out its historical place indeed did not lead us to the conclusion that the way doctors heal today is the same as two thousand years ago. The aim of Part 1 was to make both permanence and change obvious, and as we saw in Part 2, theories of health today are very different from the ones held in the classical world, although the two theoretical traditions share some basic traits with each other. My phenomenological alternative for a theory of health, as well as my hermeneutic outline of medical practice, are therefore certainly products of our own time although I try to stay *attentive* to history.

The choice of Heidegger's phenomenology as the basic platform for my health theory is important in another way than obeying the general phenomenological injunction of staying true to experience itself – in this case the experiences of health and illness. As we will see, the choice will turn out to be strategically important when we move on to medicine and hermeneutics, since Heidegger's philosophy, as we noted above, is already a form of hermeneutics – a phenomenological hermeneutics. The step from the patient's more or less direct experience and understanding of his being-in-the-world to the doctor's understanding of this being-in-the-world is therefore one which we can make sense of in the concepts of Heidegger's philosophy. Although we will find the framework of *Sein und Zeit* insufficient here, the alternative that we will choose – the philosophical hermeneutics of Hans-Georg Gadamer – is best understood as an extension of the hermeneutics of facticity laid out in Heidegger's book.

In the last section of Part 1 we reached a provisional characterization of medicine through the work of Pellegrino and Thomasma. It read: '(Medicine is) a relation of mutual consent to effect individualized well-being by working in, with, and through the body' (1981, p. 80). I have devoted a whole part of this work to the goal of this relation – well-being understood as health. The choice of health as the goal of clinical practice might not seem obvious to everyone, despite my arguments in favour of this approach in Section 8 of the first part. Do not doctors deal with the suffering and integrity of persons in addition to their diseases, for instance? My answer here is – yes, but only with the suffering and threatened integrity related to the illnesses of these persons. Happiness and integrity in general cannot be the goals of medicine, since this would expand the activities of the clinic in an absurd and even threatening way. My interpretation of health and illness – as homelike and unhomelike ways of being-in-the-world, respectively – is central here, since it gives the two phenomena a relevance and importance which extends far beyond biology, but still shows them to stay within the limits of what can reasonably be seen as the mission of medical practice. That is, the choice of health as the goal of clinical practice, and the phenomenological interpretation of it as homelike being-in-the-world, prevent both an excessively wide and an excessively narrow view of the clinical enterprise, at the same time as it shows that medicine is not the only activity of importance, when it comes to understanding and relieving illness. Health, illness and medicine can thus form the objects of research and analysis in philosophy as well as other areas within the humanities and social sciences, as I have argued and showed from the start in this work. And even more importantly, health can obviously be facilitated through other encounters than the medical one – psychoanalysis is an obvious example which we will return to.

Although, in the section in which I presented the work of Pellegrino and Thomasma, we have chosen not to adopt the rendering of the medical meeting as a 'working in, with, and through the body', as this tends to exclude important aspects and kinds of the medical meeting, I think that we would do well in addressing the primacy that the biological organism and its diseases occupy in modern medicine here at the outset. The claim that what the doctor is trying to understand and change is the patient's entire being-in-the-world and not only his diseases, will otherwise run the risk of being misread as a simple idealistic fancy which does not stay true to what doctors really *do*. In other words, we have to falsify the claim that clinical medicine is essentially mere applied science (biology), while at the same time staying true to the everyday contemporary activities of the clinic.

I have already to some extent tried to lay out the connections between disease and illness in Part 2, but in order to make this relation even more lucid I will now move on to a century-old debate about different modes of knowledge in the sciences and the humanities – the debate concerning explanation and understanding. Does the doctor explain or understand? Or if he does both, how are these different modes of knowledge related to each other in medicine?

1. EXPLANATION AND UNDERSTANDING

The dichotomy of explanation (*Erklären*) and understanding (*Verstehen*) as two different ways of attaining knowledge in science (*Naturwissenschaft*) and the humanities (*Geisteswissenschaften*), respectively, was for the first time systematically formulated by Wilhelm Dilthey more than a century ago.[183] Let me say first of all that the difference between explanation and understanding can only be made intelligible if we use the two words in a rather specialized way. In an everyday sense, to explain and to understand are clearly *both* parts of science as well as of the humanities. One explains in order to understand something puzzling, in order to bring the strange back into the normal course of events.[184] Perhaps the dichotomy can best be understood as two different ways of explaining phenomena in science and the humanities, reserving the term understanding for the everyday use we have mapped out through Heidegger's philosophy – a basic and general aspect of our being-in-the-world.

Dilthey's idea was essentially that the way we come to know cultural objects is different from the way we get to know natural objects, since the former express meaning. As an example, one does not get to know a work of art through analysing its chemical constituents, but through being attentive to the meaning it expresses. This meaning is not restricted to the meaning which the artist thought, felt, or meant to communicate in creating the artwork, but is rather a meaningful *address* of the work itself which must be taken up and interpreted by the viewer. To understand in the humanities therefore consists in interpreting in order to find out what an artifact meant to its author *and* what it means to us today.

We will return to these issues in more detail later in introducing hermeneutics, but suffice it to say for now that the objects of the humanities are *intentive* in embodying meaning in the same way as human beings do in their being-in-the-world. Having a goal, a *telos*, as we have seen, is characteristic of human actions. Having an address is characteristic of cultural objects. Both of these features are aspects of meaning embodied in ways of varying complexity. The language of artifacts in communicating meaning is to be understood as an *articulation* of a being-in-the-world addressed to other human beings. Artifacts are therefore vehicles of meaning, which cannot be understood outside the horizon of human being-in-the-world. This is particularly true of the expressions which we sometimes call allegoric or symbolic. To say of a man that 'he has a heart' is not normally intended to refer to the organ which pumps the blood in his body, but to indicate that he is a sensitive and loving person. Actions and artifacts alike must consequently be understood within the practice of a cultural lifeworld.

The objects of science are different. These objects are not artifacts, but pieces of nature which we strive to understand the ways of, and in them we obviously cannot search for or find any *meaning* intended by any human or other being. At the moment in human history when nature ceased to be the creation of God embodying his

---

[183] Countless books have been written about this dichotomy and debate from a historical as well as from a philosophical point of view. Three works that I have found very useful are von Wright (1971), presenting a very clear analysis of the relation as well as giving the necessary historical references; Hiley et al. (1991), an anthology containing many valuable texts concerning the relations between science and hermeneutics (understanding); and Nerheim (1996), a book analysing the dichotomy and synthesis of explanation and understanding with an emphasis upon our main subject here – medicine and health care.

[184] See Taylor (1970).

purposes, nature was freed from all kinds of teleology and messages. As I remarked in Section 2 in the preceding part, the heart might be thought of as having a purposeful function in pumping blood in order to supply the tissues with nutrients and oxygen, but it does not carry out any purpos*i*ve behaviour in the sense of having a goal aimed at *intentionally*. Functional explanations in biology, explaining features of nature by ascribing certain goals to them, are thus to be thought of as quasi-teleological and not genuinely teleological modes of explanation (von Wright 1971, pp. 59-60).

One explains in order to better understand. Explanation in science, like the specialized form of understanding in the humanities, therefore cannot be thought of as something excluding everyday understanding, but is rather something carried out to facilitate and enhance this understanding. Science, like all other human activities, evolves out of a lifeworld where something attracts our curiosity and wonder. Nevertheless the kind of understanding which is facilitated through science, though embedded in a lifeworld of every-day actions, takes on a certain form when it strives to understand nature. Natural events are understood not only in an everyday sense of being intelligible; they are also understood through a certain form of deductive inference called scientific explanation. Specifying certain premises we conclude that the phenomenon we want to explain follows logically. I wake up one morning and find that the street is wet. I wonder why. The explanation of this event, presented to me by a friend, has the following form: Premise A. It rained last night. Premise B. Every time it rains the street gets wet. Therefore: The street is now wet. Although this explanation is put in a far too ordinary and unspecified way to count as scientific, the basic logical form of a scientific explanation is present in it.[185] The premises consist of A – an antecedent (x) to the state (y) I want to explain – and B – a law; that is, a statement that says that *every time* x happens y will also happen. In order to make the form of scientific explanation clearer, to highlight some of its problems, and to connect it to everyday understanding, I will now proceed with one of the clinical examples I introduced in Part 2 – Peter in the grip of a bad cold.[186]

The next day – Tuesday – Peter felt equally bad. He decided to stay home from work, since he could not bear the thought of being in the book shop another stressful day. The headache was not as severe today as yesterday, but his throat was still very sore and he felt warm as if he had a slight fever. His joints and muscles felt stiff and ached when he tried to move. Since he felt sleepy he stayed in bed all day and tried to drink as much as possible. Eating was hard because of his swollen throat. On

---

[185] See von Wright (1971) and Nerheim (1996) for a detailed formulation of the pattern of scientific explanation and the many problems it gives rise to. Note that I am here restricting myself to causal explanations, since they represent the type of explanation which is most important in medicine. That is, the nomo-thetic premise is always a *causal* law in the examples I am interested in.

[186] I intend 'cold' here to have an everyday meaning, which is also quite sensible if one considers the etymology of the word. That is, by saying that Peter has a bad cold I do not stipulate anything about the aetiology of his illness, by saying, for example, that a specific virus or bacterium is causally responsible for his ailments.

Wednesday the symptoms were still there and Peter began to worry. This was probably not only a regular cold, but something which called for medical attention. The pain relievers did not do him much good and he felt really weak. One of the reasons for this was probably the fact that he had not been able to eat much during the last two days. Peter phoned his doctor. In hoarse, faint voice he spoke to the secretary and arranged for an appointment for the same afternoon. Peter took a taxi to the health-care centre, which was not very far away, and sat down in the waiting room. Dr. X was with him after a short wait and invited him to come into her office. She asked him what was the matter. Peter told her what he had felt like the last couple of days and that he thought that his condition called for medication. Dr. X asked some questions about his present situation. Peter mentioned the stressful situation in the bookshop and she asked if he had been working too much. Maybe it was time for a break? Had he felt like this on any earlier occasion this year? Peter answered that he had been feeling a bit tired lately because of his work and some 'personal' problems with his family. He did not feel that it was necessary to go into that here though, since this time it felt different and was certainly a medical and not a social problem. Worse even than the flu he had been taken ill with last year. Dr. X asked him if he knew whether anyone he had met lately had suffered from tonsillitis or epiglottitis – streptococcal infection. Peter could not recall anyone. Dr. X then performed a physical examination. She looked into Peter's throat, felt if his lymph nodes were swollen and listened to his lungs and heart with the stethoscope. She took his temperature which showed him to have a slight fever: 38.5°C. Finally she did a streptococcal antigen test with a throat swab, which gives a very fast result – one only has to wait for about five minutes. This test proved to be positive. Streptococci were present in Peter's throat and, as Dr. X told Peter, they were probably responsible for the infection. She was therefore going to give him penicillin. Peter was told to take the medicine three times a day for a week. If he did not get better he should come back. He was also told to stay home from work as long as he had a fever and sore throat.

This seems to be a fairly typical example of a modern clinical encounter. The patient comes to the doctor because he thinks that the way his life has changed character lately – in the terms of the health theory I have developed, we would say the way his being-in-the-world has taken on an unhomelike character lately – has a 'medical' reason. That is, he thinks that the doctor can help in bringing relief and cure. The doctor, searching for signs of different diseases, tries to find out why the patient feels like he does, and this involves trying to find the cause of the patient's illness. Through the dialogue with the patient and the physical examination she develops a hypothesis – streptococcal infection – and with the lab test she finally puts the hypothesis on trial and finds it to be confirmed or refuted. If the hypothesis is refuted, she will proceed and try to find some other hypothesis which can be tested. If it is confirmed, she will goe on to prescribe medication which is meant to eliminate the cause of the illness (the streptococci) and thus terminate the disease.

It is mainly the final steps of this activity – the lab test with its resemblance to scientific experiments and the powerful cure through a biochemical agent – which have given rise to the thought that medicine today is essentially applied biology. The preceding dialogue and meeting between two persons, in which the doctor expresses care and tries to help through interpretative thinking, is thought to be less essential. Possibly it is valued in terms of the generation of hypotheses which can be put to test – another typical feature of scientific activity. Let us now problematize and challenge this straight-forward picture by carrying the analysis a few steps further.

The hypothesis that Dr. X tests can be put like this: streptococci are causally responsible for Peter's sore throat. The test can be thought of as an empirical verification of a causal inference of the type, 'If streptococci are present on the throat swab it will turn red when put in the test tube'.[187] The reason it turns red is some causal relation – the streptococci (and only streptococci) will change the colour of the swab. The doctor therefore predicts that if she puts a culture from Peter's throat on the swab it will turn red. In this example the test is positive and the hypothesis is therefore confirmed.

As we can see, tests of hypotheses by way of predictions, which are generated deductively and then checked empirically, have a similar structure to scientific explanations. Explanations however go 'backwards' in time and not forward like hypothesis testing. Explanation generally comes after testing; a causal law, however, is involved in a similar way. That which we want to explain in this example is Peter's sore throat (his illness), and the explanation looks like this: Premises: A. Streptococci are present in Peter's throat. B. Every time streptococci are present in the throat their presence is accompanied by infection (soreness). Therefore: Peter has a sore throat.

But this explanation clearly cannot be right. The reason for this is that premise B is false. There is known to exist a 'carrier state' in which streptococci are present in the throat but in which their presence is not accompanied by infection.[188] Streptococci are not the only cause of sore throat, nor are they a sufficient cause of streptococcal infection.[189] So even if the test comes out positive one cannot be sure that the streptococci are really responsible for the infection.

The hypothesis Dr. X is really testing is accordingly not 'streptococci are causally responsible for Peter's sore throat', but 'streptococci are present on the throat swab'. This hypothesis could also be wrong even if the test is positive, however, since every lab test is known to result in a certain percentage of false confirmations, as well as false refutations. This is the reason why one generally performs two throat swab tests, to minimize the risk of false results. Let us assume that a certain virus is in fact responsible for Peter's sore throat, but that streptococci are simultaneously

---

[187] I here alter and simplify the circumstances – what the test really tests for are antigenes and not the bacteria themselves. But this is not essential to my analysis here.

[188] My chief source for the diagnosis of sore throat is McWhinney (1989), Chapter 11.

[189] For further analysis of the concept of causality in medicine, see King (1978) and the papers in Nordenfelt and Lindahl (1984).

present there. Or that streptococci and viruses are both responsible for his sore throat. In any of these two cases it might well happen that the penicillin will not do Peter any good even though the lab test was positive. And there is also the possibility that he will actually get well while taking the penicillin, but on account of 'natural recovery' and not on account of the penicillin.[190]

So what should the explanation of Peter's illness in this case look like? The causal law could of course be put in terms of probability: for example, 'In 75% of the cases in which streptococci are found in the throat their presence is accompanied by streptococcal infection'. But then we would no longer be dealing with a causal necessity of the sort, '*Every time* streptococci are present in the throat they are accompanied by streptococcal infection'; thus the explanation would have lost its explanatory power. The laws of probability can be used to make predictions of varying exactitude, but they are of no use to us when we seek an explanation. So we find that testing is a less certain and explanation a more complex procedure than we initially thought them to be.

To explain, as Georg Henrik von Wright puts it, is always a matter of isolating a causal system through human action (1971, p. 60 ff.). We have to choose what to look for and when. And we have to choose limited factors during a short time span, since the possible causal networks are unlimited. Indeed in every case of causal relations, the efficient cause (streptococci) is not the *only* cause of the effect in question. We cannot, however, observe in a scientific manner every cell and micro-organism in Peter's throat at the same time. And whether the streptococci we find there really are the causal antecedents of the state of infection or not, they clearly have a previous causal history of their own. How should this history be thought of? Will we not have to map it out in order to provide a true explanation of why Peter is ill? This history will clearly be related to Peter's entire physiology, the way it has been working lately and the environments it has been present in. And this in turn will have a great deal to do with the way Peter has been acting, thinking and feeling lately. This means that the history of the streptococci is ultimately related to Peter's being-in-the-world. By the same token, the unhomelikeness he is experiencing presently could have a great deal to do with the streptococci, if they are responsible for the soreness of his throat.

But on the phenomenological level of being-in-the-world we can no longer talk about causal relations and explanations in the strict scientific sense. Meaning is not analysable in the scientific terms of causal explanation, but depends on the experience and interpretation of the subject involved, in this case Peter. To be-in-the-world is not to be a closed causal system. Rather, closed causal systems, as von Wright points out, are chosen and isolated on the basis of a being-in-the-world, with the ambition to better understand and manipulate certain aspects of this world. As I pointed out in Part 2, Section 9, it is however possible to talk about a more basic, everyday

---

[190] I am, of course, simplifying: obviously, no cure achieves its effect in the absence of the organism's own recovery. What I mean here is simply that the penicillin does not contribute to the effects of these self-healing processes.

causality on the phenomenological level.[191] Bacteria and viruses of sufficient sort and number will indeed in every case lead to infection, and an infected throat is typically lived in a painful way. There is certainly a limit to the variance of how different states of the body and the world around us can be lived and interpreted. The suffering might vary; the sore throat, for instance, can still be lived and interpreted in a number of different ways, but it is probably impossible not to notice it at all. Thus a certain form of counterfactual causal pattern can be discerned in our phenomenological analysis. To take an extreme example: the pain you will experience if I chop off one of your fingers would not have come into existence if I had abstained from doing this. You could of course have suffered a number of other forms of experiences depending on the state of your body and the world and your way of interpreting these states in your lived experience, but you would not have suffered *that* kind of experience. On the other hand, nothing guarantees that chopping off another one of your fingers at a later point will release exactly the same kind of experience as last time, just as it might not lead to exactly the same kind of experience in the case of another victim. But the three experiences would probably be similar in some important aspects, and they are counterfactually related to the chopping off of fingers. The states of the body and world thus set important limits for our way of giving meaning to existence. But, as will become obvious in less extreme examples than the chopping off of fingers, they do not determine the meaningful experience of the person in any way that is possible to predict comprehensively and in detail by way of biomedical analysis. Phenomenological and hermeneutical analysis, which focus upon the meaning-structure of *lived* experience directly and not via causes, are here helpful tools in making sense of the being-in-the-world of illness.

The adherent of the view that clinical medicine is applied biology will here perhaps say that medical science may not be capable of providing perfect and complete explanations, but that biological knowledge can still be used to diagnose, predict and finally bring about cure. The test and the drug in the example involving Peter above are clearly the results of biological research, and they provide a successful way to diagnosis and cure in cases of sore throat, and this is after all what really matters. Indeed, but then the 'biologist' is no longer really saying that clinical medicine is applied biology, but that biochemistry is a highly valuable tool in the clinical encounter in the process of healing. This is a view that I would immediately endorse, as I think any sensible person living in our modern society should do. The biological knowledge could of course also be misused, and the medicine-as-applied-biology thesis would run the risk of supporting precisely such a misuse, since it tends to block out other features of medical practice than the biological as being 'unscientific'. If unscientific here means 'non-biological', the biologist would of course be right; but it seems, on the contrary, that the term is often used to mean 'unimportant', and here he is clearly wrong. Let us, in order to see why, proceed with our clinical example.

---

[191] The predominant Hempelian covering-law model of explanation, on which I base my presentation above, has indeed been called into question in the philosophy of science itself. Some of this criticism, for instance regarding counterfactuals, is of importance to my phenomenological points in this section. See for instance Needham (1988), Chapters 5 and 6.

Peter did not get well from taking the penicillin. He felt some relief after three days and tried to go back to work, but was then again plagued with the symptoms of headache, muscle and joint pain, fatigue and fever. His throat felt a little bit better, but he still had problems swallowing. He could not concentrate on the work and felt tired and lethargic. He went back to Dr. X rather frustrated and angry. Why did the penicillin not work? What was wrong with him? Why did he feel like he did at work? Peter and Dr. X had a rather long talk about his symptoms and his feelings and thoughts about what was wrong. Dr. X also asked him if he had taken the medication as prescribed and reproached him for going back to work too early. She then performed a renewed and more detailed physical examination looking into his throat and ears, listening to his lungs and heart and palpating his tender lymph nodes and muscles. She took some blood samples to send away for tests and she also took a couple of new cultures from his throat. Dr. X wrote a certificate for Peter to inform his employer that he was ill and should remain home the following week. She also told him to relax and try to rest to recover. It was probably nothing serious but just an indication that he had worked too much and needed some time off. She finally told Peter that they would get the test results within five days and that he was to come back then for a new consultation.

Peter came back to see Dr. X five days later not feeling any better. Dr. X had to tell Peter that the test-results were all negative. He did not have a streptococcal infection, so either the previous test result had been wrong or the bacteria were not responsible for his illness. The tests for Epstein-Barr virus (mononucleosis) as well as other viruses, bacteria and toxoplasma were also negative. Thus she had been unable to identify the cause of Peter's ailments, but Peter of course was still feeling as ill as before, if not worse. What was really the matter with him? Did he have cancer, AIDS or some other life-threatening disease? The doctor tried to calm him down by saying that his symptoms were not necessarily typical for any of these syndromes. However, she wanted to send Peter to a specialist, an oncologist, to rule out the possibility of lymphoma, and she also thought it was sensible to perform a test for HIV if Peter had never had one done before. After seeing several specialists in the fields of oncology, endocrinology, neurology and otorhinolaryngology, Peter was finally told that what he suffered from was called chronic fatigue syndrome. It is defined as severe fatigue accompanied by a cluster of symptoms – such as sore throat, tender lymph nodes, headaches, muscle and joint pain, impaired concentration – and no cause or cure for the illness is presently known. Peter now had a name for his suffering. Indeed it was better than nothing at all proving to some extent to others that he was not just a malingerer. But it did not make him better. Some of the drugs which Dr. X and others prescribed for him, such as strong pain relievers, muscle relaxers and anti-inflammatory medication, helped to relieve the symptoms somewhat, but they did not by any means make him well again. He could not go back to work and stayed home, becoming inactive and depressed. Dr. X tried to work together with him on his present life situation, suggesting different diets and exercise programs. She also asked about his relations to family and friends and how they had reacted to what he was going through. Did they understand him? Did he get any help from them? What about his former colleagues at work? Did they care? And did he miss his work much? She tried to get him to think about another type of job, since the one in the bookshop was obviously too physically demanding for him at the moment. They also discussed ongoing research and the possibility of finding a cause and cure in the future for what he suffered from. Peter was also told that many CFS patients had recovered spontaneously and that his condition was very much up to himself. What mattered was his attitude toward the illness and toward the things he could do to be able to live better with it.[192]

My point with this example is not to invoke a particular disease – chronic fatigue syndrome – which will forever resist scientific explanation. Maybe there exists a single, efficient agent which is causally responsible for the ailments everyone diagnosed with CFS is suffering from. It is not impossible, though rather unlikely. We might for instance be dealing with an autoimmune disease, which in the future we will be able to better explain and maybe even cure. Let us hope so. My point is rather that even if this proves to be the case, situations will continue to arise in which doctors are unable to find a causal explanation for their patients' ill health.[193] Illness is a chaotic phenomenon, on which science strives to impose causal order. But since illness – according to the argument of this study – cannot be understood exclusively on the biological level, as disease, it will probably resist this process to the bitter end.[194]

Since the Second World War we have gradually come to the insight that medicine will not find a cure or prevention for every type of illness as it seemed to do with most infectious diseases. Chronic illness has come to the focus of attention. Doctors, as we will see later, are of course still able to do a great deal for chronically ill patients to make their lives better – their being-in-the-world more homelike – although they cannot cure them. Another group of patients that will stand out increasingly, as the biological aspect of medicine beomes more and more fine-tuned and advanced, are those with whom nothing 'medically' wrong can be found. Those patients within this group who are not malingerers – and they will surely be the overwhelming majority – are ill even if they are not diseased. Their being-in-the-world is very unhomelike, and it will come to be so to an even larger extent if doctors do not take them and their problems seriously.

---

[192]My chief source for information about chronic fatigue syndrome is Fisher (1997).

[193]Some years ago researchers indeed *thought* that they had found the cause of CFS – Epstein-Barr virus – but this hypothesis proved to be false. The two groups suffering from Epstein-Barr and CFS did not overlap.

[194]Clinical medicine is *fallible* through and through. Doctors will always make mistakes, and these mistakes not only stem from incomplete biomedical knowledge, but depend on the nature of the very activity and the type of phenomena that they are dealing with. Thus every experienced clinician knows the golden rule of never taking anything for granted since *this* time with *this* patient it might always be different than the last time. See Gorovitz and MacIntyre (1976).

In such cases a basic feature of the clinical encounter – which is always present – is made visible in a sharper way. Even if the doctor cannot explain why these patients are ill he can clearly *understand* them. Dr. X can understand Peter's being-in-the-world and the way it has changed. She can try to relate this to the processes of his organism on a biomedical level. She can also, even if she with the aid of this understanding is unable to produce any scientific hypothesis which can lead to cure, meet Peter in this understanding and show that she cares for him and is interested in trying to make his situation better. The types of symptom-relieving drugs that she can give him are dependent upon her biological knowledge about Peter's organism *and* upon her understanding of his experiences on a lifeworld level. Explanation and understanding are here related to each other in a mutual way. Finally, the understanding in this case and many others is essential, because with the help of it, Dr. X can try to change some circumstances in Peter's being-in-the-world in order to make it more homelike. These actions are not primarily biomedical, but lifeworld-oriented. I am thinking about diet and exercise, but even more about Peter's work situation, his social network and the way he feels and thinks about his life – his hopes or desperation for the future.

We need to say more about understanding and the types of understanding we sometimes call interpretation or hermeneutics in order to carry on this analysis of the clinical encounter. What we can say at this point is that scientific explanation and the biological techniques for diagnosis, prognosis and cure clearly are anchored in a type of dialogic understanding forming the core mode of clinical medicine.

2. HERMENEUTICS – THE CHOICE OF GADAMER

Richard Palmer has traced the roots of hermeneutics in his book with the same title:

> The Greek word *hermeios* referred to the priest at the Delphic oracle. This word and the more common verb *hermeneuein* and noun *hermeneia* point back to the wing-footed messenger-god Hermes, from whose name the words are apparently derived (or vice versa?). Significantly, Hermes is associated with the function of transmuting what is beyond human understanding into a form that human intelligence can grasp. The various forms of the word suggest the process of bringing a thing or situation from unintelligibility to understanding. The Greeks credited Hermes with the discovery of language and writing – the tools which human understanding employs to grasp meaning and convey it to others (1969, p. 13).

Keeping this etymology in mind one can easily understand why hermeneutics started off as a part of theology referring to the principles of biblical interpretation. The holy texts needed to be deciphered in order to make full sense to the reader, and the manuals of interpretation developed in order to do this were referred to as hermeneutics. We are here able to trace one meaning of the word hermeneutics, which is still prevalent today in theology and also in other disciplines such as law and literature: methodology of interpretation. These methodologies naturally assume different forms depending upon which discipline one is working in. They also depend upon the ambitions and theoretical background of the interpreter, and they can thus generate different interpretations of the same text. Accordingly, in the interpretation of texts and other artifacts, there often arises a *conflict* between different interpretations, in which it is hard to settle which is the correct one. The settlement of this conflict clearly depends on what one means by 'correct' here; but let us at this point note that it is exactly this seemingly insoluble battle of different interpretations in the humanities that has generated a certain distrust and contempt from the side of the sciences, in which one claims to aim for objective truth and not simply for different opinions.

In the beginning of the nineteenth century – at the same time as modern scientific medicine made its early breakthroughs – a philosopher of religion, Friedrich Schleiermacher, attempted to develop a *general* hermeneutics – that is, a hermeneutics that would not be limited to a certain discipline or doctrine, but give the general rules of all interpretation. Schleiermacher's hermeneutics took off in two complementary main directions, one focusing upon the *language* of the text one is reading, and the other on empathy (*Einfühlung*) – the attempt to find out what the *author* of a document meant by trying to imagine oneself in his position. Wilhelm Dilthey, as we have seen above, adopted the hermeneutics of Schleiermacher and tried to articulate it as the method of the humanities dealing with the meaning of cultural objects in contrast to objects of nature.

The idea of hermeneutics as a method peculiar to the humanities in contrast to the sciences found sympathy in many different humanistic disciplines and was used as a theoretical basis for developing different interpretive manuals, which described methods for uncovering the intention of the author of a text (artifact) or the meaning of the text itself freed from the intentions of its author. In both these cases, however, one is dealing with hermeneutics as different *methods* for uncovering hidden meaning in artifacts through employing knowledge peculiar to the humanities in contrast to the sciences. Let me at this point say that this is *not the kind of hermeneutics* I claim is present in clinical practice. Patients are not pieces of literature, although, as we shall see, they share some important modes with the ontology of texts in their being-in-the-world. This similarity is in fact the reason why doctors can learn and improve their practice through the reading of novels and poetry. The knowledge they gain from this reading, however, is not primarily a knowledge of how texts work, but rather a knowledge about human beings and their ways of being-in-the-world.

The kind of hermeneutics which I will try to show is basic to clinical practice is the very same kind that Heidegger developed as the existential of *understanding* being-in-the-world in *Sein und Zeit*. Medical practice is to be understood as a special form of understanding, which is identical with neither explanation in science nor interpretation in the humanities. Hermeneutics is here an ontological and not a methodological concept; that is, hermeneutics is not taken as a method, but as a basic aspect of life. *Dasein* understands itself and its world in being thrown into a network of meanings referred to as its being-in-the-world. We will not here repeat the introduction to Heidegger's philosophy we gave in Section 6 of Part 2, but only remind the reader that this understanding being-in-the-world is always embodied and attuned as well as in the process of articulating itself. Articulation (*Rede*) in its most explicit form takes on the mode of being of language, as Heidegger writes in *Sein und Zeit*.

Spoken discourse, however, can also be fixed in the form of texts, which are then to be read and understood by others. Understanding here takes on a rather indirect form compared to the more immediate understanding of, for example, everyday practical activities, but the activity of reading is still tied to the same kind of being-in that is played out in the meaning-structure of the world. Hermeneutics is thus not only and not primarily a methodology for text-reading, but the basic aspect of life. To be – to exist – means to understand.

The phenomenology of being-in-the-world in Heidegger's philosophy turned out to be a hermeneutics, since the way self-understanding is performed by the everyday *Dasein* demands *uncovering*, a dismantling authentic interpretation.[195] In Part 2, Section 6, I related this necessity of systematical interpretation to the *entanglement* of inauthentic existence (*Verfallensein*), with its tendency to identify human being with an object similar to natural things lacking being-in-the-world. Authentic self-understanding, however, can not only rest on an immediate experience – the moment of anxiety – but must also develop in interpretation through language in dialogue with others. Heidegger makes clear in *Sein und Zeit* that *Dasein* is to be thought of primarily as a being with others (*Mitdasein*) (1986, p. 113 ff.). In the ensuing analysis, however, he strongly links this *a priori* trait of human existence to the inauthentic being-together of 'the they' (*das Man*), and thereby threatens to identify being-with-others with *Verfallensein*. Although there is no necessity for such an identification in *Sein und Zeit*, the emphasis on authentic understanding as a solitary phenomenon in contrast to the empty and distortive talk of the they (*Gerede*) makes his hermeneutics insufficient for developing the hermeneutics of dialogue, which I think is present in clinical medicine. Instead we will now turn to a philosopher who has developed Heidegger's hermeneutical phenomenology in the direction of a hermeneutics of being together with others: Hans-Georg Gadamer.

At first sight Gadamer's *magnum opus*, published originally in 1960 – *Wahrheit und Methode: Grundzüge einer philosophischen Hermeneutik* – might seem rather remote from the phenomenology of being-in-the-world Heidegger is working out in *Sein und Zeit*. Gadamer's book is divided into three parts; the first and second parts, which are by all means the most extensive ones, deal with the work of art and with interpretation in the humanities, respectively. The third part of *Wahrheit und Methode*, on the ontology of language, can be read as an articulation of the special pattern of understanding which Gadamer has found to be present in these disciplines.[196] As many readers have remarked, however, the title of the book should properly read 'Truth or Method' and not 'Truth and Method', since the methodological concept of hermeneutics we have introduced above with Schleiermacher and

---

[195] As Dekkers writes, the kind of understanding we normally refer to as hermeneutical is indeed the one which aims at uncovering something that is not obvious (1998, p. 278). Hermeneutics is dismantling of the 'hidden', in the sense of an uncovering that demands a focused and systematical kind of interpretation.

[196] As Gadamer acknowledges himself, however, the way of reading *Wahrheit und Methode* as an extension of the phenomenological hermeneutics of *Sein und Zeit*, which I attempt to make lucid here, is clearly the most accurate one (1990, p. 264 ff.). On this issue see also, for instance, Hoy (1993).

Dilthey is precisely the one Gadamer is trying to go beyond. Truth in *Wahrheit und Methode* is meant as a basic experience of being together with others in and through language and not as a criterion for correct interpretation. This is exactly in line with Heidegger's interpretation of truth as *a-letheia* in *Sein und Zeit*; that is, truth as an openness or disclosedness (*Erschlossenheit*) of *Dasein* for the world of meaning in which things can be found and articulated *as* such and such things (1986, p. 212 ff.). Thus, for a sentence to describe, to correspond to, a state of the world, this prior dismantling of the world as meaningful is necessary.

Truth in Gadamer's philosophy is, however, primarily to be understood as openness for the other and *his* world and not only for *my own* world. The difference, from Heidegger's point of view, would not be decisive because the world of the other is also mine – we share the same world in our being-together. Still, I think the emphasis on the world of the *other* in Gadamer's hermeneutics is important, because it brings out an aspect of being-in-the-world – an aspect that we have dealt with extensively in Part 2 in discussing health – in a new way: namely, the *alienness* of the world. As we noted in Part 2, Section 7, homelike, healthy being-in-the-world also carries with it a basic unfamiliarity, which is related to the otherness of the world and of the body (as a part of the world). This otherness becomes overwhelming and uncanny in illness in the form of the unhomelikeness of an understanding which fails to transcend in a coherent way. However, although being together with others in the world carries with it uncertainty, this alienness is not an otherness that generally makes existence unhomelike for human beings. It could do so if intersubjective understanding failed to take place – mental illness would be the paradigmatic example here; but the otherness of the other in being-together with him is generally something that, on the contrary, makes my existence homelike – precisely in understanding and being understood by the *other*. Indeed, to be at home rarely means to be alone, but rather, on the contrary, to be with others. It means to be *together* with others, sharing understanding through language and attunement.

Language in Gadamer's philosophy is emphasized as the key mode of this being together with others. The form of language he concentrates his analysis upon in *Wahrheit und Methode* is not, however, the spoken dialogue, but the reading of literature and other texts of the past. Historical texts are separated from us by a temporal distance which makes the incarnated meaning present in them more difficult to dismantle. Indeed, what does it mean to uncover the meaning of such a text? When we try to understand a historical document, our lifeworld – our horizon of meaning – is not identical with the lifeworld of the author of the document. Nevertheless, our horizons are not totally separated, but distantly united through the *Wirkungsgeschichte* – history of effects – of the document (1990, p. 305 ff.). It is consequently possible to bring the horizons closer together and reach an understanding of the document (*Horizontverschmelzung* – fusion of horizons). Gadamer is here not only referring to the necessity of learning the foreign language of the document; to understand what the words meant one must also know their historical context in the lifeworld of the person who wrote the document.

It is important to stress here that, for Gadamer, this meeting or 'fusion' of horizons is not synonymous with reaching the *same* understanding of the document as that of the person who wrote it. The distance that separates and, at the same time, unites the horizons is always a *productive* distance in the sense that we will understand the document from our point of view, with the *Vorurteile* – prejudgements – of our time (Gadamer 1990, p. 281 ff.). Interpretation, according to Gadamer, is not, however, lawless and arbitrary since we try to *meet* the horizon of the text – we submit to its authority; but at the same time we can only understand from our own point of view, and, consequently, will always reach a *different*, ideally richer, understanding of the text than the understanding reached by the author and the readers of its time.

The well-known concept of the hermeneutic circle is powerfully present here. The reader must always articulate his understanding within the horizon of his own situation: 'prejudgements' are a necessity for understanding, since interpretation is always guided by a pre-understanding of being-in-the-world. No understanding can start from scratch; understanding always evolves out of a certain historical situation. However, the circle also encompasses the horizon of the *object* – the text – since the text must be anchored within the horizon – the lifeworld – to which it belongs. Not only does every sentence of the text acquire its meaning from the whole text and vice versa (the common, more limited presentation of the hermeneutic circle), but the text itself has a horizon from within which its meaning is determined. This horizon must finally be thought of as distantly connected to the horizon of the reader; the two horizons are part of the same 'super-horizon' (1990, p. 309). That the horizons are united, belong together, although they are different, means that reading is ultimately thought of as a being-together-with-the-text, articulating difference from which togetherness in understanding can evolve (1990, p. 391).

How will it be possible to find within Gadamer's hermeneutics the essential structure of clinical practice? It seems as though his interests lie in the understanding that takes place in the humanities rather than within medicine. Before I answer this question, we should take a look at how others in various ways have proposed a role for hermeneutics in medicine. My own proposal will thereby emerge with greater sharpness and, I hope, plausibility.

3. MEDICINE AND HERMENEUTICS

To my knowledge, the first investigator to suggest that clinical practice is essentially hermeneutical was Stephen Daniel in 1986.[197] The articles and books which have

---

[197] In the survey that follows it is not my ambition to mention every paper or book which after Daniel's in some way has dealt with hermeneutics in medicine. It is, however, my aim to cover most of the ground, and I certainly hope that I have found every study that would be of relevance for my own way of approaching the subject of medicine and hermeneutics. As we have already seen in Part 1, many authors have talked about *interpretation* in medicine before Daniel suggested the more specific term 'hermeneutics'. In the end everything comes down to what one means by 'interpretation' or 'hermeneutics', which I indeed hope to make clear regarding my own proposal. Also, I should point out, that the term 'herme-

subsequently been published on the connections between medicine and hermeneutics add up to a small but very heterogeneous group. To find some system in the various proposals for how and to what end hermeneutics is or should be used in medical practice and the philosophy of medicine, I will here in a somewhat crude way organize the literature in three different groups: a first group centred around hermeneutics as an interpretive guide to different texts written and read in the clinic; a second suggesting hermeneutics as being of significance to medical ethics; and finally, a group of studies exploring hermeneutics as a model of the clinical activity itself – this is obviously the type of studies I am particularly interested in here.

The governing idea of the first group of studies is that hermeneutics could be used in order to interpret different texts that are written and read in the clinic.[198] This suggestion might not seem very revolutionary, given that hermeneutics, as we have explored above, has from the beginning been seen as the method of interpreting texts. If the Bible, works of literature, historical and legal documents can be the subject of hermeneutics, why not the medical chart or case report? The positivistic dream of a scientific language free from all interpretive difficulties is certainly not the reality of the clinic. Per Sundström, in 1987, in the study *Icons of Disease*, interpreted extracts from a medical textbook in order to show that diseases are complex, integral clinical conceptions – what he calls 'icons of disease' – rather than physiological states or processes referred to in a direct way. Since Sundström's aim with the interpretation of the textbook is to point to a hermeneutic structure of the clinical activity itself, it is certainly in a way unfair to restrict the scope of his study to a hermeneutics of the medical textbook. I will return to his book later on.

Suzanne Poirier and Daniel Brauner have, in an article from 1990, applied literary, hermeneutic methods to read the medical chart, and Kathryn Montgomery Hunter, in *Doctor's Stories* (1991), shows in a detailed way how different medical documents, such as chart, case report and case study, have a peculiar Sherlock Holmesian narrative structure. To tell a story by separating the significant facts from the insignificant, and to look for clues with a suspicious eye for the threatening as well as the treatable in developing hypotheses, seem to belong to all these genres. The medical texts are organized by a distinct type of *medical* thinking, which is learnt on the long and laborious way to becoming a good clinician. The ethnographic studies by Byron Good, carried out in Harvard Medical School, which we encountered in Part 1, Section 7, of this work, showed the powerful potential of this kind of thinking, as well as the danger of a silencing of the voices of the patients and their experi-

---

neutics' has been used by authors before Daniel in discussing paradigms restricted to *psychiatry*, mainly related to psychotherapy. See Wulff et al. (1986), Chapter 9.

[198] In addition to the works I mention here, there are also studies of medical biographies (patients who tell about their illness) using hermeneutical methods. This type of studies will not be dealt with in this survey, since these biographies are not strictly texts written *in* the clinic. They are not *medical* texts in this sense, but rather literary works. This is of course not to say that the patient's narrative is devoid of interest to a hermeneutics of medicine – as we will see in what follows, it is, on the contrary, highly significant. I will not, however, in this survey, deal directly with studies of written patient narratives.

ences and stories of their illnesses in these medical matrices. The patient's voice indeed rarely surfaces in the texts of the clinic in any direct way.

The second group of studies I will discuss here concerns medical ethics. Hermeneutics has been suggested to be a valuable tool for interpreting and judging clinical situations from an ethical point of view. Whether the point is that hermeneutics can be used in applying and balancing different ethical principles in the clinical situation (Thomasma 1994), or that a hermeneutic understanding of the clinical enterprise itself can guide ethical thinking (Carson 1990; ten Have 1994), these studies focus upon the way to the right or good action in difficult situations of medical practice.[199] My focus in this study is ontological and epistemological, rather than ethical. However, as I will reflect upon later in the closing sections of this part, these questions are clearly interrelated. The normative is in my view an unavoidable aspect of an ontological analysis of a human practice such as medicine. It is, however, too early to deal with the questions of good and right in medicine. First we have to develop the hermeneutic theory in some more detail. Let us now take a look at the third group of studies, which suggest the clinical enterprise itself to be a kind of hermeneutics.

Daniel, in the article mentioned above, claims that the patient himself is to be viewed as a text: 'I intend to show that the reader's experience of a poem, short story, or novel is similar to the physician's encounter with a patient' (1986, p. 195). Daniel then suggests interpretive models from theology, in which a text is understood on different levels as saying different things. The Bible can be understood literally and on different symbolic levels and so, Daniel claims, can the patient. The literal meaning of the patient would be the pure facts of his body and story, which are then interpreted on different symbolic levels – diagnostically, prognostically and practically – by the physician. It is, however, hard to understand in what sense these interpretations would be specifically *textual*, let alone literal, allegorical, moral or anagogical, in the way that Daniel claims.

Edward Gogel and James Terry, in an article from 1987, suggest literary methods and metaphorical readings in the humanities to be similar to what takes place in the interpretive meeting of clinical practice. But are these two types of activities really similar? Do doctors approach their patients as poems and novels and read them as texts of literature? As I have already suggested above, I do not think this is the case, although literary texts indeed share some aspects with everyday human being-in-the-world – literature consists in an articulation and sedimentation of such meaning in a specific situation. Texts, just as persons – since they are written by persons – belong to a lifeworld with a horizon of meaning in the context of which they must be understood. But to understand a person's being-in-the-world is not the same thing as understanding a text. The understanding of the patient, I therefore conclude, does not take place in the same way as the reading of literature, since the former is not pri-

---

[199] The uniting thread of these studies is the critique of 'applied ethics' in medicine. I will return to this theme in Section 9. Before these articles were published, Richard Zaner, in the book I have referred to earlier, *Ethics and the Clinical Encounter* (1988), had discussed in detail the interpretive aspect of medical ethics without, however, choosing to term his project a hermeneutical one. Another theme related to an 'interpretive ethics' is the project of casuistry; see Jonsen and Toulmin (1988).

THE HERMENEUTICS OF MEDICINE

marily tied to the understanding of *written* language, but rather to spoken language with its dialogic and attuned characteristics. Modern doctors meet their patients face-to-face and not in the form of their written statements.[200]

Drew Leder is the philosopher who, in my view, has taken hermeneutics furthest in medicine, without falling prey to a methodological understanding of the concept. Doctors, in Leder's view, are not experts on the methods developed in the humanities. Nevertheless, what they do, according to him, is to read texts. Let me here go into Leder's proposal in some detail since it merits attention and will also serve as a springboard for the hermeneutics of medicine I will try to flesh out in the following myself. In an article, *Clinical Interpretation: The Hermeneutics of Medicine* from 1990, Leder traces out four basic texts which are read in the clinical meeting: the experiential, the narrative, the physical, and the instrumental text.[201] He starts out with two basic assumptions, which are taken from Daniel's article: the concept of text is to be understood as 'any set of elements which constitutes a whole and takes on meaning through interpretation'; and the patient – 'the person-as-ill' – constitutes the primary text (1990b, p. 11). Given this very broad definition of text and the focus upon the 'person-as-ill', Leder argues that what the doctor reads in order to understand the primary text (the person-as-ill) is a set of secondary texts – the experiential, narrative, physical and instrumental texts I mentioned above.

The experiential text consists in the patient's experience of his illness – what we in this study with the aid of Heidegger have mapped out as his unhomelike being-in-the-world. This experience is often heavily embodied, given painful or distressing symptoms, but it also includes the patient's more cognitive self-understanding in reflecting upon the symptoms. This interpretation is indeed that which finally takes the patient to the doctor, since the patient interprets the experiential text as having become increasingly distressful and hard to understand and hopes that the doctor will be able to offer help in interpretation. The patient wants the doctor to help in giving expert interpretation of the experiential text – an interpretation that the patient, of course, hopes will in the end offer a possibility of healing actions, which will change the experiential text back to normal. The last point is important: the ultimate goal of

---

[200] Before the emergence of modern medicine, as we have seen in surveying the history of medical practice in Part 1, it was, however, not unusual that doctors carried out diagnosis and prescription from patients' letters alone. If the past featured the prospect of this minimal version of the medical meeting, in which the patient is only present in the form of his self-written text, the future might carry the even more threatening possibility of the doctor being present only in the form of a mechanical 'reader'. The explosive development of information technology might not only turn out to provide the doctor with helpful tools, but also carry dangers with it. The insistence upon the dialogic face-to-face meeting as basic to clinical practice seems to me of uttermost importance, given the future science-fiction scenario of computer-diagnosis, in which the computer would not form a tool for the physician (in the same way as other types of medical technologies), but indeed replace him and thereby turn medicine into something radically different from that which it previously has been – indeed, so different that, in my view, it would no longer be medicine, but rather would have become mere applied biology and information technology.

[201] For a discussion of these texts and the relations between them in Leder's article, see Dekkers (1998) and Svenaeus (1996).

the hermeneutics of medicine is obviously not truth but regained health – 'therapeutic results', in the words of Leder (1990b, p. 18).

The experiential text cannot be directly read by the physician, but must be presented to him by the patient. This story is the narrative text. It lends coherence to that which the patient experiences through a narrative organisation. It is also a text, as Leder notes, partly written by the physician, since he asks the patient about different things in the meeting. The doctor directs and channels the patient's story in a way he finds helpful for finding out why the patient is ill. Not everything having to do with the patient's life is regarded as important by the doctor, and some things are certainly found more important than others in the diagnostic search for diseases.[202]

In reading the physical text, the doctor performs his medical reading of the patient through looking at, palpating, listening to, and even smelling the patient's body. This part of clinical practice is normally called the physical examination, and it is probably here that the concept of 'text' in medicine is pressed to its uttermost limits. The patient's physical body is clearly not *written* by himself or somebody else in any elucidating sense.[203] Nevertheless, Leder says, it is *read* by the physician in a specific bodily way. The 'signs' of the patient's body are read through the understanding activities of the lived body of the physician, which has been educated to see, hear, smell and feel the pathological, on its own or aided by medical instruments such as the stethoscope. This reading is clearly more non-lingual, more perceptual, than any other textual task in medicine, but the signs of the body are still read in a systematic way. In putting his ear to the patient's chest the doctor is trying to make sense of what the patient's body 'says', and ironically, as Leder remarks, it is essential that the patient must stop *telling* his own story at this point, otherwise the doctor is not able to auscultate (1990b, p. 13).

The final text Leder names is the instrumental one. This text is produced by the modern arsenal of instruments, which are used in the clinical encounter for making the body more visible. X-ray images, ECG tracings and laboratory test results are all read and interpreted by the trained medical eye in order to better understand the illness. This text is indeed more textlike than the physical text, since it has an artifactual, separable, reproducible character. Even though the author to a large extent hap-

---

[202] Clearly it is part of the argument of this study that doctors are, and perhaps should be even more, interested in aspects of the patient's being-in-the-world which are not primarily biological. But this does not mean that every aspect of a person's life is or should be discussed in every clinical meeting. The *unhomelikeness* of the patient's being-in-the-world is that which is focused upon, and this is best done, medically, by applying a set of what Sundström (1987) calls 'icons of disease' – integral clinical conceptions directing the physician's attention towards specific features of the patient's story that are clues to underlying diseases. If a doctor is told about thirst and dizziness he will for instance suspect diabetes. However, the focus upon disease (in its integral clinical sense) does not exclude, but rather is included in, an understanding of the patient's life-situation – his being-in-the-world – as I will try to show in what follows.

[203] I will not here enter into the fascinating discussion about old and new ways to 're-write' one's own body, be it through diet and bodybuilding, or through contemporary and future scenarios of plastic surgery and cyborg technology. It clearly belongs to the philosophy of medicine, but I do no find any room for it in this work.

pens to be a machine, the image which is produced – be it in the form of a photograph, a plot, a colour, or numbers – can be reproduced and interpreted simultaneously by different people and thus intersubjectively checked. The temptingly 'objective' character of this text, when compared to other texts or aspects of the clinical meeting, as we have seen in Part 1 and in the first section of Part 3, can lead to the image of modern medicine as applied biology.

The hermeneutic circle in Leder's article is, I think, primarily articulated as a switching back and forth between the primary text and the secondary ones (Svenaeus 1996, p. 127). Not only does the primary text – the person as ill – attain its meaning through a reading of the secondary texts, but the reading also goes back and forth between the secondary texts in trying to make sense of the primary one. As Leder writes, the interpretation of the different texts is also continuously checked and revised through changing the primary text in treatment (1990b, pp. 18-19). Medical interpretation should not only make sense, but also lead to healing, and consequently the 'person-as-ill' will hopefully change into a healthy text through the interpretive readings and the therapy offered.

As I think is obvious from my presentation here, I am very sympathetic to Leder's proposal. It is clearly anchored in the same theoretical framework that I proceed from in my own analysis – Heidegger and Gadamer – even though the article format prevents Leder from adequately showing this. The key point is that hermeneutics is seen as an ontological and epistemological, and not as a methodological concept. My problem with Leder's approach lies in the concept of text he employs. As we have seen he proceeds from a very broad definition: for Leder, the text is 'any set of elements which constitutes a whole and takes on meaning through interpretation.' Is not this definition of text so broad that it threatens to render the concept of text vacuous? And even worse, is it not rather inadequate in capturing what we normally mean by a text? Are not texts always to be understood as cultural phenomena? Are not all texts *written by someone* in a way that bodies are not?[204] If the body is a meaningful phenomenon – which I have gone to some effort in the preceding part to show – this is so because it is *lived*, an aspect of our being-in-the-world, and not because it is written. And the dialogue in the clinic, the heart of medical practice, although clearly linguistic, is *spoken* rather than written and thus not textual in a normal sense.

To some extent the dispute might only be formal and not essential to the hermeneutics of medicine. The important thing is after all that one explicitly specifies what one means by the word 'text'. However, I suspect that choosing the counterintuitive definition of text also runs the risk of leading the hermeneutics of medicine in unfortunate directions. The most obvious reason for this is that the dialogic aspect of

---

[204] As I remarked in Section 1 above, when the world ceases to be authored by God(s), purpose and meaning will have to be searched for in culture and not in nature. Before this happened the body was of course a paradigmatic text corresponding to all kinds of higher purposes.

clinical practice is downplayed by the metaphor of reading. Patients are indeed partners in the medical meeting and not objects, not even textual objects.[205]

As we have seen above, nothing in Heidegger's or Gadamer's hermeneutics requires us to find any texts in medicine, other than those the average down-to-earth doctor already believes to be there, in order to develop a hermeneutics of medicine.[206] We will soon go on to explore the dialogic hermeneutics of medical practice which we have begun to develop above. Before we do this, I would, however, like to dwell for a while on other dangers of the extended metaphor of text in medicine. In using hermeneutical theories in which the concept of text is used in the narrower sense of written language, and in connecting these theories to the practice of medicine without reflecting to a satisfactory degree upon the shift in sense the concept must thereby undergo, one namely risks reaching too limited, if not false, conclusions regarding that which medicine is or ought to be about. I am thinking here particularly of the adopting of Paul Ricoeur's theories in the philosophy of medicine, which might from many angles look particularly appealing for a hermeneuticist of medicine, but which is, I will claim, in the end not so. This does not mean that I find his approach (or rather approaches) to phenomenology and hermeneutics uninteresting for a hermeneutics of medicine – indeed the opposite is rather the case – and this is also the reason for now devoting a whole section to aspects of Ricoeur's philosophy which have been made use of in this field.

4. RICOEUR – TEXTUALITY AND NARRATIVITY IN MEDICINE

It might seem paradoxical to ascribe to the influence of Ricoeur's hermeneutics in the philosophy of medicine a tendency of negligence towards dialogue. Is not Ricoeur the most communicative of all philosophers, who has continuously strived towards building bridges between different philosophical camps and cultures? Is not the dialogue with the other in a sense exactly what his philosophy is about?[207] This is certainly true, and let me therefore right from the beginning state that my objections are not directed towards Ricoeur's philosophy as such, but rather towards different ways of putting it to work in the philosophy of medicine. Ricoeur has not made the connection himself, and he will perhaps never do so, at least not in the way I will show it to have already taken place in the field. There might indeed be other ways of connecting his theories to the philosophy of medicine, which do not fall into the traps I will criticize here. Let me also say right from the start that my critique in this section might in a way be unjust also to the other authors I am dealing with, since they might not have the same aims as I have in using hermeneutics in the philosophy of medicine. They might, for instance, turn out to be interested in ethics rather than

---

[205] See Baron (1990, pp. 25-28).

[206] One strange outcome of Leder's analysis is that the phenomena which we would normally call texts in the clinical meeting – such as the chart and the medical textbook – are only 'tertiary texts' – two steps removed from the true textual level of the person-as-ill (1990b, p. 16).

[207] Kristensson Uggla has focused upon this theme as a connecting thread throughout Ricoeur's entire philosophical project in (1994).

ontology and epistemology, and they might want to focus on the nursing professions rather than on the physician. Mindful of all these disclaimers let us now turn to the points I want to highlight in Ricoeur's philosophy.

Ricoeur's philosophy is best understood as growing out of the same soil as Gadamer's; that is, the phenomenologies of Husserl and Heidegger. This is not to say that no others have been decisive for Ricoeur on his long path towards hermeneutics; the philosophies of Karl Jaspers and Gabriel Marcel, just to mention two obvious examples, are clearly of vital importance if one wants to understand Ricoeur's development. However, since this is not meant to be even an introduction to Ricoeur's vast project, but rather a descent to some of his key ideas of hermeneutics, the sections above in this work which are devoted to Husserl, Heidegger and Gadamer, will serve well as a background to my discussion. Proceeding from these introductions and the dichotomy of explanation and understanding, which we reworked in Section 1 above, I will take off rather abruptly with a well known theme in Ricoeur's philosophy – namely, that which he calls a dialectic of explanation and understanding (1991a, p. 126). This dialectic obviously means a form of reciprocal synthesis, whereby the potentialities of both paradigms can at least be voiced and cross-fertilized, if not *aufgehoben* in the strictly Hegelian sense. As Ricoeur writes: '(Understanding) *envelops* explanation. Explanation, in turn, *develops* understanding analytically' (1991a, p. 142).

At first sight, this seems very similar to the way we ourselves attempted to resolve the problem above. Ricoeur's formulations have been taken up by James Lock in an article from 1990 – *Some Aspects of Medical Hermeneutics: The Role of Dialectic and Narrative* – in which he tries to show how this dialectic is essentially at work in clinical medicine.[208] Lock neglects to mention, however, that, for Ricoeur, explanation means linguistic, structural explanation and never the nomo-thetical deductive scheme characteristic of natural science, which we encountered in Section 1 above.[209] Is this of any importance? I think it is, since the liberating power Ricoeur accords the explanatory method, in terms of its critical stance towards the understanding paradigm, hardly is pertinent in characterizing the role science plays today in clinical medicine. As we have seen in our historical survey in Part 1, it is not explanation but rather understanding that faces the threat of suffocation in the clinical enterprise of today. Ricoeur's dialectic is tied to a historical situation in the humanities and social sciences, which began in the sixties, by which structural models based on linguistic studies were offered as an antidote to naive understandings of texts as bearers of no more than their authors' intentions. This situation bears no resemblance to clinical practice today, neither in terms of methods nor objects of study.

---

[208] This paper and the book by Nerheim (1996), which I will discuss below, are both to be seen as members of the third group of studies I began to examine in the last section; that is, the group of studies which understand hermeneutics to be a characterization of the medical activity as such.

[209] This is obvious from all essays on the subject by Ricoeur which I have found: not only the one mentioned above, *Explanation and Understanding* (1991a); but also, for instance, *What is a Text? Explanation and Understanding* (1981a), and other essays in *Hermeneutics and the Human Sciences: Essays on Language, Action and Interpretation.*

For Ricoeur the dialectic of explanation and understanding is ultimately dependent upon the mode of being of the *text*. 'Text' in Ricoeur's philosophy is not understood as 'a set of elements which take on meaning through interpretation' (Daniel's and Leder's definition above), but as 'any discourse fixed by writing' (1981a, p. 145). This fixation in writing makes it possible for the text, not only to reveal a hidden world (the world of the author), but also to open up new worlds in the encounter with its reader. It is true that writing for Ricoeur is not necessarily to be understood in a literal sense, but rather as an inscription or fixation of the meaning of an *action*, be it a spoken or a written act or not.[210] Yet, for the action to be considered a text in Ricoeur's sense, it is essential that it become *sedimented* and thus be freed from its 'author'. This liberation must take place in order to enable a critical reading, which is no longer only a return to the action itself as it was intended by its subject, but develops the 'text' in new directions. This is why Ricoeur's paradigmatic example of the relation between understanding and explanation in the humanities and social sciences, when not restricted to the reading of texts in the more ordinary sense, is always historical studies. Historical evidence might come to us in the forms of the signs of language, or just as brute marks in matter, but in both these cases we cannot have a true *dialogue* with history since its subjects are long dead. For Ricoeur, precisely this more or less literal *death* of the author is vital to the being of the text in order for it to be alive for us *as a text*.

I do not think that this understanding of text as sedimented meaning, enabling critical distance for the reader, makes a connection to a hermeneutics of *medicine* suitable. The reason why Ricoeur chooses text instead of dialogue as his paradigm is obviously tied to a critique of Heidegger's and Gadamer's philosophies, based on the assumption that these philosophers exclude a critical epistemological stance towards the ontological frameworks which their hermeneutics are situated in.[211] The authority of authentic understanding and tradition needs the antidote of critical, liberating reflection, and this reflection, according to Ricoeur, is possible only when the other is encountered as inscribed, as a text. But the other is surely not encountered as such a text in medicine. The patient might be 'a set of elements which take on meaning through interpretation', but he is clearly not 'a discourse fixed by writing'. As I wrote in the preceding section, the patient's body is lived and the medical dialogue is spoken, but neither of them is written. They are not even written in the sense of being sedimented actions. What the patient says, does, or shows, in the clinic is not inscribed in a way which enables critical distancing. The way the patient's actions *are* inscribed – in the chart – does not generally produce a text which enables critical explanation and understanding, but a rather reductive understanding, in which the patient has no part. The chart is indeed not meant to liberate, but rather to report and record.

Given these reflections on Ricoeur's hermeneutics, the last part of Hjördis Nerheim's book *Vitenskap og kommunikasjon* (1996), which I have referred to above,

---

[210] See Ricoeur (1981b).

[211] See Ricoeur (1981c). See also the similar critique by Jürgen Habermas in (1971).

appears to me to be problematic. After two long, very illuminating and competent parts on the theory of science and hermeneutics and their roles in health care, Nerheim in the third part of her work comes to the conclusion that the hermeneutics of Ricoeur, and not of Heidegger and Gadamer, is most suitable for developing a philosophy of health care. I can readily understand why the existentialistic reading of Heidegger, centring around authentic anxiety, which she provides, will not bring her to the same conclusions of his value to a philosophy of medicine and health as my phenomenological reading above (1996, pp. 409-421). This is indeed a matter of interpretation, and as I made clear in Part 2 I am not interested in presenting the 'true' reading of Heidegger (there certainly according to his own standards cannot be any), but one that is enlightening and productive for my purposes. It is harder for me to understand why Gadamer's hermeneutics of dialogue is finally rejected by Nerheim, but the issue is probably connected to the apparent lack of a critical epistemological potential – in Ricoeur's and Habermas's understanding – in his philosophy, which I referred to above. Gadamer, as I have shown, certainly cannot be rejected on grounds of lacking a theory of true intersubjectivity, which might be a possible objection to Heidegger's philosophy. When Nerheim finally makes up her mind to go with Ricoeur rather than with Gadamer, it seems however to be exactly the intersubjective paradigm in the former's hermeneutics that is of importance to her. This will, however, bring her to make false inferences and reach strange consequences. She writes:

> To the extent that research and care are directed towards actions understood as texts in a health-care context, the autonomous *body* of the other will appear as 'text', that is as *expression* or *phenomenon*, not as *object* as for instance in physiology (1996, p. 423).

But the autonomous body of the other is not *sedimented* in any textual way in the clinical encounter, and since this does not take place, the whole distancing, critical, liberating point of Ricoeur's textual analysis fails to apply in medicine. The consequence of adopting Ricoeur's conceptual scheme is indeed, as Nerheim herself notes on the next page, that distance and not dialogue is central in health care. And, even more strangely, what is at stake in medicine and health care would ultimately not be the self of the patient, but the self of the doctor or nurse. This must be so because the point of textuality in Ricoeur's philosophy is the possibility it offers for the *reader* of becoming an (ethical) person.[212]

I think that the strategy of adopting Ricoeur's hermeneutics of text in the philosophy of medicine in order to save a critical distance, which is thought to be lost in the theories of Heidegger and Gadamer, is a mistake. It is so for two main reasons. The first one we have dismantled above: Ricoeur's concept of text simply does not apply in clinical medicine; and, what is worse, if adopted it brings us to strange conclusions about the structure and ends of medical practice.[213] The second reason that

---

[212] See *Oneself as Another* (1992), Chapters 5 and 6, as well as other late works by Ricoeur.

[213] I have already, in the beginning of this section, however, made a disclaimer about ethics and nursing as central to Nerheim's analysis, and by no means want to rule out the possibility of the relevance of Ri-

the choice of Ricoeur's hermeneutics is a mistake is that it rests on a false premise, which seems to exclude the possibility of adopting Gadamer's hermeneutics of dialogue: namely, that critical distance demands textuality. This is false, however, since critical distance can be found *within* dialogue. As we saw in the presentation of Gadamer's hermeneutics above, dialogue comes out of a productive distance in which the other is always understood from my point of view. Dialogue does not only imply empathy in Gadamer's philosophy.[214] We will continue the hermeneutics of medicine with the aid of Gadamer's philosophy in the next section, but first I would like to mention another aspect of Ricoeur's philosophy, which I think is of great interest to our coming analysis, and which is appropriated by both Lock and Nerheim: narrativity.

'A life *examined*, in the sense borrowed from Socrates, is a life *narrated*', writes Ricoeur in *Life: A Story in Search of a Narrator* (1991b, p. 435). Narration as the configuration of a plot in different literary genres is thus essential to our self-understanding, to our life. I think this is exactly right; life is structured as a story in many ways, and so, of course, is the ill life – in the latter case, as a story that is in the process of breaking down and falling to pieces. The homeless life of illness is characterized by a *lack* of meaning – as we tried to show in Part 2 with the aid of Heidegger's phenomenology – highlighted by the breakdown of the tool-structure of the world and the failure of coherent transcendence. The coherence of narrative is another aspect of the homelike being-in-the-world.

The way the patient is able and allowed to tell the story of his illness is essential, not only to the doctor's understanding of the illness, but also to the patient's self-understanding and identity. But the way this relation between narrative and life or self is finally envisaged in Ricoeur's philosophy does not fit easily and directly into the clinical encounter. In fact, in the essay mentioned above, *Life: A Story in Search of a Narrator* (1991b), and in *Oneself as Another* (1992), as well as in other later works by Ricoeur, life and self ultimately attain their narrative structure and identity, not through the telling of stories, but through the reading of texts:

> Let us stay for a moment on the side of the narrative, i. e., the side of fiction, and let us see how it leads back to life. My thesis here is that the process of composition, of configuration, does not realize itself in the text but in the reader, and under this condition of configuration makes possible reconfiguration of a life by the way of the narrative (1991b, p. 430).

So text, instead of dialogue, seems to be the final word in Ricoeur, also in the case of narration. Before we conclude this section on the philosophy of Ricoeur, let us mention a book in which he in fact comes close to a hermeneutics of dialogue, one which might appear very similar to a hermeneutics of medicine: *Freud and Philosophy: An Essay on Interpretation.*

---

coeur's philosophy in health care. His analysis of narrativity, for example, is very helpful in understanding the clinical encounter, as I touch upon in what follows.

[214] Ricoeur himself acknowledges this aspect of Gadamer's philosophy in (1981d, p. 87 ff.).

Ricoeur's brilliant interpretation of Freudian psychoanalysis operates with the basic aim of supplying Freud's archaeology of desire with a teleology of symbol (1970, p. 494). That is, Freud's hermeneutics of *suspicion*, revealing the play of unconscious desire and resistance beneath the patient's statements and symptoms, needs to be wedded to a hermeneutics of *revelation*, according to which the patient's language is not only the effect of unconscious forces, but actually gives birth to *new* meaning. Psychoanalysis, according to Ricoeur, is not only about the past, but also about the future – a future where the patient can reach a new self-understanding through the process and language of the analytic session.

The way Ricoeur reads Freud's energetic theory of drives as coupled to a hermeneutic *telos* of self-understanding through symbols is very helpful in making sense of psychoanalysis as something other than a science (which it obviously is not, despite Freud's and others' ambitions and intentions). The analytic session in many ways also seems similar in structure to the medical meeting, in that it is a discourse aimed at recovery. People who undergo psychoanalysis are certainly most often (but not always) ill – their being-in-the-world is unhomelike. In psychiatry, psychoanalysis – in the form of psychotherapy – is thus an important part of medicine.

The hermeneutics of psychoanalysis and the hermeneutics of medicine are, however, despite the similarities, different in structure as well as in goal. The goal of psychoanalysis is to change the patient's self-understanding and thereby – if it is absent – bring about health.[215] In the hermeneutics of medicine, recovery is not tied to self-understanding in this unequivocal way. The two phenomena – self-understanding and health – are clearly closely related to each other also in medicine, and especially in psychiatry, in the sense that regained health for the patient may require a new self-understanding. But this is indeed not always the case in medicine. The cancer patient may come to a very profound self-understanding of his situation through the medical meeting, but this does not necessarily make him well again – his being-in-the-world would in most cases still be very unhomelike.

The final goal of the hermeneutics of medicine is not the patient's self-understanding, but his regained health. And for this goal to be realized, what is necessary is the *doctor's* rather than the patient's own understanding of his being-in-the-world. The better the patient's understanding of his unhomelike being-in-the-world is, the better he will be able to tell the doctor what is wrong, and the better he will be able to adapt to new circumstances and understand their importance for recovery; but this self-understanding in medicine does not guarantee restored health. Indeed, in a sense, it is often two steps away from regained health, since it must take a detour over the doctor's understanding in order to lead to therapy and healing.

In psychoanalysis the only possibility of healing goes through the *patient's*, and not the analyst's, understanding. No matter how well the analyst understands why the patient's existence is unhomelike, this will not make any difference as long as the patient does not come to understand this himself through the session. In contrast to this univocal focus on self-understanding in psychoanalysis, in the meeting of medi-

---

[215] Regarding the goals of psychoanalysis and psychotherapy, see Jakobsson (1994).

cine the doctor need not necessarily in every case bring the patient to understand the reason behind his unhomelikeness, since diseases can be cured without any biomedical understanding whatsoever, on the part of the patient, of what is going on. Of course patients generally want to know what is wrong, and the doctor will most often try to tell them on an explanatory level that makes sense for the non-specialist. But the point is that detailed understanding on the part of the patient is not a *necessary* feature of the hermeneutics of medicine as it is in psychoanalysis, in which no healing whatsoever can take place without a radical change in the patient's self-understanding.

The patient enters analysis in order to facilitate self-understanding, but comes to the physician in order to get well. In most analytic sessions the final goal may indeed be homelike being-in-the-world, just as self-understanding for the patient in most medical meetings greatly facilitates the goal of health. But the structures of the two activities are nevertheless clearly different: medicine is not psychoanalysis and vice versa. This difference will emerge with greater clarity when we now move on in order to conceptualize the hermeneutics of medicine. For this hermeneutics will turn out to be a hermeneutics of attention and action, rather than a hermeneutics of suspicion and revelation.

5. THE MEDICAL MEETING – INTERPRETATION THROUGH DIALOGUE

In Heidegger we found understanding to be an existential – that is, an *a priori* aspect of our being-in-the-world. Medicine, then, of course, like all other human activities, must be mapped out as a kind of understanding, a form of hermeneutics. But in what way? As Leder writes: 'The key question then is not *whether* medicine is hermeneutical but *how* it is so' (1990b, p. 10). Let us sum up the clues we have found so far on our journey towards a hermeneutics of clinical medicine.

Medical practice is a form of meeting: a clinical encounter. In the first part I tried to show that this is the historical essence of medical practice, which cannot be reduced to scientific investigation. But what does it really mean to say that medicine is a *meeting* as opposed to a merely scientific investigation? A meeting takes place between persons who come to understand each other. In science it is the scientist alone, and not his object, who understands – understands, moreover, in the particular form of scientific explanation the structure of which we explicated in Section 1 above. What characterizes a meeting, in contrast to scientific explanatory understanding, is thus mutual, shared understanding. This does not mean that the understanding of the two persons who meet must be totally shared in the sense of being the *same* understanding.[216] There might exist the possibility of totally shared under-

---

[216] I concentrate here on the dyadic meeting, since this is the common form of the modern clinical encounter, and do not deal with meetings in larger groups. Indeed I do not deal with the question whether these forms of extended intersubjectivities would be *meetings* in the same sense as the dyad. See, however, Section 7 of this part, regarding the fact that patients meet with several representatives of medicine, from a variety of different professions, in the modern hospital.

standing, as in the meetings of mothers and infants or the intimate meeting of lovers, for example; but this is hardly ever the case in medicine. Indeed the medical meeting, as many have pointed out before me, is generally, despite its intimate aspects, a meeting between strangers.[217] In addition to this it seems to be a meeting that is radically *asymmetrical* in the sense that the patient is the weak help-seeking party asking for aid from the expert in health matters – the doctor, nurse or some other medical personnel.

But if, in spite of this asymmetrical estrangement, medical practice, as I claim, nevertheless *is* a meeting, this must mean that understanding is being *shared* to some extent. The doctor must understand the patient as an understanding person, through projecting himself into the patient's understanding and vice versa; and what the doctor and patient say to each other must make sense for both parties. The discourse of the meeting must indeed take place through a shared language in the sense that both parties understand what the other is saying. Language, as the medium of the meeting, must then have a mutual attunement that makes it into a dialogue – something that is shared between doctor and patient – through which their asking and answering becomes a mutual project on the way to a shared goal – homelikeness for the patient. Gestures and facial expressions – the language of the body – and intonation are often even more important than the cognitive content in establishing this shared understanding. Understanding is not only a cognitive but also essentially an emotional project. To understand in a medical meeting, as I will explore in what follows, is essentially to be understand*ing*.

The *goal* of the medical meeting is that which separates it from most other kinds of meetings, other ways of being-together-in-the-world. In contrast to everyday meetings, the clinical encounter bears certain resemblance to other meetings between professionals and clients in which the aim is specified beforehand.[218] But the medical meeting is also different from all other types of professional meetings, having health as a goal and a unique structure to accomplish this. The path from unhomelikeness to homelikeness gives the medical meeting an intense and often dramatic form of attunement. The patient, who comes looking for help, is distressed, suffering and often afraid because of what is happening to him. The dialogue and examination will have to deal with intimate parts of life, parts which one would normally only share with someone one knew very well, or perhaps with no one at all. Thus, for the meeting to take place, mutual trust and respect are needed, so that the topic of the encounter – the patient's unhomelikeness – can be shared in every necessary way.[219] Deep trust, despite estrangement and assymetry, is therefore a necessary feature of the medical meeting.

---

[217] See, for example, Zaner (1988, p. 54).

[218] Consider, for instance, meetings between lawyers and clients, in contrast to the meetings of everyday life, where the aim of the meeting is simply the enjoyment we get out of being together with the other person, sharing our being-in-the-world in different ways.

[219] See Zaner (1991).

Medical practice is not only essentially a meeting, it is also interpretation: clinical hermeneutics. I have suggested this kind of hermeneutics to be dialogic rather than based in the reading of texts. It is still, though, a hermeneutics that first and foremost takes place through language: the dialogue is spoken and it is through dialogue that physical examination and therapy are guided towards their aim. The turn that Gadamer's *Wahrheit und Methode* takes between Parts 2 and 3, moving on to an analysis of language and dialogue from the readings of texts in the humanities, is crucial to our analysis here. The claim that I will make is that Gadamer's entire hermeneutical model of *Horizontverschmelzung*, which I presented in Section 2 above, is to be found in its original form in dialogue itself, rather than in different specialized studies in the humanities. This is something which emerges clearly from a close reading of Gadamer's text, but which has not been sufficiently stressed, because of the tendency to understand *Wahrheit und Methode* as an approach to aesthetics and the humanities instead of a general ontology and hermeneutics. That the latter and not the former is the correct reading, which is explicitly stated for example on page 479, seems to be the only interpretation which makes sense, given the Heideggerian basis of Gadamer's philosophy which we laid out above. Gadamer's hermeneutics should be understood as proceeding from an ontology of being-in-the-world, in which the role of language is primarily dialogical, rather than textual. For example:

> As so often, here the interpretation remains too restricted to the special situation of the historical humanities and a 'being towards the text'. Not until in Part 3 does one explicitly encounter that which has in essence from the beginning been in my view: a broadening of the issue to language and dialogue and consequently the fundamental grasping, thereby made possible, of the concepts of distance and otherness (1990, pp. 316-317).[220]

Another feature of Gadamer's understanding of hermeneutics, which could help us to develop a hermeneutics of medicine, is his emphasis upon application (*Anwendung*) (1990, p. 312 ff.).[221] Interpretation always takes place in a certain situation and with a special aim in view – the paradigmatic example which Gadamer gives is interpretation of the law in court. With the concept of application, Gadamer amplifies a feature which we have already taken up in Section 2: understanding of the text (or the other person) always takes place from a different point of view than the originary one and is thus a new, different understanding. Interpretive understanding has a productive potential which comes from the very *distance* to the text or the other person. This pattern seems to fit the medical meeting. Understanding is here sought for healing – it is applied for a specific purpose – and it involves a critical distance – the

---

[220] See also, for instance, (1990, p. 375): 'Wir kehren also zu der Feststellung zurück, daß auch das hermeneutische Phänomen die Ursprünglichkeit des Gesprächs und die Struktur von Frage und Antwort in sich schließt. Daß ein überlieferter Text Gegenstand der Auslegung wird, heißt bereits, daß er eine Frage an den Interpreten stellt.'

[221] Application in Gadamer's philosophy is ultimately understood as *phronesis*, which is interesting given the approaches to the philosophy of medical practice we have mentioned in Part 1, Section 8. The relation of Gadamer's and Heidegger's philosophies to Aristotle, especially Book 6 of the *Nicomachean Ethics* which deals with *praxis*, will be dealt with briefly in Section 9 below.

doctor reaches a different, for the purposes of healing more complete, understanding of the patient's unhomelike being-in-the-world than the patient had before visiting the clinic.

A later work by Gadamer – *Über die Verborgenheit der Gesundheit* (1993) – which we dealt with briefly in Part 2, seems to support this interpretation.[222] Medicine is here characterized as a dialogue (*Gespräch*) by which the doctor and patient together try to reach an understanding of why the patient is ill (1993, p. 144). What is particularly obvious in the medical meeting, as I mentioned above, is the asymmetrical relation between its parties. The patient is ill and seeks help, whereas the doctor is at home – in control by virtue of his knowledge and experience of disease. This asymmetry necessitates empathy from the side of the doctor. He must try to understand the patient, not exclusively from his own point of view, but through being *understanding* – trying to put himself in the patient's situation.[223] Consequently, that the doctor attempts to reach a new, productive, different understanding of the patient's unhomlikeness in no way implies that he should avoid empathy. It is only *through* empathy that the doctor can reach independent understanding that is truly productive in the sense of shared *and* independent. We can here go back to Gadamer's model of textual interpretation, according to which the reader must understand the text as authoritative, as posing a question to him which can only be answered by meeting the text – by a 'fusion' of the two horizons of author and reader.

It is thus primarily the doctor who is the 'reader' and the patient who is the 'text'. But since the meeting is dialogic the reading is also a *mutual* process of questions and answers, though nevertheless primarily controlled and guided by the doctor. The distance between the two parties is certainly not a historical, time-related distance; but it is a distance between two lifeworld horizons, which can be narrowed down through the dialogue. This narrowing down, this 'fusion of the horizons' of doctor and patient, means that the horizons are brought in touch with each other, but nevertheless preserve their own identities in this meeting. We will return to the issues of lifeworlds and horizons in the next section, but first we need to say more about interpretation and how it is structured through the dialogue.

The medical meeting involves many different kinds of interpretations from different people (who are not all present in person in the encounter). These interpretations must be brought together and must finally result in a shared understanding that can lead to therapeutical actions, since the goal of the meeting – regained health – often demands this. The hermeneutics of medicine is fundamentally action-oriented,

---

[222]One should however note that, in the only passage in which clinical medicine is explicitly mentioned in *Wahrheit und Methode*, Gadamer identifies it with a purely non-productive type of 'dialogue', in which no truly shared understanding of the matter at hand is present (1990, p. 308). Without doubt, powerfully present in both of these works by Gadamer, and a feature to which I myself do not to the same extent subscribe, are both an exaggerated fear of science and a tendency to portray science pejoratively, as the domination (*Beherrschung*) and suffocation of language and dialogue by pure calculation and manipulation.

[223]Here and in what follows in this section regarding different forms of interpretations in the meeting and their relations to each other, the paper by Zaner (1994) has been extremely helpful.

and the kind of suspicion which guides the doctor's questions is aimed towards excluding the dangerous possibilities in terms of 'hidden' diseases and towards finding the treatable ones. As every clinician is taught, these are the two possible causes which must not be missed.

The hermeneutics of suspicion peculiar to medicine is thus very different from its psychoanalytical counterpart. The former does not adopt the basic assumption of the latter – that the patient's account is systematically distorted; rather, it simply regards the patient's account as incomplete, in the sense that the patient himself is often unaware of the ways in which a particular disease can make life unhomelike. The suspicious strain of the hermeneutics of medicine is consequently not directed toward unconsicous desire and resistance behind language. Medical hermeneutics is rather a hermeneutics of suspicion in its attention to 'the language of the body', which is largely hidden from the patient and thus unknown or incomprehensible to him. It is consequently an attentive suspicion directed towards possible therapeutic action as I hinted at in the foregoing section. The psychoanalyst can wait, indeed has to wait, since no other options are open to him, but the physician is not always given this luxury, since the disease might be rapidly progressing, literally as the dialogue transpires.

Manipulative, therapeutic action is nevertheless not always the final solution in medicine, and it must always be based on and preceded by a mutual understanding of doctor and patient.[224] In order to see this more distinctly let us go back to one of the patients we encountered in Section 9 of Part 2: Ted, who was having problems with his prostate gland. Through the clinical example we will try to map out the different kinds of interpretations present in the meeting and see how they connect to each other in the hermeneutics of medicine.

Ted went back to see the urologist – Dr. Y – a week later. The doctor invited him into his office and Ted inquired about the results of the biopsy. Dr. Y told him they were in fact positive, but of a very low grade – 3 on the so-called Gleason scale. Ted felt the horror creeping up his spine and was quiet at first. He leaned back in the chair and tried to breathe normally. Then he asked Dr. Y what three on this scale meant. Would he have to have an operation? Was he going to die from the cancer? Dr. Y said that it meant that the tumour was very small and well differentiated – that it was in an early and possibly relatively unaggressive state. Ted did not face death, the tumour was indeed treatable and the risk that it had already spread was very low – close to zero. As a matter of fact the chances that he would have gone on living with this cancer for another twenty years without ever noticing it were high indeed. But now they had to make some decisions. To treat the cancer with an operation – prostatectomy – or with radiation therapy possibly in combination with hor-

---

[224] There are possible exceptions to this, as in the case of the unconscious patient, but as we will see in Section 7 the clinical activity is in this case nevertheless based on an assumed consent on the part of the patient; that is, the actions of the health-care personnel are in this case geared towards the possibility of a future dialogue with the patient and based on the assumption that the actions are necessary in order to make this possible.

mone therapy would produce rather severe side effects. The two main possible side effects were incontinence and impotence. How did Ted feel about these issues? Was he married? Did his wife know about the examinations he had been going through and the possible results? He would have to talk things through with her although the final decision was of course up to him. Ted asked about the two different kinds of therapies and was told that prostatectomy was the safest way to proceed. With the type of local, low-grade cancer that he had, the probability, after the operation, of a total recovery from the cancer was very high – almost 100%. But this kind of treatment also produced the most severe side effects, it was very likely that he was not going to be able to have an erection after that kind of treatment, and it would indeed take some time to learn to control the urinary bladder again with risks of permanent incontinence in the future. Radiation therapy had better prospects in terms of side effects, but it was not as safe as an operation when it came to eradication of the tumour. Were there any other alternatives, Ted asked? Yes indeed, said Dr. Y, there was what is called 'watchful waiting'. This means that you go on living as normal and have your PSA level tested twice a year with renewed digital rectal exams and perhaps additional biopsies if needed. If the cancer started to grow rapidly it would obviously be time for an operation or other treatment, but if it stayed a low level, say under 5.0 ng/ml on the PSA test and under 5 on the Gleason scale, there would be no need for treatment. Of course, Dr. Y explained to Ted, this always meant a risk, since the cancer could spread at any time, even though the risk for this was not high at the moment. Anyway, Ted should think this through carefully and discuss it with his wife. There was no need to hurry. They could come back in two weeks or whenever they felt comfortable and discuss it with him to reach a conclusion. He gave Ted the name of a book that explained the process and treatment of prostate cancer and told him to call for an appointment as soon as he felt ready to make a decision.

Ted went home to discuss the issue with his wife. He was still scared of course, but did not feel shocked as before, and eventually began to see some hope around the corner. The decision was a very hard one, however. His sex life would clearly be endangered by an operation. Would his marriage survive this? Sarah – his wife – felt rather horrified at the prospect of having an incontinent and impotent husband. When she admitted this to him, however, urging him not to have the operation and thereby putting his life at risk, she clearly felt very guilty. Ted's self-image suffered a blow, as he began thinking of the side effects. He had always been the healthy, virile type. How would he survive mentally wearing diapers and being impotent? Although he was still afraid of dying, he finally made up his mind to postpone treatment and to continue being tested every sixth months. With the help of Dr. Y he made up a plan for this and tried to go back to his old life. Things would of course never be entirely normal again, he could feel death ticking within him, but in this way he thought to win some time.

We obviously in this clinical example are dealing with a multiplicity of interpretations which are inter-nested in different ways. Let us begin with Ted. He is untypical of the general structure of the hermeneutics of medicine which we have begun to develop, since his being-in-the-world is homelike when he first visits the doctor. Routine medical exams – check-ups – do not quite fit our pattern. One should notice, however, that although Ted's existence is not yet unhomelike when he first comes to the doctor, he still comes asking for *help*, and this request for help is related to illness – albeit the future possibility of illness, rather than actual illness in the present.[225] The dialogic pattern of the meeting, which we have focused on, is clearly present also in preventive medicine, but what is being discussed there is not a current condition of unhomelikeness, but rather the prevention of *future* unhomelikeness. In the case of Ted, however, his way of being-in-the-world is immediately transformed the moment he hears about the possibility of disease. The new information about his biology changes his attuned, understanding way of being-in-the-world.

Secondly, we have the doctor's interpretive understanding of Ted. Let us restrict ourselves here to the second doctor, the urologist Dr. Y. He examines Ted's prostate gland through a rectal examination and takes biopsies from it, the results of which he interprets. He also has the previous results from the prostate antigen test that he includes in his interpretation. On top of (or rather underneath) this more scientific understanding he tries to reach an understanding of Ted's being-in-the-world. He tries to calm him down, to give him hope, and inquires about his social life and how he feels. He also tries to explain the results of the medical procedures he has carried out and tell which therapeutical options are open. He tries to make Ted understand what he himself knows about prostate cancer. In addition to his scientific and everyday interpretation of Ted and his attempt to make Ted understand, he also in the dialogue interprets Ted's possible interpretations of what he is saying to him. He does not want to scare Ted, but at the same time he also wants to be frank and honest. The whole issue might indeed be complicated by the possible fact that Dr. Y wants to proceed in a certain way – say prostatectomy – but still feels it his duty to present to Ted all the alternatives and side effects, so that Ted, by considering them, might come to decide otherwise. Doctors vary, of course, in this regard – in their degree of paternalism, to put it in a popular term of modern medical ethics.

Ted, in turn, interprets what the doctor tells him in the dialogue about the test results and the treatment options. He also possibly wonders whether Dr. Y is really telling him the whole truth. Is he just trying to calm him down, in order to make him feel better? This suspicion might generate an interest in Dr. Y's being-in-the-world. What kind of person is he, how should I interpret what he is saying to me? The at-

---

[225]Other possible exceptions to the general scheme we are tracing the outlines of here, in addition to the failing unhomelikeness of the help-seeking party, are the cases of children and retarded people. These persons generally, even though their being-in-the-world has turned unhomelike, do not only meet the doctor directly but also through someone else: a parent or another assistant. But this does not mean that the clinical practice is not a meeting in these cases. It only means that two, or actually three, meetings are taking place instead of one: the meeting between child (retarded) and parent (assistant), the meeting between parent (assistant) and doctor, and finally between child (retarded) and doctor.

tunement of the dialogue is vital here, carrying trust or distrust, confidence or fear. Ted might in addition to this interpret Dr. Y's interpretation of him as fearful, and so on. These types of inter-nested interpretations are present in every dialogue, but the dialogue is nevertheless – if it is a true dialogue – not only a sum of all these interpretations, but to some extent a shared and mutual understanding occuring in the very event of speaking and listening.[226]

We also have Ted's wife and her interpretation of Ted's, and their shared, being-in-the-world and what is going to happen with them as an effect of the disease and the treatment. This interpretation clearly influences Ted's interpretation of the situation. Dr. Y, in turn, bases his interpretation, not only on Ted's and his wife's understanding of the situation, but also on expert interpretations of the disease that he gets from colleagues and their experiences with patients.

As stated above, here we obviously have a multiplicity of interpretations related to each other in different ways. And yet this web of interpretations must be wound together and result in a decision. One could say that the final decision is always Ted's, since it is his life which is at issue. In a legal sense this is of course correct. But I think this way of viewing the matter is clearly too reductive. Medical action evolves out of mutual understanding in the meeting. Few persons would go against their doctor, since he is supposed to be the expert in health matters, which is what they are dealing with at the moment.[227] And as we have seen, the doctor could indeed through his presentation of the matter influence Ted's interpretation in the way he finds suitable. Questions of paternalism and autonomy are of course lurking behind the corner here, but this is not a debate I want to take a stand on in this presentation. My point would rather be that in the significant majority of cases, what is happening, rather than the patient or doctor coming to an autonomous decision on their own, is that the network of plural interpretations is taken to a mutual, shared understanding through a meeting of the horizons of patient and doctor. Let us move on and explore these matters of lifeworlds and horizons in medicine.

6. LIFEWORLDS AND HORIZONS IN THE MEDICAL MEETING

Kay Toombs, in her work *The Meaning of Illness: A Phenomenological Account of the Different Perspectives of Physician and Patient* (1992a), has showed how the lifeworlds of doctor and patient are significantly different in clinical medicine. The doctor's world, according to Toombs, is primarily one of disease, while the patient's world is one of lived illness. We have already dealt with these two different perspectives on health in clinical medicine in some detail above, and I will not repeat all the conclusions we have reached about their difference and connection here. What I find

---

[226]The concept Gadamer makes use of in order to get hold of this mutuality in dialogue exceeding the understandings of the individuals involved is *sprachliches Spiel* – language game (1990, p. 493). Here one is naturally reminded of the late philosophy of Wittgenstein, which stresses the practical, intersubjective aspects of language with the aid of the same metaphor.

[227]What many patients do, however, if they distrust the clinical judgment of their doctor, is to go and meet with another one.

helpful in Toombs's analysis is the structuring of the clinical encounter as a meeting of two different lifeworlds with separate horizons. Toombs's theoretical background is the philosophies of Edmund Husserl and Alfred Schutz, rather than those of Heidegger and Gadamer, but as we have seen these four philosophers are members of the same phenomenological tradition.[228] Husserl's concept of lifeworld is essentially the same as Heidegger's worldliness in *Sein und Zeit*, and as Gadamer's world of the historical work in *Wahrheit und Methode*.[229] What all three philosophers are striving to articulate is that human life is embedded in a meaning-structure, a horizon of meaning that surrounds every act, action, articulation, or reading.

The doctor and the patient, although to some extent sharing the same being-in-the-world, occupy different points of perspective in the clinical meeting. The medical meeting can be viewed as a gradual coming-together of the different meaning-horizons of doctor and patient through interpretation in dialogue. The most basic difference between the horizons (or different ways of being-in-the-world) of doctor and patient can be found in the phenomenon of unhomelikeness, which we have explicated as basic to the illness experience. The patient and not the doctor experiences this unhomelikeness in his being-in-the-world, and this unhomelikeness is also the matter of the meeting. The second basic difference between the two perspectives is the doctor's expertise and mission to help in matters concerning health and disease, which is not present in the horizon of the patient.[230] In addition to this, we may find other differences, which can obstruct dialogue, such as differences due to social class, culture, gender, etc. To see how the two different horizons of doctor and patient meet (to a varying degree of course) in medical practice let us proceed with the clinical example from Part 2, Section 8: Jane, meeting with her doctor and being told that she has diabetes.

Jane came to Dr. Z's office at 9 a.m. Monday morning as agreed. She did not have any breakfast before going there, since Dr. Z had told her to abstain from this. She

---

[228] What I find problematic in Toombs's approach is her own understanding of what she is doing in relation to Husserl's philosophy. Toombs claims that what she is carrying out is a *psychological* phenomenology as opposed to Husserl's transcendental project (1992a, p. xi ff.). But if Toombs sacrifices the aspect of generality in her phenomenological analysis (a theory about the general structures of consciousness as opposed to the particular psyche) what will save her analysis from ending up being only a description of *her* experiences as ill? Given her emphasis on the phenomenology of the *body*, it also seems strange to talk about a *psychological* phenomenology. As I have indicated in Section 5 of the second part of this work, I think the difficulties with proceeding from Husserlian phenomenology in developing a theory of health lie elsewhere than in the transcendental aspect of this approach, although the problems are clearly connected to Husserl's image of transcendental philosophy.

[229] This is certainly a gross oversimplification and I do not mean to deny that there remain essential differences between the conceptual frameworks of Husserl, Heidegger and Gadamer. They nevertheless share a basic perspective on the importance of the world as a background-pattern of meaning in the phenomenological analysis, and this is not the place for a detailed investigation of the differences in question. Regarding this, see Gadamer's essays on Husserl in (1987), which make the continuity even more obvious.

[230] Unhomelikeness is even more basic than this difference in medical expertise, however, since the patient may indeed sometimes himself be a doctor who has fallen ill.

could have breakfast later, he had said, and it was essential to the tests he wanted to run that she came on an empty stomach. Jane had already told Dr. Z a great deal about what she had been through the last few months at the dinner on Saturday night, so after chatting for a few minutes and doing a regular physical examination, he went on to take blood and urine samples. Jane was then told to go and have breakfast in the cafeteria and come back after one hour for a new test. She naturally asked if this was necessary, since it meant that she would have to call the office and cancel all morning appointments and Dr. Z said it indeed was. He wanted to measure her blood glucose levels, since her symptoms fit the diagnostic pattern of diabetes. It was only a hypothesis, but he needed to do this in order to check and rule out the possibility. Jane came back after breakfast at 10 a.m. and then again at 11 a.m. to give new blood samples. Since some time was needed to analyse all the test results (not only blood glucose levels, but also other tests of blood and urine) they agreed to meet on Wednesday again. Jane was worried of course, since she had heard diabetes was a severe disease (especially the part about taking shots every day seemed revolting to her), but at the same time she felt that it was good that she had finally taken her problems to a doctor. A medical ground for the way her life had become miserable the last months at least would mean that there was possibly something that could be done about it.

When Jane came back to Dr. Z on Wednesday he told her that she had diabetes. Her fasting blood sugar was 8.2 mmol/l and the tests taken one and two hours after a meal showed 12.5 and 10.5. This meant a relatively mild diabetes, but certainly enough to produce all the symptoms of thirst, dizziness, weight loss, visual problems, etc., that she had experienced the last months. Other tests had shown her diabetes to be so-called type II diabetes, which meant that her pancreas was still producing insulin, but that the cell receptors did not respond adequately to the hormone and the glucose therefore stayed in the blood instead of being processed in the cells. Did Jane understand what he was talking about? Did she know anything about diabetes? Jane said that she did not really care that much about the details, but more about the effects of the disease and the treatment: What would this mean to her? Would she have to take shots every day? Would she become blind? Why had this happened to her? Was it genetic or had she done anything wrong? Dr. Z said that it was lucky they had discovered the diabetes at a relatively early stage because this meant that they would be able to treat it. She would not, if she followed the regulations of treatment, become blind. Indeed she would be able to live a perfectly healthy life – healthier than before – and die of old age provided she could adapt to the new circumstances. But this meant she had to take an interest in the medical aspects of diabetes, she would have to take responsibility for her own treatment and this meant knowing a great deal about the processes of the disease. Not everything of course, not even doctors know everything, as a matter of fact one thing they do not know is why the disease starts. In the case of Jane, it had, to be frank, possibly a lot to do with her life-style – she was overweight and did probably not exercise enough. Her smoking was also a significant issue. This did not rule out factors which were related to a genetic disposition, but it probably meant that these had been triggered by the fact that she was overweight and other aspects of her lifestyle, such as stress and smoking. Did any of her relatives suffer from diabetes? Jane could think of an uncle, who had died from diabetes thirty years ago, but repeated that what was really on her mind was what this would mean to her in terms of medication and change of habits. What would she need to do in order to survive and not end up like her uncle? Dr. Z said that in her case the main treatment would be a strictly regulated diet. This did not mean that she would never be able to have dessert or a glass of wine again, but it did mean that everything she ate would have to be minutely calculated to keep her blood sugar at a normal level. She would have to eat more often, and eat less fat and sugar, more long carbohydrates such as pasta and potatoes, more vegetables, and only lean meat such as chicken and fish. The diet she would be following was in fact one which everyone would feel a lot better on, only in her case it would also be designed to make her lose weight. The kilos she had lost the last few months had not been lost in a healthy way. What had happened was that the food which she had eaten had not been taken up by the cells, which meant that the body had started to use fatty tissue for energy instead. During this whole time her blood glucose levels had been much too high, which had meant severe stress on the body. The symptoms she had experienced affecting her vision were a serious signal that something needed to be done right away to get the glucose level down and prevent damage to her eyes, heart, kidneys and other organs. He would make an appointment for Jane with a dietitian, who would help her design a program for meals. She needed to learn a lot about different types of food – indeed more than he knew himself – and how they could be combined to reach optimal results in terms of keeping blood sugar levels stable and losing weight. She also needed to start exercising daily and stop smoking. She had to start watching her skin, especially her feet, for ulcers and infections, since one effect of the disease was the interference with the circulation and with immune responses. In addition to this he would prescribe medication – an oral agent – which she would take daily. She did not have to worry about shots. They would try to get the insulin up by oral medication, and only if this in combination with diet and exercise did not work would they move on to insulin therapy. Insulin was really not the problem in the first place, since Jane had type II diabetes, in which the pancreas beta cells still produce insulin, but the insulin is not taken up adequately by the body. The oral agent together with the dietary regime and exercise would probably be enough. She would also have to think through her work situation. Stress was known to be a significant factor in the onset and development of the disease. He would teach her how to measure her own blood glucose levels one day a week by using a gluco-meter, a small machine for monitoring levels of sugar within seconds with the help of a lancet prick in the finger. She would keep record of these levels as well as her weight, her meals and her exercise in a special book which they would study together. Indeed Jane was now facing big changes in her life, something he had learnt from other diabetics, but which he also realized to be the case from knowing Jane and the way she had lived before. Most of these changes were however a matter of habits and discipline *and he knew Jane could do it. Indeed she had to. He would help her and teach her everything about the disease that he thought she needed to know.*

Jane was shocked and horrified by all these changes that now faced her. At the same time she was somewhat relieved to have found out the reason for the uncanny symptoms she had suffered the last months and to have learned that something could be done about them. She wondered how hard it would be to do all this – to discipline and regulate her life in a way that seemed depressing and alien to her personality.

This clinical encounter really starts in the restaurant on Saturday night and not in the clinic on Monday morning, (see Part 2, Section 8). In the restaurant Jane tells Dr. Z what she has been through the last few months, how her life has taken on this unhomelike character. Clearly one reason for why she is doing this is that Dr. Z is a physician; she somehow suspects there to be a medical reason for the symptoms she is experiencing. Another reason in this case is that Dr. Z is an old friend with whom she feels she can share her troubles. This case is therefore untypical in two ways: it does not start in the clinic and the two parties know each other well before they meet as doctor and patient for the first time.

The first peculiarity helps us to highlight the fact that what makes the medical meeting medical is not that it takes place in the physical setting of a clinic, but that it includes the two basic differences in horizons of doctor and patient which I mentioned above (unhomelikeness versus medical expertise and mission to help), and that the meeting has the specific goal of bringing the patient's being-in-the-world back to homelikeness again. The second peculiarity of this example helps us to focus on this basic structure of medical practice as the meeting of two different perspectives *in spite of* the parties being close to each other in terms of friendship, social class, culture, etc.; that is, this basic difference of horizons will always be there in the medical meeting and is consequently simply further pronounced and harder to bridge if there exist additional differences pertaining to class, culture and gender.

What this example brings out nicely is that the medical encounter is a *mutual* meeting of two horizons. As I have said above, the doctor is of course the essential interpreter, but if the goal of the meeting is to be attained it is not only necessary that the doctor is able to put himself in the patient's situation; the patient too must come to see things from the medical viewpoint of the doctor. This is obvious in the case of Jane. For Dr. Z it is maybe not so hard to put himself in Jane's situation, since he knows her habits, thoughts and feelings from before. Jane, however, has never been interested in medical matters, but now she has to learn, since she is the very person who is suffering from these biomedical processes and will have to control them through her own behaviour. In a few months she will be an expert in matters of diet, blood glucose levels and other aspects of her disease. Indeed, she does not have a choice if she wants to stay alive and homelike in her being-in-the-world.

Will Jane through the treatment be able to regain health – homelike being-in-the-world? Or is she doomed to unhomelikeness for the rest of her life? Diabetes is indeed a chronic disease – on the physiological level Jane will always be malfunctioning. But on the level of the lifeworld – and this is indeed the level which is important since it is the level experienced and lived by the patient – things might turn out differently. Provided Jane has the strength and will to adjust to the new controlled regime, homelikeness might be a future possibility, just as in the case of some handicaps we mentioned in Section 10 of Part 2. Things here depend both on the person and the development of the disease. If the disease becomes severe enough it might be impossible to bring back a homelike existence no matter how determined Jane is to do this, since the symptoms and strict regime will simply be too much to bear for her. Even if this happens, the unhomelikeness can, one hopes, be kept on a 'lower level' with the help of therapy. If Jane, on the other hand, makes no effort to change her life-style and accept the regulations, homelikeness will not come back no matter how many insulin shots the doctor gives her. Jane has to change *her* understanding of the situation to regain homelike attunement. This includes knowledge, attitude, feelings and actions. Jane will not be alone here – her new understanding is established in meetings with others – aside from Dr. Z, the dietitian, Jane's husband and other close friends will be of importance. I will now proceed to examine further the possibilities of attaining the goal of the clinical encounter – homelike being-in-the-world – through an example of even more severely changed conditions.

7. THE GOAL OF THE MEDICAL MEETING(S)

The goal of the medical meeting is to facilitate health – homelike being-in-the-world. This, as I have pointed out, is one of the basic factors that separates the clinical encounter from other types of meetings between persons. The doctor strives to attain this goal together with the patient through dialogue in a meeting that can be thought of as the interpretive coming-together of the horizons of two different lifeworlds. In some medical cases such a meeting between the horizons might be very hard to establish. One cannot meet with unconscious persons and it is hard to meet with persons who have had main functions of movement and speech destroyed through injury or disease. Meetings in clinical medicine might take place to a large extent through representatives, as is typical for example in the case of children. And the medical meeting is not always a singular meeting; the patient indeed often meets with several different persons from other professions than the physician's during his time in the clinic.

These encounters are, however, still *meetings*, ways of being together which can be understood within the basic structure of dialogic interaction that I have set up with the aid of Gadamer's hermeneutics. The variations will all be taken up and analysed in the next clinical example – one which, just like the others, we began analysing in Part 2: Mary, who, having suffered a stroke, is struggling to come back to a homelike life again. But this example is also chosen in order to discuss a case in which the goal of total recovery might indeed be an illusion. That disease is not always possible to cure is clear. Homelike being-in-the-world, however, is still a possibility in many cases of chronic disease, like in the case of Jane we discussed in the previous section. But homelikeness itself might also in several cases be a goal impossible to fully attain. If the return to homelike being-in-the-world – being healthy as I have analysed it – is hard to imagine, the doctors and the other professions of the clinic must, however, still strive to come as far in this direction as possible. It is in this way that the goal of medicine is to be understood – as an ideal which is strived for, but not always fully within reach.

When Mary wakes up her life has taken on a very uncanny character:

Mary was driven to the emergency unit of the nearby hospital in an ambulance. As she opened her eyes, the medical team gathered en masse around her, checking her responses, determining her reactions, trying to determine the extent of the injury. An oxygen mask lay on Mary's face and fluid was dripping into her arm. She felt disoriented and worried and began to thrash her head. She wanted to say 'What has happened?' and 'Help me!', but did not have the strength. A nurse tried to calm her and she fell back to sleep.

Over the next three days several diagnostic tests were performed on Mary such as a CT scan, an MRI, an echocardiogram and an angiogram. Mary was also given an anticoagulant – heparin – through the cannula in her arm to prevent additional clot formations in the blood vessels. In this way she was also given nutrients and fluid. The tests showed that Mary had suffered a stroke – a cerebral infarction – because of a thrombus – a clot – in her right middle cerebral artery. Damage had been done in her right middle temporal and frontal lobes, and possibly in the thalamus region of her brain as well. The left side of Mary's body was paralysed as the result of this and she had problems communicating with the persons around here. Indeed, she spent the first few days in the hospital for the most asleep, slowly coming back to a life after the infarction.

The way doctors, nurses and others take care of Mary these first few days in the hospital does not seem very dialogic. It rather seems to be a case of applied biology given the impressive display of medical technology which surveys her and keeps her alive. Yet all these machines are in the hands of different persons who use them in order to help Mary. And the way they help her is of course not restricted to the monitoring of high-technology devices, but includes more everyday things such as washing Mary, changing her bedclothes, sitting beside the bed talking to her although they are not sure that she understands, or simply stroking her forehead in order to calm her down and make her feel better. Heidegger in *Sein und Zeit* lays out this basic mode of the togetherness (*Mitdasein*) of being-in-the-world as *Fürsorge* – concern for others:

> Even 'taking care' of feeding and clothing, the nursing of the sick body is concern (*Fürsorge*). . . . With regard to its positive modes, concern has two extreme possibilities. It can, so to speak, take the other's 'care' away from him and put itself in his place in taking care, it can *leap in* for him (für ihn *einspringen*). Concern takes over what is to be taken care of for the other (1986, pp. 121-122).

This is the type of care which is currently given to Mary. Since she is prevented from doing everyday things like washing herself and going to the bathroom; others have to do it for her. The 'leaping in place of Mary' is however provisional and aimed at a future, fuller sense of being-with, namely 'leaping ahead of Mary' (*ihr vorausspringen*):

> In contrast to this, there is the possibility of a concern which does not so much leap in for the other as *leap ahead* of him (ihm *vorausspringt*) in his existential possibility to be. Not in order to take 'care' away from him, but in the first place to give it back to him as such (1986, p. 122).

This is the mode of helping togetherness which, as we shall see, is typical of rehabilitation. 'Leaping ahead of' means teaching the patient to do things himself, not doing them for him. Both these modes of concern for the other (*einspringen* and *vorausspringen*) are, however, to be understood, not as excluding dialogue, but as privative modes of the full dialogue with the other. They do not exclude dialogue, but represent togetherness in a more primitive sense. Mary will still *respond* to her caregivers through the expression of her face and body, not being able to talk to them in a normal way. And as she gets better the dialogue will emerge in a more and more articulated sense, as she returns towards a more homelike being-in-the-world. As I pointed out in part two, even her unconscious body is not treated as a thing, as a part of a big laboratory where experiments are performed, but as the body of an other human being who we want to help.

The stroke which Mary suffered destroyed many functions which were located in the damaged area of her brain. This had profound consequences for Mary's being-in-the-world: for the moods she is now thrown into, for the experience of her own embodiment, for her way of dealing with things around her, for her ability to communicate with others and experience their presence, for her relation to the future and the past – to put it succinctly, for her whole pattern of understanding.

After a few days Mary regained her ability to talk. But her speech had lost the usual inflection and tone, making a machine-like and dead impression. It was hard for Mary's daughter to recognize her warm and humorous mother behind this new voice. Mary was slowly regaining the ability to move her left arm and leg, but the left part of her face was still paralysed which added to her altered appearance. In addition to this the very phenomenon of a left side seemed to have stopped existing for her. She neglected everything on her left side. She ate food only from the right side of her dinner plate, did not notice anyone who approached her from the left, etc. But these were not the worst things for Mary and her relatives. The worst thing was that Mary did not remember the persons who had been closest to her. Sometimes she seemed to remember for a few seconds, only to forget immediately afterwards with whom she had been talking. Mary's whole personality seemed to have changed – not only did she have problems remembering and speaking, but she had turned extremely moody, swinging from manically impulsive, energetic states to deep lethargy several times a day. She was also unpredictable and careless in a way that was totally alien to the old Mary, sometimes refusing to eat and throwing the food on the floor, or using the armchair in her room as a toilet. Mary as well as her relatives were all in despair and wondered what to do in this new and unfamiliar situation.

Mary is clearly very ill and needs help to come back to a healthier life. How is this help set up and carried out in the hospital clinic? The doctor responsible for Mary – Dr. W – is a neurologist who is a specialist on stroke and rehabilitation. She has ordered and analysed all the examinations we mentioned above – computed tomography and magnetic resonance imaging of Mary's brain, echocardiogram and angiography to visualize Mary's heart and cerebral arteries in order to look for blood clots, measurements of her blood pressure, and other tests on Mary's blood. She has also prescribed anticoagulants – heparin and aspirin – for Mary. In addition to this she has carried out several neurological examinations on Mary, which involve communicating with her, asking her to lift her hand, count from ten to one backwards, etc. Dr. W has also tried to find out as much as possible about Mary's earlier life talking to Mary and her relatives. This dialogue will have touched upon her age, job, social situation, history of eating, drinking, smoking, exercise and other relevant issues. The discussion will also, of course, have dealt with Mary's present situation and despair, as the doctor attempts to comfort, explain, predict and plan for the future.

Dr. W is the central figure in the medical meeting with Mary, but she is by no means the only one that Mary meets with. Dr. W is surrounded by a medical team consisting of specialists on stroke rehabilitation which will guide Mary on her way back to a more homelike existence. First, there are the nurses who take care of Mary, helping her with washing, eating, going to the toilet, giving her medication, talking to her and comforting her. They will spend more time with Mary than Dr. W, who has several patients she is responsible for, and they will keep up a dialogue with Mary as well as with Dr. W (just as the other persons responsible for Mary's care, whom we will mention in what follows, will) about her condition.

Secondly, we have the physical therapist, who will help Mary to regain strength and mobility on her left side of the body, which was paralysed by the stroke, through exercise and massage. With the help of the therapist Mary will after four months be able to use her left arm, hand and leg again – not as well as before, but well enough to walk around with crutches. Together with the physiotherapist Mary will also try to regain the left side of her perceptual field with the aid of different exercises.

Thirdly, we have the speech therapist, who helps Mary to regain abilities pertaining to language. The disabilities which the speech therapist deals with may be mainly physical, as in the case of Mary's facial paresis, but they may also pertain to more cognitive skills of language use. It is common after stroke to have problems understanding and responding adequately through language. Words, expressions, logical and grammatical structures are typically lost in left-hemisphere stroke. Since the damage in Mary's brain was located on the right side, she did not have many of these problems, but instead suffered the strange flattening of her voice which we mentioned above. She also had problems with concentration and interaction with others in dialogue and constantly forgot what had just been dealt with in the discussion. Mary's problems recognizing her loved ones and the dramatic mood changes she constantly went through resulted in a very painful situation for her and the relatives. Since Mary suffered from anxiety and feelings of meaninglessness a psychiatrist was consulted, who prescribed an antidepressant medication to relieve her of these symptoms. Unfortunately this medication did not help, but rather made Mary more absent-minded and tired.

After six months it was agreed to move Mary to a nursing home. She clearly could not return to her job, but at sixty-five, she was about to retire anyway. It was also thought unsuitable to take her back to her old apartment, since she could not look after herself, and her closest relative – a daughter – felt she could not take full responsibility for her mother's care. Mary's husband had died ten years earlier, and the other close relatives, two brothers and a sister and their children, felt just as the daughter did. Mary's changed appearance had been very hard for them to accept, and although they certainly still felt very warmly for her, they could not imagine living together with her and devoting their lives to her care. They still hoped for a recovery, but thought the nursing home was the right way to proceed at this point.

Mary herself did not seem to care much; it was as if she was closing off the outer world. The occupational therapist – a representative of another important profession in this type of case – had made great progress with Mary in terms of everyday activities, such as washing and dressing herself, eating, even cooking and washing the dishes, but Mary still seemed disoriented while doing these familiar things. She had found the old patterns in terms of movements and the order of actions, but she was strangely unable to plan ahead and do things in new ways. If spoken to, she would often stop in the middle of a movement simply unable to proceed, and she often forgot vital things, such as, for instance, to turn off the oven, and would go on to watch television while the food turned black and began to burn. It was clear that she was not able to live by herself at the present time.

At this point we leave Mary, although her rehabilitation, successful or not, will go on for a long time. Whether it is successful or not – that is, whether it is able to bring back homelikeness or not – clearly depends on several factors, as we mentioned in the last section. It depends on her doctor and all other medical and paramedical personnel that treat and meet with Mary. It depends on her relatives and the time and commitment they are willing to put in in their relationship with her. And, finally, it depends on Mary herself and her understanding of her own situation and future. *She* must find the way to a regained homelikeness in her being-in-the-world; although guided in dialogue and action by others, it remains *her* way.

As I touched upon briefly in the section on Ricoeur, this new understanding of her own life, just like her former understanding, has a basic narrative structure. Mary makes sense of her life in terms of decisive moments in her history and in terms of the things and persons surrounding her. To understand her life is to understand a story with a plot and time sequence. Obviously the stroke will now be part of this story; there will be a before and after the stroke. Whether Mary is going to be able to return to a homelike existence or not clearly depends on her understanding of this event and how it transformed everything into a before and after. It is not a matter of forgetting all of the past (though Mary, as a matter of fact, as a result of the stroke, has already forgotten a great deal), but rather of finding a new place for the past in the story of her life – a place which does not make the future unattractive and impossible.[231]

By this I do not mean to say that it is Mary who has the last say on the matter of her health; it might indeed be that the neurological damage is too severe for her to be able to find this way back, no matter how good the care of others is and how strong her own will is. Mary's being-in-the-world is not to be understood only as her thoughts and will, but also includes the more opaque domains of attunement and embodiment, which are parts and aspects of her understanding. But no healing can take place if the 'personal' aspect of the case is left unattended to. Dr. W and her colleagues must come to understand Mary and her situation in the dialogue with her in order to be able to help her, and Mary must come to understand and re-evaluate her own situation in order to change it. The meeting must take place in order for this mutual understanding to emerge, for just as Dr. W's medical understanding of Mary must take her perspective into account, Mary's understanding of her new situation can only develop through the meeting with Dr. W and other caregivers. The medical dialogue itself has indeed often been said to have a healing effect, and it is *out of* this dialogue that healing actions come.

8. THE HERMENEUTICS OF MEDICINE – A RECAPITULATION AND DISCUSSION

Let us sum up the analysis of the structure of medical practice which we have carried out so far. Part 1 showed the central feature of this practice to be a *meeting* between doctor (as well as representatives of other professions of the clinic) and patient geared towards regained health for the ill and help-seeking party. After analysing this goal of the clinical encounter in Part 2, we have then in Part 3 endeavoured to understand this meeting as a form of hermeneutics – that is, as interpretive understanding taking place through the meeting. The kind of hermeneutics we have chosen is not a methodology of text reading, but Heidegger's hermeneutics of being-in-the-world, in which understanding is an existential – that is, an *a priori* aspect of the being-together of human beings in the world. Gadamer's hermeneutics was then explicated in order to find a dialogic model for this togetherness of doctor and patient. Understanding as the core mode of the clinical encounter was also shown to *envelop* biological knowledge in the forms of explanation and testing. On the other hand, the biological state of the organism sets certain limits for and typically directs the experiences of the patient's being-in-the-world in a characteristic way in different diseases. Thus, scientific causal explanation, to speak the language of Ricoeur, *develops* understanding (but in a different sense than his type of structural explanation) (1991a, p. 142).

Medical practice has here been found to consist in an interpretive, attentive dialogue geared towards healing actions. To heal means to bring back lost health, a

---
[231] On the topic of narrativity and chronic illness, see Kleinman (1988).

concept which we have analysed in Part 2 as homelike being-in-the-world. With the help of Gadamer's hermeneutics we can understand this interpretive dialogue as the fusion of two horizons – the patient's perspective of unhomelikeness and the doctor's perspective of medical expertise and mission to help the ill. The meeting of the two horizons as the inter-nesting of interpretations means that both parties must come to see things from the other party's point of view in order to reach a new more productive understanding. The doctor must understand the patient's perspective and vice versa, and this can only happen in the shared language of a dialogue. The two parties of the meeting must also through this process of fusion of horizons ultimately reach a to some extent shared understanding which results in a therapeutic decision. The hermeneutics of medicine is thus, to put it in the terminology of Gadamer, an applicative hermeneutics – a kind of understanding and interpretation put to work in a certain setting with a specific goal. The dialogic interpretation is consequently a shared project that contains more than the sum of the two perspectives and which is put to work in the service of healing.

To understand in medicine from the point of view of the physician or of some other member of the medical personnel means to be understand*ing*, which implies the attempt to put oneself in the patient's situation. This situation is always the situation of a particular individual experiencing a particular kind of unhomelikeness in his being-in-the-world. Thus the patient's story – narration – of the illness is a central part of the meeting, offering the best way to such individualized knowledge. The impersonal, case-like aspect of medical practice, especially pronounced in the scientific explanation of diseases we explicated in Section 1 above, is consequently always placed in an understanding dialogue between individuals. This dialogue is marked by different kinds of attunements that are shared to a varying degree in the meeting – unhomelikeness, despair, urge to help, trust, hope, etc. – which reflect the basic asymmetry and estrangement which must be bridged in the meeting. This bridging takes place through a kind of empathy – to be understand*ing* – but the empathy does not exclude a critical, productive distance through which the doctor's (and patient's) understanding takes on a new positive character marked by the professional horizon carrying its specific kind of medical expertise and mission. The meeting between doctor and patient as a fusion of their lifeworld horizons thus includes a productive difference in perspectives which is preserved in the very coming-together of the horizons, which consequently remain distinct although united.

In Section 7 we saw how clinical practice often takes place in the form of the patient's meeting with *several* persons, rather than with just one. These encounters are related to each other – most often through the central place of the physician, who coordinates the medical team and meets the patient in a bundling together of the different clinical perspectives, which are all geared towards healing. The interpretive perspectives that can be of importance in the clinical meeting also include the understanding of relatives or other persons close to the patient, which might have significant impact upon the patient's understanding of his illness and how he is able to change the situation through this understanding. To regain health – homelike being-in-the-world – in many cases demands altered self-understanding, a different interpretation of a radically new situation in life. We also saw how more limited forms of the meeting can be understood as different types of concern (*Fürsorge*), which are dialogic in a restricted sense and aimed towards the possibility of a dialogic meeting in a more complete sense. Health and illness – homelikeness and unhomelikeness in our being-in-the-world – as the end and starting point of the meeting must finally be seen as graded phenomena. The total absence of the unhomelikeness of illness is thus the ideal goal of the medical meeting, but it is a goal that cannot always be fully attained.

Medical practice encompasses a very vast and diverse area. It has been my aim to cover as much as possible of this area with my clinical examples. Through choosing common types of encounters strategically placed in different paradigmatic corners of the clinical territory – streptococcal infection, chronic fatigue syndrome, prostate cancer, diabetes and stroke – I hope to have succeeded in this. But I see no possibility here of dealing with every type of activity and encounter in the clinic, and thus the possibility remains of finding exceptions to the structure I have found typical and essential for medical practice.

One area of medicine which I have purposely abstained from plunging into in this work is psychiatry. The most obvious reason for this is that the hermeneutic structure here is easier to discern than in somatics, and that I consequently have found it more important and challenging to analyse other examples of clinical work than psychiatry. The mental aspects of illness are, however, in no way absent in my examples, but are rather integrated in the somatic scenario. This mirrors the conclusion of the phenomenological analysis in Part 2, that body, feeling, thinking and talking must be seen as inter-nested phenomena, joined together in an attuned understanding bodying forth and articulating itself in the meaning patterns of the world. 'Mental illness' is thus present in the story about Mary (stroke), and mental factors play a significant role in all the other examples in different ways.

In the introduction to this book I declared that my focal point was the generalist rather than the specialist, and that the activities of the latter might embody only parts of the hermeneutical pattern explicated in my analysis. Given this disclaimer the reader might still wonder if it is appropriate to talk about a hermeneutics of medicine in the case of, for example, a broken leg that is put back in position through operation. The patient might hardly see, much less *meet*, the surgeon, who takes care of the fracture. The physician in such a case seems closer to a craftsman than a dialogue partner in life issues. In much the same way as I did in the concluding section of Part 2, I would here like to point out that my phenomenological analysis strives towards explicating the essential, central structure of medical practice, rather than providing an all-inclusive definition of the concept in question. We might have to live with exceptions; the important thing is that they are not central and my examples marginal in the clinical enterprise.

That examples from clinical practice fail to fit my hermeneutical pattern might, however, have another reason than the incompleteness of my analysis: they may be examples of *defective* clinical practice – that is, medicine which fails to live up to parts of its inherent goal and structure. Oliver Sacks, in his autobiographical, clinical story *A Leg to Stand On* (1984), suffers an injury to his leg on a hike in Norway and is subsequently taken to a hospital in England, where he is treated. The surgeon refuses to meet and talk with Sacks about the latter's experiences of his leg being 'dead'. The surgeon does not believe what Sacks is telling him about not being able to feel and move his leg, since this is impossible given physiological data (it later turns out to have a neurophysiological explanation, of course). He has done his job and fixed the leg and the personal problems of Mr. Sacks do not concern him – he has got work to do. Thus he refuses to discuss aspects of the diagnosis, prognosis, or Sacks's experiences of his injured leg with the patient. The portrait of Dr. Swan in Sacks's book is certainly a caricature of a type of physician we can only hope is not too common in the clinic today. Nevertheless it makes obvious that the image of the doctor as only a skilled craftsman or scientist is false even in the case of a broken leg. Most certainly this is true of the *good* physician and of *good* medical practice. But is this reference to ideals rather than facts really a possible counterargument to the examples of clinical practice which fail to live up to the hermeneutical pattern explicated by my analysis? We have now reached a point where the question of the normativeness of this analysis, mentioned in passing several times in the text, can no longer wait.

9. BETWEEN FACTS AND NORMS – DESCRIPTIVE AND NORMATIVE ANALYSIS IN THE PHILOSOPHY OF MEDICINE

This section is designed to treat a possible objection to my analysis of medical practice in this work which might have been on the reader's mind for some time now. The counterargument goes something like this: What the hermeneutical theory of medical practice aims at carrying out is an ontological and epistemological analysis – that is, a descriptive analysis defining the essential forms and limits of medical practice. But what in reality has been carried out above is not a descriptive but a normative analysis, stating not what medical practice *is* but what it *ought to be*. My analysis would thus be defective since it confuses and merges the boundaries of two fundamentally different types of philosophical analysis, dealing with facts on the one hand and norms on the other. Thus, for instance, my understanding of the medical meeting as a dialogue between two persons and not only as a scientific investigation, or of the goal of this meeting as regained homelikeness in the patient's being-in-the-world instead of merely absence of disease, would represent ideals of clinical practice – norms – which are seldom given consideration in contemporary medicine.

I think this counterargument is faulty, but not only for the simple reason that dialogue and a striving towards regained homelikeness really are present (to a varying degree, of course) in contemporary medical practice. My defence against the accusation of having co-mingled descriptive and normative analysis goes much deeper than this and involves the counterargument to the counterargument that the ideal of a neat border between facts and norms is an illusion in the case of medicine as in many other areas. Hume's famous dictum that from an 'is' never follows an 'ought' can be taken as the starting point for this modern view, which has been shown to be illusory and criticized by many before me – notably by Alasdair MacIntyre in the influential work *After Virtue* (1985). The illusion of a sharp border between facts and norms is still very much alive, however, and built into the culture of Western enlightenment, which has been constitutive for medicine as well as for philosophy during the last two hundred years. It is a very powerful illusion, which has undoubtedly produced significant results in both areas, but which has nevertheless begun to be called into question during the last decades of this century. One aspect of this calling into question of the idea of a sharp border between facts and norms is indeed the rebirth of philosophy within medicine which we traced the outlines of in Section 8 of Part 1 above. The philosophy of medicine as a self-sufficient discipline cannot consist in the simple adding together of the philosophies of science, mind and ethics, but will have to find its way through an analysis of medical practice itself. This analysis will involve ontological, epistemological *and* ethical aspects of the activity as parts of the same philosophy. Ethics is not something which can be added as a separate system of norms once the descriptive analysis has been carried out, but will have to form part of the same analysis.

Consequently, the questions of existing medical practice and good medical practice respectively cannot be considered separately as different areas of inquiry. The two questions are obviously *different* questions, but the very possibility of discussing and defining good medical practice rests on an understanding of what medicine *is* in its essence.[232] Only through an ontological analysis can the structures and goals that are to be striven towards in good medicine be found. Still, there is of course something very convincing about Hume's argument. It is indeed hard to see how any new facts about for instance the make-up of the human brain on its own could provide an argument for how we ought to live. New scientific results only alter our view of actions as good or bad *when combined with* some kind of norm that cannot be deduced from science itself. For instance, once we learned that the newborn infant can feel pain in the same way that grown-ups do, we came to look upon some aspects of traditional neonatal care as cruel. But this was only so because we already subscribe to a norm according to which the infliction of pain on human beings is bad.

Bernard Williams has argued for a rewording of Hume's dictum as a contrast between science and ethics rather than between facts and norms (1985, p. 135). Thus his conclusion is that even if ethical norms cannot be directly deduced from scientific research, the only way a conceivable ethics could be developed is by starting with an investigation and analysis of *human nature*. This analysis would deal with the social nature of our being and would consequently not be carried out with the help of the natural sciences, but would take into consideration the results of psychological and social science (Williams 1985, pp. 154-155). I do not think Williams has to limit himself to psychology and sociology here. It would indeed be sensible to include apects of the humanities, anthropology and even ethology, which all deal with the social being of (pre-) human nature. But above all such a research project could

---

[232] I share this perspective with Pellegrino and Thomasma (1981, p. 170 ff.), with whom I began my analysis in Part 1, Section 8.

profit immensely from the disciplines of phenomenology and hermeneutics, which deal with human being-in-the-world as subjective, factual and sociocultural constitution of meaning. The world of human being is a world of meaning, and ethics is clearly part of this sphere of analysis.

As I have tried to show above, medical practice as a form of meeting has a certain goal which separates it from other human activities and meetings – regained homelikeness in the patient's being-in-the-world. This goal is attained through an interpretive dialogue, and the structure of the meeting as this particular form of dialogue depends on the activity having the very goal which it has. Medicine as a human practice thus carries its goal, its essence, inside itself as something that develops and controls the structure of the very activity. Medical ethics – the question of the good in medicine – can thus only be approached through an analysis of the clinical practice itself. The idea of an 'applied ethics' in medicine will always be a mistake if it is merely modelled on principles taken from existing ethical systems which are then simply applied to individual clinical cases in exactly the same manner that they are applied outside the clinic.[233] Utilitarian or deontological ethics in this handbook form will not make us any wiser when facing difficult decisions in the clinic.[234] What is needed in medical ethics is not an old or new supersystem of norms to apply to a value-neutral description of clinical situations, but an ontology and epistemology of medical practice which can guide our thinking when we consider what good means in medicine.

This Aristotelian torch used to illuminate and set alight theories of applied medical ethics in modern analytical philosophy obviously needs further argument and grounding in order to be effective. What is also needed rather than a conflagration in applied ethics is an alternative view which will prove more helpful than earlier ones in the clinic. I will not be able to meet this need in any satisfying way in this work. To a certain extent, however, I think that the analysis of health and medicine, carried out in this study, in itself provides the beginnings of such a theory in taking a few

---

[233] See Pellegrino and Thomasma (1981, p. 170 ff.) and Zaner (1988, p. 6 ff.).

[234] One of the obvious signs of this failure of doctrinary applied medical ethics is, I think, that one of the most influential, and also maybe the best, book in the field, Tom Beauchamp's and James Childress's *Principles of Biomedical Ethics* (1994), articulates different prima facie rules rather than one ethical system. Indeed, these rules cannot be weighed against each other with the help of any normative supersystem such as some version of utilitarianism or deontological ethics. This set-up with different prima facie rules or principles reflecting different ethical systems and ideas (the four main principles in the book are, beneficence, non-maleficence, autonomy and justice), and the absence of a manual enabling us to decide between them, rather than a set-up with one absolute principle for decision-making, mirrors the shortcoming of modern ethical theories when applied in the complex environment of the clinic. The compromise of Beauchamp and Childress brings us back to the original problem of application, of having to choose between these principles in reaching a decision in the concrete clinical situation. If this choice is not to be made through a preexisting ethical theory it must evolve out of a knowledge of and a feeling for the clinical situation itself. As I mentioned in Section 3 above, some authors have suggested hermeneutics as a valuable tool in weighing the principles against each other in the concrete clinical situation. My vision is rather that an ontology of medical practice as a form of hermeneutics in itself provides the way to a feasible clinical ethics. This is, however, a view which I will not be able to develop and defend in any sufficient detail in this work.

steps towards a plausible philosophy of medical practice. Norms have here been found *through* the explication of phenomena and have not been added subsequent to a value-neutral description. But this analysis needs further explication precisely concerning the relation in my phenomenological and hermeneutical theory between facts and norms. In what sense is it possible, indeed necessary, for such a theory to stay *between* facts and norms, without falling prey to a simple confusion of boundaries?

In order to see why the counterargument against my view, accusing it of having confused descriptive and normative analysis, is faulty, let us try to work out what would have to be the case if the objection were correct. The first thing to point out here is that my discussion above in this section has been greatly simplified by focusing exclusively on *ethical* norms and their relation to factual analysis. There are, of course, many other types of norms than ethical ones that one might want to take into consideration in an ontological analysis: scientific norms, rational norms, aesthetic norms, just to mention a few. But in addition to these different fields of norms, there also exists another form of basic normativeness in factual, descriptive analysis which Hume and his followers would not deny the existence and importance of. Indeed, it is not possible to dispute that ontology and epistemology are in themselves normative activities in the sense of explicating borders, of supplying definitions concerning that which ought to be considered, for instance, medicine and medical knowledge and that which ought not. But is this the only kind of normativeness our analysis in this work reveals? I think not. It seems to me that health and medicine are indeed 'thick' phenomena in the sense of embodying many different kinds of normativeness. Thus our analysis of health was not only a characterization of its core mode and limits, but also revealed the normativeness of health as an evaluative concept in the sense of being something *good*, something we want to maintain. This goodness, in turn, is clearly related to an ethical 'ought' in the clinic – health is something which we ought to bring back when it is gone – that is, the person experiencing and communicating unhomelikeness ought to be guided home to health.

In a more specified and less ethically-centered version than I have laid out above, the counterargument against my analysis which I am dicussing here rests on the presumption that one can isolate the description of a phenomenon from its essence. Indeed, it rests on the presumption that there is no other essence to phenomena than the essences that we choose them to have in our descriptions and uses of them. Nominalism and nihilism are undoubtedly features of modern Western society. But what the proponents of these views often seem to blind themselves to is the fact that language and actions are embedded in historical, cultural and social horizons through which they attain their meaning. I have analysed these networks of meanings with the aid of Husserl's concept of lifeworld and Heidegger's concept of being-in-the-world. The claim I am making through this analysis is rather obvious and straightforward. It is clear, for instance, that one cannot arbitrarily decree what the word 'scalpel' will mean, or claim to be auscultating when one is in fact operating on the patient with the aid of one. That which one says and does attains its meaning through being recognized by people in one's community as a specific statement or activity.[235]

To give a description of clinical activity without referring to any goals or essence inherent in this activity would mean to give a description of it in terms of abilities, skills or competences of the persons involved. One cannot give a description of it in terms of actions, since to give a full description of an action also entails the specification of some goal of the action in question.[236] The idea of this type of analysis would be that the specified competence could be used to attain any goal in medicine; that is, the norms as goals to be attained could be added afterwards to the purely descriptive analysis and definition of what medical practice is. How the competence is to be used would be decided by doctors, patients, politicians, or any other persons found suitable.[237] But how could it be possible to describe a competence – an ability – without referring to an action that is goal-determined? As we have seen in Part 2, Section 3, that which is constitutive for an action is exactly that it has a goal aimed at by the agent, and furthermore, any ability must be defined in relation to a specific action. To be able is always to be able to *do* something.

It is indeed possible to give relatively goal-devoid descriptions of abilities to perform very *basic* actions, such as lifting one's hand or even cutting through skin, where the goals of the actions referred to are clearly subgoals which are always aimed for in order to attain more final goals.[238] But as soon as one discusses competence for carrying out more complex actions – such as, for instance, the performance of an appendectomy – it seems like the goal is already embedded in the description of the very ability to carry out the action. And as one reaches the level of the clinical encounter itself it will clearly not be possible to describe the activity in terms of competence which is used in order to bring about goals that can freely be chosen by some agent. Such a description would not be a truthful description of what is going on in clinical practice. The dialogue is not only a putting to work of the doctor's skills in an appropriate way (however the appropriateness is thought to be determined subsequently here), but is also made possible by the *dyadic* setting of doctor and patient. This intersubjective setting, in turn, has a goal which depends on the

---

[235] This is not only a phenomenological insight, but a truth as old as modern philosophy itself which has been expressed in many different theoretical settings. See, for example, von Wright (1971, p. 114) for a Wittgensteinian formulation of this thesis.

[236] See Section 3 of Part 2 above.

[237] For such a view, see Nordin (1996).

[238] See Liss (1996) for a very helpful analysis of the relation between subgoals and final goals in activities as well as of other aspects of the concept of goal in medicine. The question is also, however, whether descriptions of actions on a very basic plane are ever true to what is really being done. The relation between the goals of an action described on a basic and on a more generated plane is indeed not a causal one. The different goals are just different points of view on the same action. In the end, it seems somehow more sensible to describe doctors as carrying out healing actions and not only as uttering phrases, listening through stethoscopes and cutting through skin, at the very least it seems more sensible to include both types of descriptions and their relation to each other in one's analysis, than to leave either of them out.

historical lifeworld that surrounds and determines its meaning – the history of medical practice.

It is not that the individual – doctor or patient – is never able to *choose* what to do in medicine. As we have seen, clinical practice is indeed to a great extent geared towards choices which have to be made in order to bring about healing actions. It is rather that this very freedom is made possible by constraining norms which are inherent in the activity as an intersubjective and historical practice.[239] *Geworfenheit* (thrownness) is what makes *Entwurf* (individual projection) possible, as we have seen in the presentation of Heidegger's philosophy in Part 2. The goals that I choose to strive for through my actions are dependent upon a basic facticity of embodiment and attunement which I did not choose, but which is necessary for an individual choice to be possible. I can only choose freely as *me*, and my individuality depends upon having been thrown into the world of nature and culture. Embodiment represents the 'natural' side of facticity, language its cultural side, with actions stretched out between these extremes as the always-attuned, existential pattern of understanding. Thus my body, the scalpel, the activity of appendectomy, and finally the use of the word 'scalpel', are all played out in the understanding network-pattern of tools that make up my being-in-the-world. This totality of relevance among tools (*Bewandtnisganzheit*) can be appropriated in order to attain different subgoals by which I through my individual understanding (*Entwurf*) can choose what to do and say. But my choices are always determined to a certain extent by my facticity, involving embodiment, history and sociality, which envelops my understanding. Thus the goals are not set only by myself, but also through the historical and social horizon of the lifeworld itself.[240] Medical practice carries such an inherent structure and goal inside itself as the helping of the ill back to health through a interpretive and dialogic therapeutic pattern of healing.

Although many of my arguments in this section have an Aristotelian flavour to them – and we have in Part 2 indeed noted the importance of Aristotle's philosophy of *praxis* for Heidegger's hermeneutics of being-in-the-world[241] – it is certainly not meant as a return to metaphysical biology. As we pointed out, invoking von Wright, above, the purposefulness of the heart must not be misunderstood as purpos*ive* behaviour which demands an acting agent. The goal inherent in medicine is therefore not meant as a potential form inherent in *nature*, in the same manner as the seed bears the form of the tree. The essence of medicine, as it has been explicated in this work, is indeed a goal inherent in *culture*, and it thus expresses the purposiveness of

---

[239] See Brandom (1985), which traces this sort of analysis back to the philosophies of Kant and Hegel.

[240] That human intersubjective practices have goals that are not the sum of the participating agents' aims is not a thesis unique to Heidegger's philosophy. Nor is it a thesis which must rest on a pantheistic philosophy of a *Weltgeist*. See, for example, von Wright (1971), Chapter 4, and MacIntyre (1985), Chapter 14.

[241] See Franco Volpi, *Dasein as praxis: The Heideggerian Assimilation and Radicalization of the Practical Philosophy of Aristotle* (1996). In the case of Gadamer, as I have pointed out, the firm relation to the *praxis*-based philosophy of the *Nicomachean Ethics* becomes at once obvious from a reading of *Wahrheit und Methode* itself (1990, pp. 317-323).

human beings as thinking, feeling, acting and talking creatures expressing meaning in their being-in-the-world. The phenomenological analysis is thus neither physical nor metaphysical. Let us, before closing this section, return one more time to the status and nature of such a phenomenological analysis.

As we have seen in Part 2, Husserl in searching for the *eidos* of experience as *noemata* – constituted by consciousness – became the founder of phenomenology – an attempt to find essence in human cultural being without ascribing this essence a place outside of culture itself. The noematic pattern of the lifeworld does not come from a Platonic otherworldly realm of ideas, from a Christian God, or a from a Hegelian *Geist*, which are thought to embody the purpose and meaning of human existence, but from experience itself. In the same way, the goal and structure of medical practice do not come from 'nature', whatever kind of metaphysics that would involve, but from facticity and intersubjectivity. The purposiveness of medical practice as an inherent normativeness is thus of the same type as the purposiveness of the individual acting agent. But it is a purposiveness which – far from being an unbounded, arbitrary will – is constrained by the meaning-patterns of being-in-the-world as embodied, attuned and social existence; that is, medicine is an intersubjective, historical practice, the structure and goal of which are not determinable in any direct way by any individual person inside or outside of medicine. The practice, the meetings, do, however, certainly involve individuals, and the way they think, act and feel will have an impact on the practice in the long run. This is indeed the only way the practice *could* change: through doctors, nurses, patients, politicians, maybe even philosophers, articulating new ideas and expressing new wishes and wants about the clinical activity.[242] But since medical practice embodies feelings and needs as old as human being itself, it is not only a cognitive, political and scientific business, which we can choose to reshape however we want – at least not if we want to stay true to the ethical demands it places upon us. To fulfil the inherent goal of medical practice means to stay attentive to its hermeneutical structure, which is to a large extent given not only in the form of thoughts and actions, but in the form of feelings and moods. In the concluding section of this work I will focus upon this opaque and essential aspect of clinical practice – its attunement.

---

[242] One must also take into account the embeddedness of clinical activity in a political context, which influences the structure of medicine. I tried to make some sense of this relationship in Section 7 of Part 1, but it is obvious that what I said there has to be integrated with the rest of my analysis in a much more thorough way. This is yet another need I will not be able to meet here. I think, however, that the analysis would have to be carried out on the lifeworld level by studying the interconnection between the more specific meaning patterns of clinical activity and the sociopolitical pattern of, for example, the organisation of health care. See here as a good example of such an analysis the third part of Wifstad (1997), which investigates the lifeworld of modern psychiatry and its relations to science and politics in a very elucidating way by paying close attention to the works of Foucault and Habermas.

10. CONCLUDING REMARKS AND FUTURE PROJECTS – TO APPROACH MEDICAL ETHICS FROM ATTUNEMENT

The reason that I choose to focus upon the attunement of the clinical meeting in this last section is not only that I think this opens up a promising ground for medical ethics, but also that it will enable me to sum up the conclusions I have reached about the structure of medical practice in this work in a somewhat different and, I hope, lucid way. As I have made clear above, what I will say here about medical ethics remains very provisional and tentative – perhaps it would be better to remain silent – and must only be considered a modest outline for a project that would demand another book than this one. It has, nevertheless, struck me in my work on this book, that the attunement of medicine seems to be a, to a large extent, neglected field, at least when considered as something vital and central to the structure and goal of clinical practice.

The biomedical model of health and clinical practice forms an obvious starting point for my critique here. In conceptualizing illness as merely disease and the clinical encounter as merely applied biology, the experience of illness and the unique attunement of the clinical encounter are downplayed as secondary phenomena, which are not essential to the understanding of medicine. What remains of this attunement in the analysis is, if anything at all, a focus upon the pain experienced by the patient as something to be mitigated. Many of the theories of applied medical ethics – particularly utilitarian theories – suffer from the same weakness on this point as the applied biomedical theories. They likewise reduce the vast territory of feelings in medicine to pain as the experience to be minimized and pleasure as the experience to be maximized, and in the same manner as the applied biologists the applied ethicists do not link these experiences conceptually to the worlds and thoughts of patient and doctor. Feelings in these theories carry no meaning but rather are reduced to pure sensations. These sensations are then thought to be evaluated by the rational agent as painful or pleasurable. Such a cognitivist approach is bound to overlook the fact that our understanding, our thoughts and actions, are largely predetermined by our feelings and moods in being attuned. Feeling and thought are indeed inter-nested as attuned understanding in our being-in-the-world, as was pointed out through the presentation of Heidegger's phenomenology above.

In Part 2 I chose to conceptualize health as homelike being-in-the-world in trying to stay attentive to the very experience of being ill and thus regarding the moods of disorientedness, alienness, helplessness and suffering as central to illness. This was not an explication of illness as pure 'subjective feeling' as opposed to objective biological malfunctioning or inability to act, but a theory of attuned, embodied, articulated *understanding*, which included action, thought and language. The latter phenomena, however, were found to be attuned in illness by an unhomelikeness in the person's being-in-the-world and were thus envisaged *by way of* the mood of illness. Moods and feelings in Heidegger's philosophy are not something reflected upon and evaluated by the person as a rational agent, but rather parts of the person's being which shape his thoughts. Indeed, doctors in the clinic do not meet with agents who evaluate their pain and take a rational stand upon what they want to have done with their biological processes, but with worried, help-seeking persons, who need care and understanding in order to be brought back to a homelike being-in-the-world again. *Unhomelikeness*, I think, is the first type of attunement which needs to be emphasized by an ontology and ethics of medicine.

The second type of attunement which I want to emphasize here is primarily embodied by the doctor (or by representatives of other professions in the clinic). I am thinking here of the urge to help the help-seeking by making their lives better, more homelike, again. All the way through this work I have highlighted this aspect of medical practice through my focus upon the meeting and my refusal to identify medicine with science. Medicine as a helping interaction between persons is not aimed primarily at truth, but at guiding the ill back to health again. Science is here an immensely important tool, but nevertheless only a tool and not the basis of the activity. I will readily admit that this one-sided stand, forced upon me by the present historical situation, has lead to a certain negligence in my characterization of clinical activity: it could very well be the case that the doctor in the clinic embodies not only helping attunement but also a certain curiosity and awe in the face of the phenomenon of human being which is most characteristically expressed in medical science and research. The *urge to know* might very well play a more important role in medical practice than I have been able to make apparent here. This attunement of curiosity and wonder must however clearly be wedded to the attunement of helping if it shall not lead to perverted behaviour in the clinic. The patient is always first and foremost a person to help and not a research object.

The interpretive aspect of the meeting as a dialogue aimed at regained health for the patient clearly expresses this dialectic between curiosity and the desire to help on the part of the doctor. To understand the unhomelikeness of the patient's being-in-the-world the doctor needs to both understand and be understand*ing*. As we have seen this understanding envelops scientific explanation and testing in reaching a conclusion regarding the reason for the patient's illness. Understanding also involves empathy and trust, in the way we have developed it with the help of Gadamer's hermeneutics of fusion of horizons in the dialogic meeting between two lifeworlds. And it finally involves a certain form of suspiciousness and openness for the unexpected in the unique constellation of clinical hermeneutics, whereby one diagnoses the individual person through a set of 'icons of disease' (Sundström 1987).

The way from unhomelikeness to regained homelikeness in the patient's being-in-the-world can thus be described through a number of attunements which are typically present in the understanding dialogue between doctor and patient. These attunements are of two primary kinds. The first kind – expressed in unhomelikeness on the part of the patient and the urge to help and know on the part of the doctor – are typically, at least initially, embodied by only one of the parties in the meeting. They are tied to the individual person in his experience and understanding of himself and the surrounding world. Attunements of the second kind are typical of the very dialogue *between* the parties; that is, they are shared in an intersubjective manner which is not reducible to the participants as individuals. Trust is a paradigmatic example here. The trust between doctor and patient which attunes, or to a certain extent fails to attune, the dialogue is a mutual trust. Trust may begin as one-sided, but if it is to last it must always pertain to a mutuality. The urge to know, the curiosity concerning how things *really are*, is another example of an attunement that might gradually become more and more shared as the dialogue continues. The doctor wants to understand why the patient is ill right from the beginning, and so does the patient of course, but their perspectives and tools for reaching this understanding may be quite different. The meeting of the horizons of their lifeworlds means that these different forms of understanding gradually 'tune in' to one another.

As is obvious from this short outline of a philosophy of the attunement of clinical practice, which could be valuable in working out a medical ethics, I have chosen a different starting point than the main proponents of the critique against applied ethics which I referred to in the last section. MacIntyre as well as Pellegrino and Thomasma propound an ethics based in the Aristotelian or Christian notions of virtues and the good and rightful life.[243] I think a phenomenological and hermeneutical analysis of attunement opens up a more promising scenario, given the possibility of individually *and* intersubjectively attuned understanding. Exactly how the different forms of significant attunements which are found in the analysis (and there are obviously more of them than I have been able to uncover in a systematic way here) are to be related to an *ought* is a question that will have to be dealt with elsewhere. If given the opportunity in the future to attempt to answer this question, I would begin by examining the traces of existing analyses of this sort – analyses formulated primarily within the phenomenological tradition – through a study of the works of authors such as Max Scheler, Paul Ricoeur, Emmanuel Lévinas, Knud Løgstrup, Werner Marx, Hans Jonas and Herbert Spiegelberg.[244] I would also study carefully and systematically the structure and attunement of spoken dialogue in a way that has not been possible in this work.[245] But this is a future project. For the time being I and the reader will have to be satisfied with the ontological and epistemological steps taken here towards a philosophy of medical practice as a particular form of hermeneutics. They might not represent a full-blown theory, but they are nevertheless, I hope, significant steps further on the path to a sound philosophy of medical practice.

---

[243] See MacIntyre (1985), and Pellegrino and Thomasma (1993).

[244] With two exceptions I do not find it necessary to enumerate famous and well-known titles here: in Jonas's case I am not thinking of his philosophical biology that I dealt with in Part 1, but of his later works, notably *Das Prinzip der Verantwortung* (1979); and in the case of Spiegelberg I do not mean his more scholary work on the phenomenological tradition, but the less well-known *Steppingstones Toward an Ethics for Fellow Existers* (1986). It is important to stress and remember the expression 'traces of an analysis of attunement' when I refer to these authors as possible sources for a medical ethics. What I do not intend is, of course, some kind of impossible synthesis of their different theories and points of view, but a critical reading gathering thoughts (or rather feelings) for an independent analysis. It seems highly likely to me that such an analysis will not end up abandoning all principles of the applied ethics which I have criticized above, but rather will return to many of them in a new way on the basis of a different theory of human nature.

[245] Here works such as Cassell (1985) and Mishler (1984), mentioned in Part 1, are exemplary in their approach to the *spoken* language of medicine.

SUMMARY

This study has been an attempt to develop an ontology and epistemology of medicine with the aid of the philosophical theories of phenomenology and hermeneutics. Medicine has in this work been considered to be a particular form of practice with a certain intersubjective structure, rather than an assembly of scientific theories and technologies applied in the clinic. To be more precise, medicine has been suggested to be an interpretive, helping meeting between two persons (doctor or other health-care professional and patient) aimed at bringing about health for the ill, help-seeking party. Phenomenology and hermeneutics have then been used to more fully understand what is meant by an interpretive, helping meeting and by its goal – health.

As we have seen, modern science and technology are indeed put to work today in this medical meeting in order to guide diagnosis and therapy (and most often certainly for the best), but, in spite of this, medical practice cannot be understood as applied biology only. The tendency to identify medical practice with applied medical science and technology – investigation and manipulation of the biological organism – in contemporary medicine runs the risk of making the ill person, the subject of the scientific investigations and therapies, invisible, since he is thereby reduced to a biological organism *only* and not focused upon as a person suffering and expressing an illness as a meaningful phenomenon with significance in his everyday world.

Consequently, rather than being regarded as the essence of medical practice, modern medical science should be understood within the context of the interpretive, healing meeting between doctor and patient; the task of applied medical science is thus to subserve the goal of this meeting – regained health for the patient. In order to see this more clearly, a historical survey of the practice of medicine was provided in Part 1 of this work. Before the advent of modern medicine around 1800 the meeting aspect of medical practice – its status as an encounter between persons – is more easily discernible, since the interpretive matrices employed in order to understand health and illness are connected to a cosmology of lifeworld characteristics and not to modern biology. Humoral pathology is the most obvious example of this, since according to that doctrine, an excess of a certain fluid is thought to cause an illness which also expresses the temperament of the individual in question. The meeting between doctor and patient in pre-modern medicine thus in an obvious way involved a dialogue with the ill person which took into consideration his personality, feelings and thoughts about illness and life.

The dawning of modern medicine in Paris around 1800 and the slowly emerging influence on medical practice exerted by the new scientific attitude led to a change in the relationship between doctors and patients. A new trust for the medical profession, fostered by the success of medical science in diagnosing and curing disease, was eventually joined by a distrust caused by the marginalization of the dialogue between doctor and patient. Modern medical science and technology tend to promote a conceptualization of the patient as an object instead of a subject, and, despite the scientific success of this attitude, the practice of medicine as a consequence faces new problems.

To paint a picture of this state of modern medical practice I surveyed influential research carried out in medical psychology, sociology and anthropology, and called attention to several symptoms of a crisis. These symptoms were the awareness of a threatened 'art of medicine' in contrast to medical science within the medical establishment; the influence of psychoanalysis on general practice; the difficulty to deal with chronic illness and illness without disease; problems with patient compliance; patients' interest in alternative medicine influenced by other world views than the Western scientific one; the exploding interest for medical ethics; and patient autonomy movements. Finally, in the last section of Part 1, I presented the 'rebirth' of the philosophy of medicine, which has taken place during the last three decades, with a focus on the philosophy of medical practice. I adopted the definition of Pellegrino and Thomasma – 'Medicine is a relation of mutual consent to effect individualized well-being by working in, with, and through the body' – as a framework and starting point for my own theory of medical practice, and thus established that a characterization of health as the goal of the medical meeting ('individualized well-being') is crucial in working out a philosophy of medicine.

Part 2 of this work was accordingly devoted to health theory. I first presented some main strains of ancient health theory and then moved on to the modern scientific alternative in the form of the biostatistical theory of Boorse, based on statistical normality of biological functions, which ultimately serve the survival and reproduction of the organism. I considered the main weakness of this theory to be that it looks upon human beings exclusively as biological organisms – as sophisticated machines – and not, in addition to this, as persons. Organisms have diseases, and these are certainly in most cases the cause of ill health, but only human beings living in the world are ill or healthy. Health and illness are consequently not phenomena analysable exclusively in the terms of science, but are evaluative concepts referring to the experiences, ambitions and abilities of human beings situated in certain contexts – lifeworlds.

In order to find a health concept for the clinician rather than the pathologist I then turned to the holistic theory of Nordenfelt, according to which health is defined as the ability of an individual to realize vital goals given standard circumstances. The focus upon goals to be realized by acting in the world brings out the significance of purposiveness and environment as crucial in developing a theory of health. My own alternative, based on the phenomenology of Heidegger, works within such a meaning-centred perspective, by highlighting the life of the person as an understanding being-in-the-world. The concept of attunement (*Befindlichkeit*) was chosen as the starting point for an explication and characterization of the phenomena of health and illness as, respectively, homelike and unhomelike ways of being-in-the-world. The attunement of understanding, which takes on the character of unhomelikeness in illness, was then further examined and exemplified through case studies of different types of diseases. The concepts of defective transcendence, coherence, rhythm and balance were used to develop and better understand the unhomelikeness played out in the ill person's being-in-the-world. The phenomenological outline was compared to the holistic theory of Nordenfelt, and similarities were found in the focus upon being-in-the-world as an action pattern of the person. The emphasis upon *attuned* understanding, however, also highlights the central position of the feeling of illness in the phenomenological alternative for a theory of health.

Finally the lived body (*Leib*) was integrated into the existential pattern Heidegger lays out in *Sein und Zeit* and linked to his analysis of the totality of relevance of tools (*Bewandnisganzheit*). The status of the lived body as belonging to this structure of the world, and yet at the same time being a projective aspect of *Dasein*, brings out the basic alienness of human life, which manifests itself in illness, in a new way. Not only is the world alien in illness, but the body as a part of this world also reveals itself as having a life of its own, which one is not able to control. In a concluding section of Part 2 I then tried to defend my characterization of illness as unhomelike being-in-the-world against several types of objections, and related my phenomenological outlines of illness and health to the mission of clinical medicine, the goal of which is thus, according to my proposal, *homelikeness* in the being-in-the-world of the patient.

In Part 3 I attempted to develop a hermeneutical theory of clinical practice through a philosophical analysis of the structure of the clinical encounter between health-care professional and patient. Medical practice has here been found to consist in an interpretive, attentive dialogue geared towards healing actions. To heal means to restore lost health – that is, homelike being-in-the-world. Interpretive understanding of the patient's being-in-the-world was thus shown to be central to the medical diagnosis, and biomedical explanation and prediction were shown to form specialized parts of this pattern of understanding. To quote Ricoeur: 'Understanding *envelops* explanation, explanation, in turn, *develops* understanding'.

In Sections 3 and 4 of Part 3 I examined earlier attempts to develop a hermeneutics of medicine – the most important one being the work of Leder – based on different conceptualizations of text reading. The tradition of hermeneutics I have chosen to work within in this work is not a methodology of text reading, but Heidegger's phenomenological hermeneutics of being-in-the-world, according to which understanding is an existential – that is, an *a priori* aspect of the being-together of human beings in the world. Gadamer's hermeneutics – evolving out of the soil of Heidegger's philosophy – was explicated in Part 3 in order to find a dialogic model for this togetherness of doctor and patient.

With the help of Gadamer's hermeneutics we can understand the interpretive dialogue of the medical meeting as the gradual fusion of two horizons – the patient's perspective of unhomelikeness and the doctor's perspective of medical expertise and mission to help. The meeting of the two horizons as the inter-nesting of interpretations means that both parties must come to see things from the other party's point of view in order to reach a new, more productive understanding. The doctor must understand the patient's perspective and vice versa, and this can only happen in the shared language of a dialogue. The two parties of the meeting must also, through this process of gradual fusion of horizons, ultimately reach a, to some extent, shared understanding, which results in a therapeutic decision. The hermeneutics of medicine is thus, to speak the language of Gadamer, an applicative hermeneutics – a kind of understanding and interpretation put to work in a certain setting with a specific goal. The dialogic interpretation is consequently a shared project which contains more than the sum of the two perspectives and which is put to work in the service of healing.

To understand in medicine from the doctor's, or other medical professional's, point of view implies to be understand*ing*, which means attempting to put oneself in the patient's situation. This situation is always the situation of a particular individual experiencing a particular kind of unhomelikeness in his being-in-the-world. Thus the patient's story – narration – of the illness is a central part of the meeting, offering the best way to such individualized knowledge. The impersonal, case-like aspect of modern medical practice, especially pronounced in the scientific explanation of diseases, is consequently always placed in an understanding dialogue between individuals. This dialogue is marked by different kinds of attunements, which are shared to a varying degree in the meeting – unhomelikeness, despair, the urge to help, trust, hope, etc. – which reflect the basic asymmetry and estrangement to be bridged in the meeting. This bridging takes place through a kind of empathy – through the doctor being understand*ing* – but the empathy does not exclude a critical, productive distance through which the doctor's understanding takes on a new, positive character marked by the professional horizon manifesting its specific kind of medical thinking. The meeting between doctor and patient as a fusion of their lifeworld horizons thus includes a productive difference in perspectives which is preserved in the very coming-together of the horizons, which consequently remain distinct although united.

In Section 7 of Part 3 we saw how clinical practice often takes place in the form of the patient's meeting with *several* persons, rather than with just one. These encounters are related to each other – most often through the central place of the physician who co-ordinates the medical team and meets with the patient in a synthesis of the different clinical perspectives, which are all geared towards healing. The interpretive perspectives that can be of importance in the clinical meeting also include the understanding of relatives or other persons close to the patient, which might have significant impact upon the patient's understanding of his illness and how he is able to change the situation through this understanding. To regain health – homelike being-in-the-world – in many cases demands altered self-understanding, a different interpretation of a radically new situation in life. We also saw how more limited forms of the meeting can be understood as different types of concern (*Fürsorge*), which are dialogic in a restricted sense and aimed towards the possibility of a dialogic meeting in a more complete sense. Health and illness – homelikeness and unhomelikeness in our being-in-the-world – as the end and starting point of the meeting must finally be seen as graded phenomena. The total absence of the unhomelikeness of illness is thus

SUMMARY

the ideal goal of the medical meeting, but it is a goal that cannot always be fully attained.

Medical practice encompasses a very vast and diverse area. It has been my aim to cover as much as possible of this area with my clinical examples. Through choosing common types of encounters strategically placed in different paradigmatic corners of the clinical territory – streptococcal infection, chronic fatigue syndrome, prostate cancer, diabetes and stroke – I hope to have succeeded in this.

The two last sections of Part 3 have dealt with the question of the normative status of my analysis. Clearly the hermeneutical structure of medical practice, which I have uncovered in this work, is not only related to a description of existing medical practice, but also to a pattern which is claimed to be constitutive of *good* medical practice. Thus the ontological and epistemological analysis is linked to the questions of medical ethics. The structure and goal of medical practice are thus inherent to the activity itself as a historically determined essence to be realized, and also, within certain confining limits, changed, by the participants in the medical enterprise. Finally, the different attunements of the medical meeting were proposed as an interesting starting point for examining the facticity of medical practice and the demands it places on an ethical analysis.

REFERENCES

Ackerknecht, Erwin H. (1967) *Medicine at the Paris Hospital 1774-1848*, Baltimore: Johns Hopkins University Press.
Ackerknecht, Erwin H. (1982) *A Short History of Medicine*, Baltimore: Johns Hopkins University Press.
Amundsen, Darrel W., and Ferngren, Gary B. (1983) 'Evolution of the Patient-Physician Relationship: Antiquity Through the Renaissance', in *The Clinical Encounter: The Moral Fabric of the Patient-Physician Relationship*, ed. Shelp, Earl E., Dordrecht: Reidel Publishing.
Antonovsky, Aaron (1987) *Unravelling the Mystery of Health*, San Francisco: Jossey-Bass Corp.
Aristotle, Works translated into English, Oxford University Press.
Balint, Michael (1972) *The Doctor, His Patient and the Illness*, New York: International Universities Inc.
Baron, Richard J. (1990) 'Medical Hermeneutics: Where is the "Text" We are Interpreting?', *Theoretical Medicine*, vol. 11: pp. 25-28.
Beauchamp, Tom L., and Childress, James F. (1994) *Principles of Biomedical Ethics*, 4th ed., Oxford University Press.
Bernet, Rudolf, Kern, Iso, and Marbach, Eduard (1989) *Edmund Husserl: Darstellung seines Denkens*, Hamburg: Felix Meiner Verlag.
Binswanger, Ludwig (1962) *Being-in-the-World: Selected Papers of Ludwig Binswanger*, New York: Basic Books.
Boorse, Christopher (1975) 'On the Distinction Between Disease and Illness', *Philosophy and Public Affairs*, vol. 5: pp. 49-68.
Boorse, Christopher (1976) 'What a Theory of Mental Health Should Be', *Journal for the Theory of Social Behaviour*, vol. 6: pp. 61-84.
Boorse, Christopher (1977) 'Health as a Theoretical Concept', *Philosophy of Science*, vol. 44: pp. 542-573.
Boorse, Christopher (1997) 'A Rebuttal on Health', in *What is Disease?*, eds. Humber, J., and Almeder, R., New Jersey: Humana Press.
Borck, Cornelius (1996) 'Anatomien medizinischer Erkenntnis: der Aktionsradius der Medizin zwischen Vermittlungskrise und Biopolitik', in *Anatomien medizinischen Wissens, Medizin, Macht, Moleküle*, ed. Borck, Cornelius, Frankfurt am Main: Fischer Verlag.
Borell, Merriley (1993) 'Training the Senses, Training the Mind', in *Medicine and the Five Senses*, eds. Bynum W. F., and Porter, Roy, Cambridge University Press.
Boss, Medard (1975) *Grundriss der Medizin und der Psychologie*, Bern: Hans Huber Verlag.
Bracegirdle, Brian (1993) 'The Microscopical Tradition', in *Companion Encyclopedia of the History of Medicine*, vol. 1, eds. Bynum W. F., and Porter, Roy, London: Routledge.
Brandom, Robert B. (1985) 'Freedom and Constraint by Norms', in *Hermeneutics and Praxis*, ed. Hollinger, Robert, University of Notre Dame Press.
Buytendijk, F. J. J. (1958) *Mensch und Tier: ein Beitrag zur vergleichenden Psychologie*, Hamburg: Rohwolt.
Buytendijk, F. J. J. (1962) *Pain: Its Modes and Functions*, University of Chicago Press.
Buytendijk, F. J. J. (1974) *Prolegomena to an Anthropological Physiology*, Pittsburgh: Duquesne University Press.
Bynum, W. F., and Porter, Roy (eds.) (1993a) *Medicine and the Five Senses*, Cambridge University Press.
Bynum, W. F., and Porter, Roy (eds.) (1993b) *Companion Encyclopedia of the History of Medicine*, London: Routledge.

REFERENCES

Byrne, Patrick S., and Long, Barrie E. L. (1976) *Doctors Talking to Patients: A Study of the Verbal Behaviour of General Practitioners Consulting in their Surgeries*, London: HMSO.

Canguilhem, Georges (1991) *The Normal and the Pathological*, New York: Zone Books.

Cannon, Walter B. (1932) *The Wisdom of the Body*, New York: Norton.

Carson, Ronald A. (1990) 'Interpretive Bioethics: The Way of Discernment', *Theoretical Medicine*, vol. 11: pp. 51-59.

Cassell, Eric J. (1976) *The Healer's Art*, New York: Lippincott.

Cassell, Eric J. (1985) *Talking with Patients*, Cambridge, Mass.: MIT Press.

Cassell, Eric J. (1991) *The Nature of Suffering*, Oxford University Press.

Childress, James F., and Siegler, Mark (1984) 'Metaphors and Models of Doctor-Patient Relationships: Their Implications for Autonomy', *Theoretical Medicine*, vol. 5: pp. 17-30.

Conrad, Lawrence I. (1995a) 'The Arab-Islamic Medical Tradition', in *The Western Medical Tradition 800 B.C. to A.D. 1800*, eds. Conrad, Lawrence I. et al., Cambridge University Press.

Conrad, Lawrence I., et al. (eds.) (1995b) *The Western Medical Tradition 800 B.C. to A.D. 1800*, Cambridge University Press.

Cunningham, Andrew, and Williams, Perry (eds.) (1992) *The Laboratory Revolution in Medicine*, Cambridge University Press.

Daniel, Stephen L. (1986) 'The Patient as a Text: A Model of Clinical Hermeneutics', *Theoretical Medicine*, vol. 7: pp. 195-210.

Davis, F. Daniel (1997) '*Phronesis*, Clinical Reasoning, and Pellegrino's Philosophy of Medicine', *Theoretical Medicine*, vol. 18: pp. 173-195.

Dekkers, Wim (1998) 'Hermeneutics and the Experiences of the Body: The Case of Low Back Pain', *Theoretical Medicine and Bioethics*, vol. 19: pp. 277-293.

Dreyfus, Hubert L. (1991) *Being-in-the-World: A Commentary on Heidegger's Being and Time, Division 1*, Cambridge, Mass.: MIT Press.

Dreyfus, Hubert L., and Rabinow, Paul (1982) *Michel Foucault: Beyond Structuralism and Hermeneutics*, University of Chicago Press.

Edelstein, Ludwig (1967) *Ancient Medicine: Selected Papers of Ludwig Edelstein*, eds. Temkin Owsei, and Temkin C. Lilian, Baltimore: Johns Hopkins University Press.

Eisenberg, Leon (1977) 'Disease and Illness: Distinctions Between Professional and Popular Ideas of Sickness', *Culture, Medicine and Psychiatry*, vol. 1: pp. 9-23.

Engel, George (1977) 'The Need for a New Medical Model: A Challenge for Biomedicine', *Science*, vol. 196, no. 4286: pp. 129-136.

Engelhardt, H. Tristram, Jr. (1984) 'Clinical Problems and the Concept of Disease', in *Health, Disease, and Causal Explanation in Medicine*, eds. Nordenfelt, Lennart, and Lindahl, Ingemar B., Dordrecht: Reidel Publishing.

Engelhardt, H. Tristram, Jr., and Spicker, Stuart F. (1975) *Evaluation and Explanation in the Biomedical Sciences: Proceedings of the First Trans-Disciplinary Symposium on Philosophy and Medicine Held at Galveston, May 9-11, 1974*, Dordrecht: Reidel Publishing.

Feinstein, Alvan R. (1967) *Clinical Judgement*, Baltimore: Williams and Wilkins.

Fisher, Gregg Charles (1997) *Chronic Fatigue Syndrome: A Comprehensive Guide to Symptoms, Treatments, and Solving the Practical Problems of CFS*, New York: Warner Books.

Fitzpatrick, Ray, and Scambler, Graham (1984) 'Social Class, Ethnicity and Illness', in *The Experience of Illness*, ed. Fitzpatrick, Ray, New York: Tavistock Publications.

Fleck, Ludwik (1980) *Entstehung und Entwicklung einer wissenschaftlichen Tatsache: Einführung in die Lehre vom Denkstil und Denkkollektiv*, Frankfurt am Main: Suhrkamp Verlag.

Foucault, Michel (1972) *Histoire de la folie à l'âge classique*, Paris: Editions Gallimard.

Foucault, Michel (1974) *Surveiller et punir*, Paris: Editions Gallimard.

Foucault, Michel (1984) *Histoire de la sexualité*, vols. 2, and 3, *L'usage des plaisirs* and *Le souci de soi*, Paris: Editions Gallimard.

Foucault, Michel (1994a) *The Birth of the Clinic: An Archaeology of Medical Perception*, New York: Vintage Books.

Foucault, Michel (1994b) *The Order of Things: An Archaeology of the Human Sciences*, New York: Vintage Books.

REFERENCES

French, Roger (1993) 'The Anatomical Tradition', in *Companion Encyclopedia of the History of Medicine*, vol. 1, eds. Bynum, W. F., and Porter, Roy, London: Routledge.

Freud, Sigmund (1919) *Das Unheimliche*, in Gesammelte Werke, vol. 12, London: Imago Publishing.

Fulford, K. W. M. (1989) *Moral Theory and Medical Practice*, Cambridge University Press.

Fulford, K. W. M. (1993) 'Praxis Makes Perfect: Illness as a Bridge Between Biological Concepts of Disease and Social Conceptions of Health', *Theoretical Medicine*, vol. 14: pp. 305-320.

Gadamer, Hans-Georg (1987) *Hegel, Husserl, Heidegger*, Tübingen: J. C. B. Mohr.

Gadamer, Hans-Georg (1990) *Wahrheit und Methode: Grundzüge einer philosophischen Hermeneutik*, 6th ed., Tübingen: J. C. B. Mohr.

Gadamer, Hans-Georg (1993) *Über die Verborgenheit der Gesundheit*, Frankfurt am Main: Suhrkamp Verlag.

Gatens-Robinson, Eugenie (1986) 'Clinical Judgement and the Rationality of the Human Sciences', *Journal of Medicine and Philosophy*, vol. 11: pp. 167-178.

Gelfand, Toby (1993) 'The History of the Medical Profession', in *Companion Encyclopedia of the History of Medicine*, vol. 2, eds. Bynum, W. F., and Porter, Roy, London: Routledge.

Goffman, Erving (1974) *Stigma: Notes on the Management of Spoiled Identity*, New York: J. Aronson.

Gogel, Edward L., and Terry, James S. (1987) 'Medicine as Interpretation: The Uses of Literary Metaphors and Methods', *Journal of Medicine and Philosophy*, vol. 12: pp. 205-217.

Good, Byron J. (1977) 'The Heart of What's the Matter: The Semantics of Illness in Iran', *Culture, Medicine and Psychiatry*, vol. 1: pp. 25-58.

Good, Byron J. (1994) *Medicine, Rationality and Experience: An Anthropological Perspective*, Cambridge University Press.

Good, Byron J., and Good, Mary-Jo DelVecchio (1981) 'The Meaning of Symptoms: A Cultural Hermeneutic Model for Clinical Practice', in *The Relevance of Social Science for Medicine*, eds. Eisenberg, Leo, and Kleinman, Arthur, Dordrecht: Reidel Publishing.

Gorovitz, Samuel, and MacIntyre, Alasdair (1976) 'Toward a Theory of Medical Fallibility', *Journal of Medicine and Philosophy*, vol. 1: pp. 51-71.

Graninger, Ulrika (1997) *Från osynligt till synligt: bakteriologins etablering i sekelskiftets svenska medicin*, Linköping Studies in Arts and Science.

Granshaw, Lindsay (1993) 'The Hospital', in *Companion Encyclopedia of the History of Medicine*, vol. 2, eds. Bynum, W. F., and Porter, Roy, London: Routledge.

Guignon, Charles B. (1991) 'Pragmatism or Hermeneutics? Epistemology after Foundationalism', in *The Interpretive Turn: Philosophy, Science, Culture*, eds. Hiley, David R., et al., Ithaca: Cornell University Press.

Guignon, Charles B. (1993) 'Authenticity, Moral Values, and Psychotherapy', in *The Cambridge Companion to Heidegger*, ed. Guignon, Charles B., Cambridge University Press.

Guthrie, Diana W., and Guthrie, Richard A. (1997) *The Diabetes Sourcebook*, Los Angeles: Lowell House.

Habermas, Jürgen (1971) *Hermeneutik und Ideologiekritik*, Frankfurt am Main: Suhrkamp Verlag.

Hardy, Robert C. (1978) *Sick: How People Feel about Being Sick and what They Think of Those who Care for Them*, Chicago: Teach'em Inc.

Harrington, Anne (ed.) (1997) *The Placebo Effect: An Interdisciplinary Exploration*, Cambridge, Mass.: Harvard University Press.

Have, Henk ten (1994) 'The Hyperreality of Clinical Ethics: A Unitary Theory and Hermeneutics', *Theoretical Medicine*, vol. 15: pp. 113-131.

Heidegger, Martin (1954a) 'Bauen Wohnen Denken', in *Vorträge und Aufsätze*, Pfullingen: Neske.

Heidegger, Martin (1954b) 'Die Frage nach dem Technik', in *Vorträge und Aufsätze*, Pfullingen: Neske.

Heidegger, Martin (1983) *Grundbegriffe der Metaphysik: Welt – Endlichkeit – Einsamkeit*, Gesamtausgabe, vol. 29-30, Frankfurt am Main: V. Klostermann.

Heidegger, Martin (1986) *Sein und Zeit*, 16th ed., Tübingen: Max Niemeyer Verlag.

Heidegger, Martin (1988) *Phänomenologische Interpretationen zu Aristoteles: Einführung in die phänomenologische Forschung*, Gesamtausgabe, Bd. 61, Frankfurt am Main: V. Klostermann.

Heidegger, Martin (1989) *Nietzsche I*, Pfullingen: Neske.

Heidegger, Martin (1994) *Zollikoner Seminare*, Frankfurt am Main: V. Klostermann.

REFERENCES

Held, Klaus (1993) 'Fundamental Moods and Heidegger's Critique of Contemporary Culture', *Reading Heidegger: Commemorations*, ed. Sallis, John, Bloomington: Indiana University Press.

Hellström, Olle (1994) *Vad sjukdom vill säga: om patienters uttryck och läkares svar, om dialogmedicin och skapande möten*, Örebro: Libris.

Helman, Cecil G. (1990) 'Gender and Reproduction', in *Culture, Health and Illness*, London: Wright Butterworth Scientific.

Hiley, David R., Bohman, James F., and Shusterman, Richard (eds.) (1991) *The Interpretive Turn: Philosophy, Science, Culture*, Ithaca: Cornell University Press.

Horgby, Ingvar (1995) 'Begreppet person: en essä om en kristen uppfinning', in *Hälsosamma tankar*, eds. Liss, Per-Erik, and Petersson, Bo, Nora: Nya Doxa.

Hoy, David Couzens (1993) 'Heidegger and the Hermeneutic Turn', in *The Cambridge Companion to Heidegger*, ed. Guignon, Charles B., Cambridge University Press.

Hunter, Kathryn Montgomery (1991) *Doctors' Stories: The Narrative Structure of Medical Knowledge*, New Jersey: Princeton University Press.

Husserl, Edmund (1976a) *Ideen zu einer reinen Phänomenologie und phänomenologischen Philosophie. Erstes Buch: Allgemeine Einführung in die reine Phänomenologie*, Husserliana III, Den Haag: Nijhoff.

Husserl, Edmund (1976b) *Die Krisis der europäischen Wissenschaften und die transzendentale Phänomenologie*, Husserliana VI, Den Haag: Nijhoff.

Hydén, Lars-Christer, and Mishler, Elliot G. (1999) 'Language and Medicine', *Annual Review of Applied Linguistics*, vol. 19: pp. 174-192.

Jakobsson, Einar (1994) *Psykoterapins uppgift: hälsa, bot och självförbättring i modernt psykoanalytiskt tänkande*, Linköping Studies in Arts and Science.

Jensen, Uffe Juul (1983) *Sygdomsbegreber i praksis*, København: Munksgaard.

Jewson, N. D. (1975) 'The Disappearance of the Sick-Man from Medical Cosmology 1770-1870', *Sociology*, vol. 10: pp. 225-244.

Johannisson, Karin (1994) *Den mörka kontinenten: kvinnan, medicinen och fin-de-siècle*, Stockholm: Norstedts.

Johannisson, Karin (1997) *Kroppens tunna skal*, Stockholm: Norstedts.

Jonas, Hans (1966) *The Phenomenon of Life: Toward a Philosophical Biology*, New York: Harper & Row.

Jonas, Hans (1979) *Das Prinzip der Verantwortung: Versuch einer Ethik für die technologische Zivilisation*, Frankfurt am Main: Insel Verlag.

Jonsen, Albert R., and Toulmin, Stephen (1988) *The Abuse of Casuistry: A History of Moral Reasoning*, Berkeley: University of California Press.

Kantoff, Philip, and McConnell, Malcolm (1996) *Prostate Cancer: A Family Consultation*, Boston: Houghton Mifflin Company.

Kass, Leon R. (1975) 'Regarding the End of Medicine and the Pursuit of Health', in *The Public Interest*, no. 40: pp. 11-42.

Khushf, George (1997) 'Why Bioethics Needs the Philosophy of Medicine: Some Implications of Reflection on Concepts of Health and Disease', *Theoretical Medicine*, vol. 18: pp. 145-163.

King, Lester S.(1978) 'The Cause of Disease', in *The Philosophy of Medicine: The Early Eighteenth Century*, Cambridge, Mass.: Harvard University Press.

Kisiel, Theodore (1986-87) 'Das Entstehen des Begriffsfeldes "Faktizität" im Frühwerk Heideggers', *Dilthey Jahrbuch*, vol. 4, Göttingen: Vandenhoeck und Ruprecht.

Kisiel, Theodore (1993) *Genesis of Heidegger's Being and Time*, Berkeley: University of California Press.

Klein, Ernest (ed.) (1966) *A Comprehensive Etymological Dictionary of the English Language*, vol. 1, Amsterdam: Elsevier.

Kleinman, Arthur (1980) *Patients and Healers in the Context of Culture: An Exploration of the Borderland between Anthropology, Medicine, and Psychiatry*, Berkeley: University of California Press.

Kleinman, Arthur (1988) *The Illness Narratives: Suffering, Healing and the Human Condition*, New York: Basic Books.

Kleinman, Arthur (1995) *Writing at the Margin: Discourse Between Anthropology and Medicine*, Berkeley: University of California Press.

Koprowski, Hilary, and Oldstone, Michael (eds.) (1996) *Microbe Hunters, Now and Then*, Bloomington: Medi-Ed Press.
Krell, David Farrell (1992) *Daimon Life: Heidegger and Life-Philosophy*, Bloomington: Indiana University Press.
Krell, David Farrell (1996) *Infectious Nietzsche*, Bloomington: Indiana University Press.
Kristensson Uggla, Bengt (1994) *Kommunikation på bristningsgränsen: en studie i Paul Ricoeurs projekt*, Stockholm: B. Östlings bokförlag Symposion.
Kuhn, Thomas S. (1970) *The Structure of Scientific Revolutions*, 2nd enl. ed., University of Chicago Press.
Lachmund, Jens (1996) 'Die Erfindung des ärztlichen Gehörs: zur historischen Soziologie der stetoskopischen Untersuchung', in *Anatomien medizinischen Wissens, Medizin, Macht, Moleküle*, ed. Borck, Cornelius, Frankfurt am Main: Fischer Verlag.
Lain Entralgo, Pedro (1969) *Doctor and Patient*, London: Weidenfeld and Nicolson.
Lain Entralgo, Pedro (1970) *The Therapy of the Word in Classical Antiquity*, New Haven: Yale University Press.
Larsson, Ullabeth Sätterlund (1989) *Being Involved: Patient Participation in Health Care*, Linköping Studies in Arts and Science.
Latour, Bruno (1987) *Science in Action: How to Follow Scientists and Engineers through Society*, Cambridge, Mass.: Harvard University Press.
Leder, Drew (1984-85) 'Toward a Phenomenology of Pain', *Review of Existential Psychology and Psychiatry*, vol. 19: pp. 255-266.
Leder, Drew (1990a) *The Absent Body*, University of Chicago Press.
Leder, Drew (1990b) 'Clinical Interpretation: The Hermeneutics of Medicine', *Theoretical Medicine*, vol. 11: pp. 9-24.
Leder, Drew (1995) 'Health and Disease: The Experience of Health and Illness', in *Encyclopedia of Bioethics*, vol. 2, ed. Reich, W. T., New York: Simon & Schuster Macmillan.
Lévinas, Emmanuel (1961) *Totalité et infini: essai sur l'extériorité*, La Haye: Nijhoff.
Lindeboom, G. A. (1979) *Descartes and Medicine*, Amsterdam: Editions Rodopi.
Liss, Per-Erik (1996) 'On the Notion of a Goal: A Conceptual Platform for the Setting of Goals in Medicine', in *The Goals and Limits of Medicine*, eds. Nordenfelt, Lennart, and Tengland, Per-Anders, Stockholm: Almqvist & Wiksell International.
Lock, James D. (1990) 'Some Aspects of Medical Hermeneutics: The Role of Dialectic and Narrative', *Theoretical Medicine*, vol. 11: pp. 41-50.
MacCormack, Carol (1993) 'Medicine and Anthropology', in *Companion Encyclopedia of the History of Medicine*, vol. 2, eds. Bynum W. F., and Porter, Roy, London: Routledge.
MacDonald, Michael (1981) *Mystical Bedlam: Madness, Anxiety, and Healing in Seventeenth-Century England*, Cambridge University Press.
MacIntyre, Alasdair (1985) *After Virtue, a Study in Moral Theory*, 2nd ed., London: Duckworth.
McWhinney, Ian R. (1989) *A Textbook of Family Medicine*, Oxford University Press.
Merleau-Ponty, Maurice (1962) *Phenomenology of Perception*, London: Routledge.
Mishler, Elliot G. (1984) *The Discourse of Medicine: Dialectics of Medical Interviews*, Norwood, New Jersey: Ablex Cop.
Moscucci, Ornella (1990) *The Science of Woman: Gynaecology and Gender in England, 1800-1929*, Cambridge University Press.
Myerscough, Philip R., et al. (1992) *Talking with Patients: A Basic Clinical Skill*, Oxford University Press.
Needham, Paul (1988) *Law and Order: Issues in the Philosophy of Science*, Uppsala: Philosophical Studies published by the Philosophical Society and the Department of Philosophy.
Nerheim, Hjördis (1996) *Vitenskap og kommunikasjon: paradigmer, modeller og kommunikative strategier i helsefagenes vitenskapsteori.*, 2nd ed., Oslo: Universitetsforlaget.
Nicolson, Malcolm (1993a) 'The Art of Diagnosis: Medicine and the Five Senses', in *Companion Encyclopedia of the History of Medicine*, vol. 2, eds. Bynum W. F. and Porter, Roy, London: Routledge.
Nicolson, Malcolm (1993b) 'The Introduction of Percussion and Stethoscopy to Early Nineteenth-Century Edinburgh', in *Medicine and the Five Senses*, eds. Bynum, W. F. and Porter, Roy, Cambridge University Press.

REFERENCES

Nietzsche, Friedrich (1973) *Die fröhliche Wissenschaft,* Kritische Gesamtausgabe, div. 5, vol. 2, Berlin: Walter de Gruyter & Co.

Nikku, Nina (1997) *Informative Paternalism: Studies in the Ethics of Promoting and Predicting Health,* Linköping Studies in Arts and Science.

Nordenfelt, Lennart (1987, rev. ed. 1995) *On the Nature of Health: An Action-Theoretic Approach,* Dordrecht: Reidel Publishing.

Nordenfelt, Lennart (1993) *Quality of Life, Health and Happiness,* Aldershot: Avebury.

Nordenfelt, Lennart (1996) 'On Medicine and Other Species of Health Enhancement', in *The Goals and Limits of Medicine,* eds. Nordenfelt, Lennart, and Tengland, Per-Anders, Stockholm: Almqvist & Wiksell International.

Nordenfelt, Lennart, and Lindahl, Ingemar B. (eds.) (1984) *Health, Disease, and Causal Explanation in Medicine,* Dordrecht: Reidel Publishing.

Nordenfelt, Lennart, and Twaddle, Andrew (1993) *Disease, Illness and Sickness: Three Central Concepts in the Theory of Health: A Dialogue Between Andrew Twaddle and Lennart Nordenfelt,* Linköping: Studies on Health and Society.

Nordin, Ingemar (1996) 'On the Rationality of Medicine', in *The Goals and Limits of Medicine,* eds. Nordenfelt, Lennart, and Tengland, Per-Anders, Stockholm: Almqvist & Wiksell International.

Nussbaum, Martha C. (1994) *The Therapy of Desire: Theory and Practice in Hellenistic Ethics,* New Jersey: Princeton University Press.

Nutton, Vivian (1993) 'Galen at the Bedside: The Methods of a Medical Detective', in *Medicine and the Five Senses,* eds. Bynum, W. F., and Porter, Roy, Cambridge University Press.

Nutton, Vivian (1995a) 'Medicine in the Greek World, 800-50 B.C.', in *The Western Medical Tradition 800 B.C. to A.D. 1800,* eds. Conrad, Lawrence I., et al., Camridge University Press.

Nutton, Vivian (1995b) 'Medicine in Late Antiquity and the Early Middle Ages', in *The Western Medical Tradition 800 B.C. to A.D. 1800,* eds. Conrad, Lawrence I., et al., Cambridge University Press.

Nutton, Vivian (1995c) 'Medicine in Medieval Western Europe, 1000-1500', in *The Western Medical Tradition 800 B.C. to A.D. 1800,* eds. Conrad, Lawrence I., et al., Cambridge University Press.

Ong, L. M. L., et al. (1995) 'Doctor-Patient Communication: A Review of the Literature', *Pergamon,* vol. 40, no. 7: pp. 903-918.

Ottosson, Per-Gunnar (1984) *Scholastic Medicine and Philosophy: A Study of Commentaries on Galen's Tegni (ca. 1300-1450),* Napoli: Bibliopolis.

Palmer, Richard E. (1969) *Hermeneutics: Interpretation Theory in Schleiermacher, Dilthey, Heidegger, and Gadamer,* Evanston, Illinois: Northwestern University Press.

Peabody, Francis W. (1987) 'The Care of the Patient', in *Encounters between Patients and Doctors,* ed. Stoeckle, John D., Cambridge, Mass.: MIT Press.

Pellegrino, Edmund D., and Thomasma, David C. (1981) *A Philosophical Basis of Medical Practice: Toward a Philosophy and Ethics of the Healing Professions,* Oxford University Press.

Pellegrino, Edmund D., and Thomasma, David C. (1993) *The Virtues in Medical Practice,* Oxford University Press.

Pendleton, David, et al. (1984) *The Consultation: An Approach to Learning and Teaching,* Oxford University Press.

Petersson, Bo (1995) 'Platon, hälsan och läkarna', in *Hälsosamma tankar,* eds. Liss, Per-Erik, and Petersson, Bo, Nora: Nya Doxa.

Plato, Collected Works, London: Loeb Classical Library.

Plügge, Herbert (1962) *Wohlbefinden und Missbefinden,* Tübingen: Max Niemeyer Verlag.

Pocai, Romano (1996) *Heideggers Theorie der Befindlichkeit,* München: Karl Alber Verlag.

Poirier, Suzanne, and Brauner, Daniel J. (1990) 'The Voices of the Medical Record', *Theoretical Medicine,* vol. 11: pp. 29-40.

Porter, Dorothy (1993) 'Public Health', in *Companion Encyclopedia of the History of Medicine,* vol. 2, eds. Bynum W. F., and Porter, Roy, London: Routledge.

Porter, Dorothy, and Porter, Roy (1989) *Patient's Progress: Doctors and Doctoring in Eighteenth-Century England,* Cambridge: Polity Press.

Porter, Roy (1992) *Doctor of Society: Thomas Beddoes and the Sick Trade in Late-Enlightenment England,* London: Routledge.

REFERENCES 189

Pörn, Ingmar (1984) 'An Equilibrium Model of Health', in *Health, Disease, and Causal Explanations in Medicine*, eds. Nordenfelt, Lennart, and Lindahl, Ingemar B., Dordrecht: Reidel Publishing.

Pörn, Ingmar (1993) 'Health and Adaptedness', *Theoretical Medicine*, vol. 14: pp. 295-303.

Rattner, Josef, and Danzer, Gerhard (1997) *Medizinische Anthropologie: Ansätze einer personalen Heilkunde*, Frankfurt am Main: Fischer Verlag.

Rawlinson, Mary C. (1982) 'Medicine's Discourse and the Practice of Medicine', in *The Humanity of the Ill: Phenomenological Perspectives*, ed. Kestenbaum, Victor, Knoxville: University of Tennessee Press.

Raymond, Didier (ed.) (1999) *Nietzsche ou la grande sante*, Paris: Éditions L'Harmattan.

Reiser, Stanley J. (1978) *Medicine and the Reign of Technology*, Cambridge University Press.

Reiser, Stanley J. (1993) 'Technology and the Use of the Senses in Twentieth-Century Medicine', in *Medicine and the Five Senses*, eds. Bynum, W. F., and Porter, Roy, Cambridge University Press.

Richardson, William J. (1993) 'Heidegger Among the Doctors', in *Reading Heidegger: Commemorations*, ed. Sallis, John, Bloomington: Indiana University Press.

Richt, Bengt (1992) *Mellan två världar: om konflikten mellan livets krav och doktorns önskningar: lärdomar från familjer med diabetessjuka barn*, Linköping Studies in Arts and Science.

Ricoeur, Paul (1970) *Freud and Philosophy: An Essay on Interpretation*, New Haven: Yale University Press.

Ricoeur, Paul (1981a) 'What is a Text? Explanation and Understanding', in *Hermeneutics and the Human Sciences: Essays on Language, Action and Interpretation*, Cambridge University Press.

Ricoeur, Paul (1981b) 'The Model of the Text: Meaningful Action Considered as a Text', in *Hermeneutics and the Human Sciences: Essays on Language, Action and Interpretation*, Cambridge University Press.

Ricoeur, Paul (1981c) 'The Task of Hermeneutics', in *Hermeneutics and the Human Sciences: Essays on Language, Action and Interpretation*, Cambridge University Press.

Ricoeur, Paul (1981d) 'Hermeneutics and Critique of Ideology', in *Hermeneutics and the Human Sciences: Essays on Language, Action and Interpretation*, Cambridge University Press.

Ricoeur, Paul (1991a) 'Explanation and Understanding: On Some Remarkable Connections between the Theory of Texts, Action Theory, and the Theory of History', in *From Text to Action: Essays in Hermeneutics, II*, Evanston, Illinois: Northwestern University Press.

Ricoeur, Paul (1991b) 'Life: A Story in Search of a Narrator', in *A Ricoeur Reader: Reflection and Imagination*, University of Toronto Press.

Ricoeur, Paul (1992) *Oneself as Another*, University of Chicago Press.

Ritter, Joachim, and Gründer, Karlfried (eds.) (1971-) *Historisches Wörterbuch der Philosophie*, Basel: Schwabe & Co.

Roter, Debra L., and Hall, Judith A. (1992) *Doctors Talking with Patients /Patients Talking with Doctors*, Westport, Conn.: Auburn House.

Sachs, Lisbeth, and Uddenberg, Nils (1984) *Medicin, myter, magi: ett annorlunda perspektiv på vår sjukvård*, Stockholm: Akademilitteratur.

Sacks, Oliver W. (1984) *A Leg to Stand On*, New York: Summit Books.

Sacks, Oliver W. (1985) *The Man Who Mistook His Wife for a Hat and Other Clinical Tales*, New York: Summit Books.

Scarry, Elaine (1985) *The Body in Pain*, Oxford University Press.

Seedhouse, David (1986) *Health: The Foundations for Achievement*, Chichester: Wiley.

Senelick, Richard C., and Rossi, Peter W. (1994) *Living with Stroke: A Guide for Families*, Chicago: Contemporary Books.

Shakespeare, William (1985) *Hamlet, Prince of Denmark*, Cambridge University Press.

Shorter, Edward (1985) *Bedside Manners: The Troubled History of Doctors and Patients*, New York: Simon & Schuster.

Shorter, Edward (1992) *From Paralysis to Fatigue: A History of Psychosomatic Illness in the Modern Era*, New York: Free Press.

Shorter, Edward (1997) *A History of Psychiatry: From the Era of the Asylum to the Age of Prozac*, New York: John Wiley & Sons, Inc.

Shryock, Richard Harrison (1948) *The Development of Modern Medicine*, London: Victor Gollancz LTD.

REFERENCES

Siegler, Mark (1981) 'The Doctor-Patient Encounter and its Relationship to Theories of Health and Disease', in *Concepts of Health and Disease: Interdisciplinary Perspectives*, eds. Caplan A. L., Engelhardt, H. T., Jr., and McCartney, J. J., Reading Mass.: Addison Wesley.

Singer, Peter (1993) *Practical Ethics*, 2nd ed., Cambridge University Press.

Spiegelberg, Herbert (1972) *Phenomenology in Psychology and Psychiatry*, Evanston, Illinois: Northwestern University Press.

Spiegelberg, Herbert (1982) *The Phenomenological Movement: A Historical Introduction*, 3d rev. ed. Den Haag: Nijhoff.

Spiegelberg, Herbert (1986) *Steppingstones Toward an Ethics for Fellow Existers: Essays 1944-1983*, Dordrecht: Kluwer.

Spitzack, Carole (1992) 'Foucault's Political Body in Medical Practice', in *The Body in Medical Thought and Practice*, ed. Leder, Drew, Dordrecht: Kluwer.

Starr, Paul (1982) *The Social Transformation of American Medicine*, New York: Basic Books.

Steinbock, Anthony J. (1995) *Home and Beyond: Generative Phenomenology after Husserl*, Evanston, Illinois: Northwestern University Press.

Stewart, Moira (1995) 'Effective Physician-Patient Communication and Health Outcomes: A Review', *Journal of the Canadian Medical Association*, vol. 152, no. 9: pp. 1423-1433.

Straus, Erwin (1966a) 'Norm and Pathology of I-World Relations', in *Phenomenological Psychology*, New York: Basic Books.

Straus, Erwin (1966b) 'The Upright Posture', in *Phenomenological Psychology*, New York: Basic Books.

Straus, Erwin (1969) 'Psychiatry and Philosophy', in *Psychiatry and Philosophy*, ed. Natanson, Maurice, New York: Springer-Verlag.

Sundström, Per (1987) *Icons of Disease: A Philosophical Inquiry Into the Semantics, Phenomenology and Ontology of the Clinical Conceptions of Disease*, Linköping Studies in Arts and Science.

Svenaeus, Fredrik (1996) 'The Hermeneutics of Medicine', in *The Goals and Limits of Medicine*, eds. Nordenfelt, Lennart, and Tengland, Per-Anders, Stockholm: Almqwist och Wiksell International.

Svenaeus, Fredrik (1997) 'Heideggers stämningsbegrepp', in *Fenomenologiska perspektiv*, eds. Orlowski, Alexander, and Ruin, Hans, Stockholm: Thales.

Svenaeus, Fredrik (1999a) 'Alexithymia: A Phenomenological Approach', *Philosophy, Psychiatry, and Psychology*, vol. 6: pp. 71-107.

Svenaeus, Fredrik (1999b) 'Freud's Philosophy of the Uncanny', *Scandinavian Psychoanalytic Review*, vol. 22: pp. 239-254.

Szasz, Thomas S., and Hollender, Marc H. (1956) 'Contribution to the Philosophy of Medicine: The Basic Models of the Doctor-Patient Relationship', *American Medical Association – Archives of Internal Medicine*, vol. 97: pp. 585-592.

Taylor, Charles (1970) 'The Explanation of Purposive Behaviour', in *Explanation in the Behavioural Sciences, Confrontations*, eds. Borger, Robert, and Cioffi, Frank, Cambridge University Press.

Taylor, Charles (1989) *Sources of the Self: The Making of the Modern Identity*, Cambridge University Press.

Tegern, Gunilla (1994) *Frisk och sjuk: vardagliga föreställningar om hälsan och dess motsatser*, Linköping Studies in Arts and Science.

Temkin, Owsei (1977) *The Double Face of Janus*, Baltimore: Johns Hopkins University Press.

Tengland, Per-Anders (1998) *Mental Health: A Philosophical Analysis*, Linköping Studies in Arts and Science.

Theunissen, Michael (1966) 'Skeptische Betrachtungen über den anthropologischen Personbegriff', in *Die Frage nach dem Menschen*, ed. Rombach, Heinrich, München: Karl Alber Verlag.

Thomasma, David C. (1994) 'Clinical Ethics as Medical Hermeneutics', *Theoretical Medicine*, vol. 15: pp. 93-111.

Toombs, S. Kay (1990) 'The Temporality of Illness: Four Levels of Experience', *Theoretical Medicine*, vol. 11: pp. 227-241.

Toombs, S. Kay (1992a) *The Meaning of Illness: A Phenomenological Account of the Different Perspectives of Physician and Patient*, Dordrecht: Kluwer.

Toombs, S. Kay (1992b) 'The Body in Multiple Sclerosis', in *The Body in Medical Thought and Practice*, ed. Leder, Drew, Dordrecht: Kluwer.

REFERENCES

Toombs, S. Kay, Barnard, David, and Carson, Ronald A. (eds.) (1995) *Chronic Illness: From Experience to Policy*, Bloomington: Indiana University Press.
Tuckett, David, et al. (1985) *Meetings Between Experts*, London: Tavistock.
Verwey, Gerlof (1987) 'Toward a Systematic Philosophy of Medicine', *Theoretical Medicine*, vol. 8: pp. 163-177.
Volpi, Franco (1996) 'Dasein as *praxis*: The Heideggerian Assimilation and Radicalization of the Practical Philosophy of Aristotle', in *Critical Heidegger*, ed. Macann, Christopher, London: Routledge.
von Wartburg, Walther (ed.) (1964) *Französisches etymologisches Wörterbuch*, vol. 11, Basel: Zbinden.
von Wright, Georg Henrik (1971) *Explanation and Understanding*, Ithaca, New York: Cornell University Press.
Waldenfels, Bernhard (1997) *Grenzen der Normalisierung: Studien zur Phänomenologie des Fremden 2*, Frankfurt am Main: Suhrkamp Verlag.
Wear, Andrew (1995) 'Medicine in Early Modern Europe, 1500-1700', in *The Western Medical Tradition 800 B.C. to A.D. 1800*, eds. Conrad, Lawrence I., et al., Cambridge University Press.
Whitbeck, Caroline (1981) 'A Theory of Health', in *Concepts of Health and Disease: Interdisciplinary Perspectives*, eds. Caplan A. L., Engelhardt, H. T., Jr., and McCartney, J. J., Reading Mass.: Addison Wesley.
Widdershoven-Heerding, Ineke (1987) 'Medicine as a Form of Practical Understanding', *Theoretical Medicine*, vol. 8: pp. 179-185.
Wifstad, Åge (1997) *Vilkår for begrepsdannelse og praksis i psykiatri: en filosofisk undersøgelse*, Oslo: Tano Aschehoug.
Williams, Bernard (1985) *Ethics and the Limits of Philosophy*, Cambridge, Mass.: Harvard University Press.
Wulff, Henrik R., Pedersen, Stig Andur, and Rosenberg, Raben (1986) *Philosophy of Medicine: An Introduction*, London: Blackwell.
Zahavi, Dan (1994) 'Husserl's Phenomenology of the Body', *Études Phénoménologiques*, vol. 19: pp. 63-84.
Zaner, Richard M. (1964) *The Problem of Embodiment: Some Contributions to a Phenomenology of the Body*, Den Haag: Nijhoff.
Zaner, Richard M. (1970) *The Way of Phenomenology: Criticism as a Philosophical Discipline*, New York: Pegasus.
Zaner, Richard M. (1981) *The Context of Self: A Phenomenological Inquiry Using Medicine as a Clue*, Athens: Ohio University Press.
Zaner, Richard M. (1988) *Ethics and the Clinical Encounter*, New Jersey: Prentice Hall.
Zaner, Richard M. (1991) 'The Phenomenon of Trust in the Patient-Physician Relationship', in *Ethics, Trust, and the Professions: Philosophical and Cultural Aspects*, eds. Pellegrino, Edmund D., Veatch, Robert M., and Langan, John P., Washington D. C.: Georgetown University Press.
Zaner, Richard M. (1993) *Troubled Voices: Stories of Ethics and Illness*, Cleveland: The Pilgrim Press.
Zaner, Richard M. (1994) 'Phenomenology and the Clinical Event', in *Phenomenology of the Cultural Disciplines*, eds. Daniel, M., and Embree, L., Dordrecht: Kluwer.

INDEX OF NAMES

Ackerknecht, Erwin H. 12, 22
Amundsen, Darrel W. 13
Antonovsky, Aaron 97
Aristotle 15, 28, 35, 52-54, 60-62, 72, 87, 107, 114, 148, 168, 171, 175
Auenbrugger, Leopold 30
Bacon, Francis 19
Balint, Michael 40, 41, 43
Baron, Richard J. 140
Bayle, Gaspard L. 30
Beauchamp, Tom L. 168
Beddoes, Thomas 28
Benedict, Ruth 46
Bentham, Jeremy 72
Bernard, Claude 64, 67
Bernet, Rudolf 76, 81
Bichat, M. F. X. 23, 31
Binswanger, Ludwig 41, 80, 91, 93
Boas, Franz 46
Boerhaave, Hermann 27
Boissier de Sauvages, François de 25
Boorse, Christopher 62-68, 74-75, 79, 99, 114, 178
Borck, Cornelius 65
Borell, Merriley 32
Boss, Medard 41, 80, 91-92, 110
Bracegirdle, Brian 31
Bramwell, Edwin 36
Brandom, Robert B. 171
Brauner, Daniel J. 135
Buber, Martin 41
Buytendijk, F. J. J. 41, 92, 98, 103, 109
Bynum, W. F. 20
Byrne, Patrick S. 42
Canguilhem, Georges 11, 46, 64, 66-67, 69, 99
Cannon, Walter B. 64
Carson, Ronald A. 136
Cassell, Eric J. 52, 55, 175
Childress, James F. 44, 168
Comte, Auguste 67
Conrad, Lawrence I. 18
Cullen, William 25
Cunningham, Andrew 32
Daniel, Stephen L. 134-137, 142
Danzer, Gerhard 41
Davis, F. Daniel 54
Dekkers, Wim 132, 137

Democritus 15
Descartes, René 19, 63
Dilthey, Wilhelm 84, 122, 131, 133
Dreyfus, Hubert L. 25, 82
Dubois, Paul 36
Edelstein, Ludwig 13-14, 16, 39, 51
Eisenberg, Leon 48
Engel, George 48
Engelhardt, H. Tristram 52, 66
Feinstein, Alvan R. 41-42
Ferngren, Gary B. 13
Fisher, Gregg Charles 78, 129
Fitzpatrick, Ray 44
Fleck, Ludwik 45
Foucault, Michel 22-29, 31, 35, 45, 61, 172
French, Roger 18
Freud, Sigmund 36-37, 93, 111, 144-145
Fulford, K. W. M. 66, 69
Gadamer, Hans-Georg 6, 8, 38, 79-80, 84, 92, 94, 98, 119, 121, 130, 132-134, 139-144, 148-149, 153-154, 158, 163-164, 171, 174, 179
Galen 16-19, 29, 32, 51, 60
Galileo 32
Gatens-Robinson, Eugenie 54
Gelfand, Toby 19
Goffman, Erving 112
Gogel, Edward L. 136
Good, Byron J. 46, 47, 49, 50, 135
Good, Mary-Jo DelVecchio 50
Gorovitz, Samuel 129
Graninger, Ulrika 32
Granshaw, Lindsay 18-19
Gründer, Karlfried 4, 68
Guignon, Charles B. 84, 91
Guthrie, Diana W. 78, 113
Guthrie, Richard A. 78, 113
Habermas, Jürgen 84, 142-143, 172
Hall, Judith A. 39
Hardy, Robert C. 78, 96
Harrington, Anne 35
Harvey, William 20
Hegel, G. W. F. 141, 171-172
Heidegger, Martin 6-8, 59, 76, 80, 83-98, 100-104, 106-111, 114-116, 118, 120, 122, 131-133, 137, 139-140, 144, 146, 148, 154, 159, 163, 169, 171, 173, 178-179

193

INDEX OF NAMES

Held, Klaus 87
Hellström, Olle 41
Helman, Cecil G. 44
Hempel, Carl Gustav 127
Hiley, David R. 122
Hippocrates (Hippocratic Corpus) 13-19, 39, 44, 51, 60, 120
Hollender, Marc H. 43
Holmes, Oliver W. 34
Homer 15
Horgby, Ingvar 68
Hoy, David Couzens 132
Hume, David 166-167, 169
Hunter, Kathryn Montgomery 135
Husserl, Edmund 6-7, 45, 48, 64, 75-78, 80-84, 86-90, 106-108, 141, 154, 169, 172
Hydén, Lars-Christer 44
Hölderlin, Friedrich 107
Jakobsson, Einar 145
Jaspers, Karl 41, 141
Jensen, Uffe Juul 65
Jewson, N. D. 27-28
Johannisson, Karin 18, 36, 50
Jonas, Hans 19, 23, 31, 175
Jonsen, Albert R. 136
Kant, Immanuel 63, 77, 171
Kantoff, Philip 78, 106
Kass, Leon R. 69, 111
Khushf, George 56
King, Lester S. 125
Kisiel, Theodore 84, 87, 114
Klein, Ernest 68
Kleinman, Arthur 46-50, 78, 163
Koch, Robert 32
Koprowski, Hilary 32
Krell, David Farrell 84, 90, 103
Kristensson Uggla, Bengt 140
Kuhn, Thomas S. 28
Lacan, Jacques 80
Lachmund, Jens 30
Laënnec, R. T. H. 23, 30, 34
Lain Entralgo, Pedro 14-15, 17-18, 55
Larsson, Ullabeth Sätterlund 44
Latour, Bruno 45
Leder, Drew 19, 80, 97-98, 103, 109, 112, 137-140, 142, 146, 179
Leeuwenhoek, Antoni van 20, 27, 31
Lévinas, Emmanuel 92, 175
Lindahl, Ingemar B. 125
Lindeboom, G. A. 20
Linnaeus, Carolus 25
Liss, Per-Erik 170
Lock, James D. 141, 144
Locke, John 63
Long, Barrie E. L. 42
Louis, P. C. A. 23
Løgstrup, Knud E. 175

MacCormack, Carol 46
MacDonald, Michael 28
MacIntyre, Alasdair 61, 129, 167, 171, 175
Macquarrie, John 87
Marcel, Gabriel 141
Marx, Karl 39
Marx, Werner 175
McConnell, Malcolm 78, 106
McWhinney, Ian R. 38, 125
Merleau-Ponty, Maurice 82, 92, 103, 107-108, 110
Mishler, Elliot G. 44, 175
Morgagni, Giovanni Battista 23
Moscucci, Ornella 27, 36
Myerscough, Philip R. 39
Napier, Richard 28
Needham, Paul 127
Nerheim, Hjördis 122-123, 141-144
Nicolson, Malcolm 20-21, 34
Nietzsche, Friedrich 90
Nikku, Nina 44
Nordenfelt, Lennart 53, 61, 66, 68-76, 78-80, 82, 94, 99, 100-104, 112, 115, 125, 178
Nordin, Ingemar 170
Nussbaum, Martha C. 15, 51, 61-62
Nutton, Vivian 13, 15-18, 31
Oldstone, Michael 32
Ong, L. M. L. 39
Ottosson, Per-Gunnar 18
Palmer, Richard E. 130
Paracelsus 19
Peabody, Francis W. 38
Pellegrino, Edmund D. 52-56, 121, 167-168, 175, 178
Pendleton, David 39
Petersson, Bo 60-61
Pinel, Philippe 23, 35
Plato 2, 5, 14-15, 59-61, 172
Plügge, Herbert 41, 95
Pocai, Romano 87
Poirier, Suzanne 135
Porter, Dorothy 20-21, 28, 39
Porter, Roy 20-21, 28, 34, 39
Pörn, Ingmar 61, 69
Rabinow, Paul 25
Rattner, Josef 41
Rawlinson, Mary C. 109
Raymond, Didier 90
Reiser, Stanley J. 20, 29-33, 38, 40
Richardson, William J. 80
Richt, Bengt 78
Ricoeur, Paul 37, 100, 140-145, 162-163, 175, 179
Ritter, Joachim 4, 68
Robinson, Edward 87
Rossi, Peter W. 78, 102
Roter, Debra L. 39

INDEX OF NAMES

Röntgen, Wilhelm C. 31
Sachs, Lisbeth 40
Sacks, Oliver W. 115, 165
Sartre, Jean-Paul 91, 108
Scambler, Graham 44
Scarry, Elaine 109
Scheler, Max 175
Schelling, F. W. J. 63
Schleiermacher, Friedrich D. E. 131, 133
Schutz, Alfred 48, 154
Seedhouse, David 69
Senelick, Richard C. 78, 102
Shakespeare, William 1
Shorter, Edward 20-21, 24, 28-29, 31, 34-36, 42
Shryock, Richard Harrison 16, 22-24, 32, 34, 51
Siegler, Mark 44, 53
Singer, Peter 68
Spengler, Oswald 84
Spicker, Stuart F. 52
Spiegelberg, Herbert 75, 80, 175
Spitzack, Carole 27
Stambaugh, Joan 83, 87
Starr, Paul 39
Steinbock, Anthony J. 82
Stewart, Moira 41
Straus, Erwin 41, 92-93, 95, 108, 116
Sundström, Per 135, 138, 174
Svenaeus, Fredrik 54, 87, 104, 107, 111, 137, 139
Sydenham, Thomas 19, 25, 27
Szasz, Thomas S. 43
Taylor, Charles 21, 89, 122
Tegern, Gunilla 94
Temkin, Owsei 13, 15, 24, 60
ten Have, Henk 136
Tengland, Per-Anders 74
Terry, James S. 136
Theunissen, Michael 68
Thomasma, David C. 52-56, 121, 136, 167-168, 175, 178
Toombs, S. Kay 38, 80, 109, 112, 116, 153-154
Toulmin, Stephen 136
Tuckett, David 44
Twaddle, Andrew 79
Uddenberg, Nils 40
Verwey, Gerlof 52
Vesalius, Andreas 19
Virchow, Rudolf 32
Volpi, Franco 87, 114, 171
von Gebsattel, V. E. 41
von Wartburg, Walther 68
von Weizsäcker, Viktor 41
von Wright, Georg Henrik 65, 122-123, 126, 170-171
Waldenfels, Bernhard 82
Wear, Andrew 21
Whitbeck, Caroline 69
Widdershoven-Heerding, Ineke 54
Wifstad, Åge 172
Williams, Bernhard 32, 167
Wittgenstein, Ludwig 153, 170
Wulff, Henrik R. 135
Wunderlich, Carl 33
Young, Allan 50
Zahavi, Dan 82
Zaner, Richard M. 17, 31, 43, 54, 76, 78, 80, 82, 89, 100, 107, 111, 136, 147, 149, 168

INDEX OF SUBJECTS

a priori, 17, 54, 93, 132, 146, 163, 179
ability, 46, 65-66, 69-74, 79-80, 92, 99-103, 112, 115, 160, 170, 178
action theory, 69-70
ageing, 98-99
alienness, 49, 93, 98, 111, 116-118, 133, 157, 160, 173, 179
analytical, 6, 41, 44, 49, 66, 85-86, 91-92, 145-146, 168
anatomy, 16-17, 19, 22-23, 27, 29, 31, 34-35, 43, 49, 62
animals, 19-20, 27, 65, 103, 110
anthropology (see also medical anthropology), 50, 79, 89, 167, 178
antibiotics, 24, 37, 124, 126, 128
anxiety, 46, 50, 87, 90, 92-93, 104, 106-108, 132, 143, 162
art, 1, 5, 12, 14, 20, 38, 40-41, 54, 61, 78, 122, 132, 178
articulation, 5, 6, 86-88, 122, 131-132, 134, 136, 154
artifact, 122, 131
asymmetrical, 147, 149
attunement, 81-82, 86-88, 92, 94-111, 113-116, 118, 131, 133, 137, 147, 152-153, 157-158, 163, 165, 171-175, 178-179
authenticity, 87, 89-93, 106-108, 116, 132, 142-143
autobiographical, 135, 165
autonomy, 21, 26, 29, 38-39, 42-44, 52, 71, 91-92, 143, 153, 168, 178
availableness, 85
bacteria (see also micro-organisms), 20, 31, 124-128
balance (see also homeostasis), 13-14, 51, 60-62, 64, 74, 87, 94-95, 98-100, 114, 136, 179
being at home (see also homelikeness), 92-93, 118
being-in-the-world, 85-87, 89, 93-95, 97-105, 109, 112-117, 120-122, 127, 129-133, 136, 138, 145, 152, 154, 158-159, 163, 165, 172-173, 178-180
being-there (see also Dasein), 83, 93, 97, 106, 110
being-with (see also intersubjectivity and togetherness), 104, 132, 160
biological function, 64-66, 68

biology, 6-7, 12, 24, 26, 37-38, 46, 51, 54, 63-66, 68, 75, 79, 84, 87, 90, 99, 108-109, 111-112, 114, 121, 123, 125, 127, 129-130, 137-139, 152, 159, 163, 171, 173, 175, 177-178
broken tool, 108-109
cancer (see also prostate cancer), 63, 105-106, 128, 145, 150, 152, 165, 181
chart, 34, 49, 105, 135, 140, 142
children, 34-35, 43, 47, 103, 152, 158, 162
chronic fatigue syndrome, 98, 128-129, 165, 181
chronic illness, 38, 48, 55, 113, 129, 163, 178
clinical encounter (see also doctor-patient relationship and medical meeting), 1, 6-7, 9, 11, 16-17, 28, 32-33, 39-40, 52-53, 78, 105, 114, 124, 127, 130, 136, 138, 143-144, 146-147, 154, 157-158, 163, 170, 173, 179
clinical judgement, 41-42
coherence, 16, 52, 97, 99-100, 103, 112, 114-115, 133, 138, 144, 179
coma (see also unconscious), 101-104, 107, 117
communication, 9, 41-42, 47, 49, 93, 100, 122, 160
compliance, 39, 41-42, 50, 178
concern, 159-160, 165-166, 180
consciousness (see also inner-time consciousness and unconscious), 68, 76-77, 82-86, 104, 110, 154, 172
consent, 52, 56, 121, 150, 178
constitution, 14, 23, 27, 45, 48-49, 73, 76-78, 88-89, 93, 109-110, 114, 137, 139, 168, 172
conversation (see also dialogue), 18, 33, 36, 47
cosmology, 12, 22, 27, 45, 114, 177
crisis, 33, 37, 39, 52, 116, 178
culture, 6, 25-26, 31, 38, 44-50, 60, 71, 84, 90, 92-93, 125, 139, 154, 157, 167, 171-172
cure (see also healing), 6, 12-15, 17-18, 21, 29-30, 34, 38, 42, 55, 56, 113-114, 124-130, 146, 158, 177
das Man (see also inauthenticity), 90, 132
Dasein, 80, 83-86, 88-89, 92-94, 103, 106, 108-109, 131-133, 171, 179
death, 18-19, 23, 38, 50, 76, 79, 82-83, 88, 90-91, 99, 102, 105, 107, 111, 142, 148-151, 155-156, 162

197

definition, 3, 27, 52-56, 71-72, 75, 114-115, 137, 139, 142, 165, 170, 178
diabetes, 96-97, 111, 113, 138, 154-155, 165, 181
diagnosis, 1, 20-22, 27, 29-30, 32-33, 35, 38, 41-42, 49-50, 106, 116, 125, 127, 130, 137, 166, 177, 179
dialectic, 44, 141-142, 174
dialogue (see also conversation), 2, 5, 9, 28, 56, 124-125, 130, 132-133, 137, 139-140, 142-144, 147-154, 158-166, 168, 170-171, 174-175, 177-180
disability, 56, 71, 74, 78, 100-103
disclosedness, 87, 133
discourse, 15, 25-28, 44, 86, 88, 132, 142, 145, 147
disease, 3, 5-6, 12-13, 17, 19, 23-25, 27, 30, 33-34, 38, 40-42, 45-49, 56, 63, 65-67, 71, 74-75, 79, 97-98, 103, 105-106, 111-113, 116, 121, 125, 128-129, 135, 138, 149-150, 152-155, 157-158, 166, 173-174, 177-178
distance, 30, 66, 133-134, 142-143, 148-149, 164, 180
distrust, 20, 29, 31, 52, 131, 153, 178
doctor-patient relationship (see also clinical encounter and medical meeting), 14-16, 20, 24, 28-29, 36, 39-43, 46-47, 53
domination, 21, 36, 149
dualism, 19, 43, 61, 79, 109, 111
dyad, 146, 170
education, 14, 19, 35, 37, 49, 138
ego, 76
eidos, 59, 76-77, 172
embodiment (see also Leib and lived body), 6-7, 19, 43, 75, 82, 91, 98, 117, 122-123, 131, 137, 160, 163, 165, 169, 171-174
emotion (see also attunement and feeling), 50, 62, 72
empathy, 28, 43, 104, 131, 144, 149, 164, 174, 180
episteme, 25, 27, 53, 64
epistemology, 4-5, 25-26, 39, 45, 51, 83, 136, 139, 141-143, 166-169, 175, 177, 181
epoche, 48, 76-77
estrangement, 147, 164, 180
ethics (see also medical ethics), 15, 17, 44, 51-54, 56, 61-62, 91, 136, 140, 143, 148, 167-168, 171, 173-175
everydayness, 83, 89, 91
existential, 84-86, 88, 90-93, 100, 110-112, 114-118, 131, 146, 160, 163, 171, 179
existentialism, 91
explanation, 21, 26, 46, 50, 65, 102, 116, 121-123, 125-127, 129-131, 141-142, 146, 163-164, 166, 174, 179-180
explication, 2, 4, 6-7, 24, 55, 64, 67, 69, 71, 73, 75, 79, 82, 85, 88, 91-92, 99, 104, 107-108, 115, 118, 146, 154, 163-166, 169, 171, 173, 178-179
facticity, 86, 107, 117, 121, 171-172, 181
facts and norms, 166-167, 169
feeling (see also attunement and emotion), 18, 20-21, 30-32, 35, 38, 41-42, 47, 62, 66, 72-73, 75, 78-82, 84-87, 93, 94-97, 100-101, 104-107, 114, 117, 124, 126, 128, 130, 138, 151-152, 156-159, 162, 165-168, 172-173, 175, 177, 179
finitude, 88, 90, 93, 111
free fantasy variation, 78, 107
freedom, 69, 91-92, 171
function (see also biological function), 3-5, 20, 23, 26, 30, 48-49, 56, 63-69, 80, 85, 99, 103, 108-109, 111-113, 123, 130, 158, 160, 178
fundamental ontology, 83-84, 87, 89
fusion of horizons, 133, 164, 174, 180
general practice, 1, 6-7, 36, 38, 40, 53, 178
genetics, 76, 81, 155
goal of medical practice, 8, 172, 181
goal of medicine, 55-56, 159
hammer, 85, 108-110
handicap, 112-113, 158
happiness (see also minimal happiness and well-being), 55, 72-73, 94, 100
healing (see also cure), 2, 6, 11-16, 18-19, 28, 34, 44-48, 52-53, 60, 114, 120, 126-127, 137, 139, 145, 148, 163-164, 170-171, 177, 179-180
health, 1-6, 8-9, 13-14, 16, 32, 34, 36, 39-46, 48-57, 59-76, 78-82, 87, 90-95, 97-101, 103-104, 107, 109, 111-122, 124, 129, 133, 138-139, 143-147, 149-151, 153-155, 157-159, 163-164, 168-169, 171-174, 177-180
health care, 2, 48-49, 52, 143
health theory, 8, 53, 56, 59, 63, 67, 118, 120, 124, 178
helplessness, 78, 81, 115, 173
hermeneutic circle, 134, 139
hermeneutic method, 135
hermeneutics (see also interpretation), 4-8, 19, 28, 37, 45, 50, 55, 64, 75, 83, 87, 89, 91, 114, 119-120, 122, 130-146, 148-150, 152, 158, 163-165, 168, 171, 174-175, 177, 179
hermeneutics of medicine, 1, 8, 37, 135, 137-140, 142, 144-146, 148-150, 152, 163-165, 179-180
hermeneutics of psychoanalysis, 37, 145
hermeneutics of suspicion, 145-146, 150
history of effects, 133
history of medicine, 5, 11, 22, 25, 28-29
homelessness (see also unhomelikeness), 81, 93, 104, 116-117
homelikeness (see also being at home), 92, 94-95, 97-100, 113-118, 121, 129-130, 133,

INDEX OF SUBJECTS

144, 146-147, 152, 157-162, 164-166, 168, 173-174, 178-180
homeostasis (see also balance), 64-65, 94
horizon (see also fusion of horizons), 7, 46, 122, 133-134, 136, 149, 153-154, 164, 169, 171, 175, 179-180
humanities, 4, 7, 121-123, 131-132, 134, 136-137, 141-142, 148, 167
humoral pathology, 19, 24, 177
hypothesis, 124-125, 129-130, 155
idealism, 108
illness (see also mental- and somatic illness), 2, 4-6, 8, 12-14, 17, 20-24, 27, 30, 36, 38, 40-41, 45-48, 50, 52, 55-57, 59-60, 64, 67-69, 73-75, 78-82, 89-91, 93-95, 97-107, 109, 111-118, 120-121, 123-129, 133, 135, 137-138, 144, 152-154, 164-165, 173-174, 177-180
inauthenticity (see also das Man), 90-91, 132
induction, 78
inner-time consciousness, 76
institutions, 1-2, 26-27, 48, 68
integrity, 28, 121
intentionality, 76-77, 80, 82, 85, 89
interpretation (see also hermeneutics), 2, 11-14, 17, 27, 34, 36-37, 45, 50-51, 63, 76, 78, 83, 87, 89-90, 93, 98, 104, 106, 114, 117, 120-121, 125-126, 130-132, 134-137, 139, 142-143, 145, 148-149, 152-154, 158, 163-165, 168, 171, 174, 177, 179-180
intersubjectivity (see also being-with and togetherness), 29, 83, 86, 88, 92, 102-103, 115, 133, 143, 153, 170-172, 174, 177
laboratory test, 32, 124-125, 138
law, 53, 123, 125-127, 130, 135, 148, 153
Leib (see also embodiment and lived body), 84, 90, 108, 110, 179
lifeworld, 6-7, 19, 44-46, 48-49, 64, 68, 70, 79, 84, 88, 93, 115, 117, 122-123, 130, 133-134, 136, 149, 153-154, 158, 164, 169, 171-172, 174-175, 177-178, 180
literature, 130-131, 133, 135-136
lived body (see also embodiment and Leib), 82, 103, 108, 110, 115, 117, 138, 179
malady, 102
materialism, 43, 79
meaning-pattern, 45, 88, 101-103, 105-106, 108-109, 114-115, 117, 172
meaning-structure, 64, 77, 83-90, 92, 94, 100, 106-108, 110, 115-118, 120, 127, 132, 154
measurement, 32, 54, 84-85, 155-156, 161
medical anthropology, 46, 50
medical ethics, 4-5, 16, 52, 135-136, 152, 168, 173, 175, 178, 181
medical history, 24, 27, 29
medical meeting (see also clinical encounter and doctor-patient relationship), 1, 7-8, 11-12, 14, 16, 20-22, 29, 31, 33, 35-37, 39, 41-44, 48, 50, 53, 121, 137, 140, 145-149, 153-154, 157-158, 161, 165-166, 177-179, 181
medical practice, 1-2, 4-7, 11, 14-16, 19-20, 22, 28-29, 31-35, 37, 39, 42-44, 46, 52-56, 100, 119-121, 127, 135-137, 139-140, 143, 146-148, 154, 157, 163-175, 177-178, 180-181
medical psychology, 178
medical science, 5, 7, 11, 29, 36-38, 41, 46, 51-54, 56, 63-64, 75, 100, 127, 174, 177-178
medical technology, 29, 31-33, 159
medical therapy, 15, 17, 21, 33-34, 36, 42, 47, 55, 139, 145, 148, 150-151, 156, 158, 177
mental illness, 35, 47, 74, 93, 104, 117, 133, 165
metaphor, 1, 4, 30-31, 94, 98, 136, 140, 153
metaphysical, 19, 27, 63, 86, 171-172
method, 1, 4, 7, 26, 30, 52-53, 78, 102, 130-132, 135, 141, 163, 179
micro-organisms (see also bacteria and virus), 32, 46, 126
minimal happiness, 72, 73
misunderstanding, 1, 9, 50, 63, 91
modern medicine, 4, 7, 11, 15-16, 20-24, 28-29, 31-33, 35-39, 41-42, 44, 46, 50-52, 54, 56, 60, 62-63, 105, 121, 137, 139, 177
mood (see also attunement), 86-87, 90, 92-95, 97-100, 102-104, 107-108, 116, 160, 162, 172-173
mutual understanding, 150, 153, 163
narrative, 48, 135, 137-138, 144, 162, 164, 180
natural attention, 90
nature, 2-4, 17, 19-20, 24, 27, 29, 33, 39, 54-55, 59, 64-65, 71, 79, 84, 93, 110-112, 123, 129, 131, 139, 167, 171-172, 175
nihilism, 34, 169
noemata, 77, 88, 172
nominalism, 75, 169
normality, 29, 32, 59, 63-68, 71, 76, 82, 90, 95-96, 98-99, 105, 113, 118, 122, 137, 139, 151, 156, 160, 178
normative, 5, 54, 56, 61, 70, 75, 119, 136, 166, 168-169, 181
nursing, 7, 53, 141, 143, 147, 159, 161-162, 172
ontic, 84, 87, 89, 118
ontological (see also fundamental ontology), 4, 11, 19, 23, 39, 45-46, 51-52, 54, 56, 76, 83, 85, 90, 118, 131, 136, 139, 142, 166-167, 169, 175, 181
ontology, 5, 53-54, 90, 131-132, 141, 148, 168-169, 174, 177
openness, 85, 97, 99, 103, 133, 174

INDEX OF SUBJECTS

organism, 3-4, 37-38, 46, 49, 61-66, 68-69, 88, 92, 102, 108-109, 111, 121, 126, 130, 163, 177-178
organs, 19, 23, 30, 65-67, 110, 122, 156
otherness, 93, 111, 133, 148
pain, 12, 22, 29, 45, 74, 78, 80-82, 90, 96-97, 101-102, 104, 109, 111, 124, 127-128, 137, 162, 167, 173-174
paternalism (see also autonomy), 42, 152, 153
pathology, 11, 16, 22-23, 27, 31-32, 34-35, 41, 43, 46, 62-63, 67, 98, 105, 138
perception, 3, 77, 82, 101, 107-108
person (see also self), 2, 6, 11, 16, 20-21, 27, 29, 31, 33, 35-38, 45-46, 50, 52-54, 56, 64-66, 68-74, 76, 79, 82, 89, 92, 97, 99-104, 106-107, 109, 112-118, 121-122, 125, 127, 134, 136-140, 143, 146-149, 152-153, 157-162, 164, 166, 169-170, 172-174, 177-178, 180
phenomenological reduction, 77, 89-90, 101, 106-107
phenomenology, 1-2, 4-8, 19, 28, 40-41, 48, 50-52, 55, 57, 59, 64, 75-77, 79-84, 86-90, 92, 94, 97, 100, 104-105, 108-109, 112, 114-117, 120, 132, 140, 144, 154, 168, 172-173, 177-178
philosophy of medicine, 2, 4, 8, 51-53, 55-56, 63, 135, 138, 140, 143, 167, 178
philosophy of mind, 51, 87
phronesis, 13, 35, 53-54, 61, 148
physiology, 20, 26, 29, 35, 37-38, 40-41, 63-65, 67-68, 70-71, 94, 98, 100, 103, 105, 112, 126, 135, 143, 158, 166
politics, 56, 64, 172
power, 12, 15, 26-27, 36, 42-44, 48, 64, 109, 118, 126, 141
praxis, 28, 60, 148, 171
prediction, 30, 102, 125-127, 161, 179
pregnancy, 98
prejudgements, 134
pre-understanding, 134
prevention, 32, 55-56, 63, 129, 152
primary text, 137, 139
profession, 6-7, 11, 14, 16-17, 19, 28, 31, 34, 37, 39, 49, 53, 73, 97, 118, 141, 146-147, 158-159, 162-164, 174, 177, 179-180
prognosis, 13, 32, 42, 49, 130, 166
projection, 88, 97, 171
prostate cancer, 105, 150-152, 165, 181
prosthesis, 109
psychiatry, 35-36, 40, 46, 55, 91, 135, 145, 165, 172
psychoanalysis, 35-37, 40, 43, 91, 121, 145-146, 178
psychology (see also medical psychology), 3, 50, 64, 79, 87, 89, 115, 167
psychosomatics, 35, 38, 40-41, 52, 91

psychotherapy, 91-92, 135, 145
reductionism, 19, 37, 109, 111
reflection, 1, 63, 75, 78, 90, 118, 142
rehabilitation, 113, 160-162
relativism, 84
rhythm, 80, 94, 98-99, 118, 179
sedimentation, 136, 142-143
self (see also person), 7, 20-22, 34, 36, 41, 46, 48, 61, 68, 75-76, 80, 82-83, 86, 88-89, 92, 97-98, 100, 109, 111, 114, 116-119, 126, 132, 137, 143-146, 151, 164, 167, 180
self-understanding, 83, 89, 132, 137, 144-146, 164, 180
semantics, 47, 50
signs, 20, 23, 25, 31, 124, 138, 142, 168
social construction, 36, 64
social sciences, 121, 141-142
sociology, 44, 50, 64, 79, 167, 178
somatic illness, 36, 74
specialist, 38, 128, 146, 161, 165
standard circumstances, 71, 72, 115
statistical, 32, 38, 63-64, 66, 68, 71, 75, 178
stroke, 102, 104, 158-162, 165, 181
structuralism, 29
suffering, 7, 15, 17-18, 28, 31, 33, 38, 45, 48, 55, 62, 74, 97, 98, 101-104, 112, 121, 127-129, 147, 156-157, 166, 173, 177
surgery, 5, 12, 15-16, 18-21, 24, 29, 34, 36, 56, 138, 165-166
symbolic, 47, 122, 136, 145
sympathy, 35, 131
symptom, 20, 23, 25, 27, 31, 34, 37-38, 40-41, 45-46, 50, 66, 98, 105-106, 124, 128, 130, 137, 145, 155, 157-158, 162, 178
synthesis, 75, 122, 141, 175, 180
techne, 13, 53-54
technology (see also medical technology), 4, 11, 22, 24, 29, 33, 37, 40, 51, 53, 137-138, 159, 177-178
teleology, 19, 65, 69, 122-123, 145
text (textuality, see also primary text), 130-144, 148-149, 163, 179
theory of medicine (see also philosophy of medicine), 12, 51-53, 59
thrownness, 88, 92, 97, 171
time (temporality), 73, 77, 81, 85, 88, 94, 96, 98-99, 105-107, 111, 113, 116, 125, 129, 133, 149, 151, 156, 160, 162
tiredness, 96-99, 116-117, 124, 128, 162
togetherness (see also being-with and intersubjectivity), 134, 159-160, 163, 179
tool (see also broken tool), 19, 24, 31, 33, 35, 37, 40, 44, 50, 53, 63, 85-86, 88, 106, 108-111, 115, 117-118, 127, 130, 136-137, 144, 168, 171, 174-175, 179
totality of relevance, 85, 87-88, 90, 92, 106-109, 171, 179

INDEX OF SUBJECTS

transcendence, 86-89, 95, 97, 99-100, 103, 107, 110-112, 114-115, 117-118, 144, 179
transcendental, 76-77, 81-82, 84, 86, 154
transplantation, 4, 110
trust, 12, 15, 24, 34, 147, 153, 164, 174-175, 177, 180
uncanny, 93, 97, 111, 116, 133, 157, 159
unconscious, 37, 41, 43, 71, 73, 102-103, 145, 150, 158, 160
uncover, 6, 37, 78, 115, 131-133, 175
unhomelikeness (see also homelessness), 93, 95, 97-101, 104, 107, 111-118, 121, 124, 126, 130, 133, 137-138, 145-147, 149-150, 152, 154, 157, 164-165, 169, 173-174, 178-180
utilitarianism, 168, 173
well-being (see also happiness), 24, 51-52, 55, 72, 79, 94, 101, 111, 121, 178
virus (see also micro-organisms), 102, 123, 126-129
vital goals, 69-74, 92, 99, 101, 103, 112, 115, 178
worldliness (see also being-in-the-world), 83-85, 101, 103, 107-108, 110, 154
writing (see also sedimentation and text), 18, 112, 130, 142

International Library of Ethics, Law, and the New Medicine

1. L. Nordenfelt: *Action, Ability and Health.* Essays in the Philosophy of Action and Welfare. 2000
ISBN 0-7923-6206-3
2. J. Bergsma and D.C. Thomasma: *Autonomy and Clinical Medicine.* Renewing the Health Professional Relation with the Patient. 2000
ISBN 0-7923-6207-1
3. S. Rinken: *The AIDS Crisis and the Modern Self.* Biographical Self-Construction in the Awareness of Finitude. 2000
ISBN 0-7923-6371-X
4. M. Verweij: *Preventive Medicine Between Obligation and Aspiration.* 2000
ISBN 0-7923-6691-3
5. F. Svenaeus: *The Hermeneutics of Medicine and the Phenomenology of Health.* Steps Towards a Philosophy of Medical Practice. 2001
ISBN 0-7923-6757-X

KLUWER ACADEMIC PUBLISHERS – DORDRECHT / BOSTON / LONDON

Printed by Publishers' Graphics LLC